T0293386

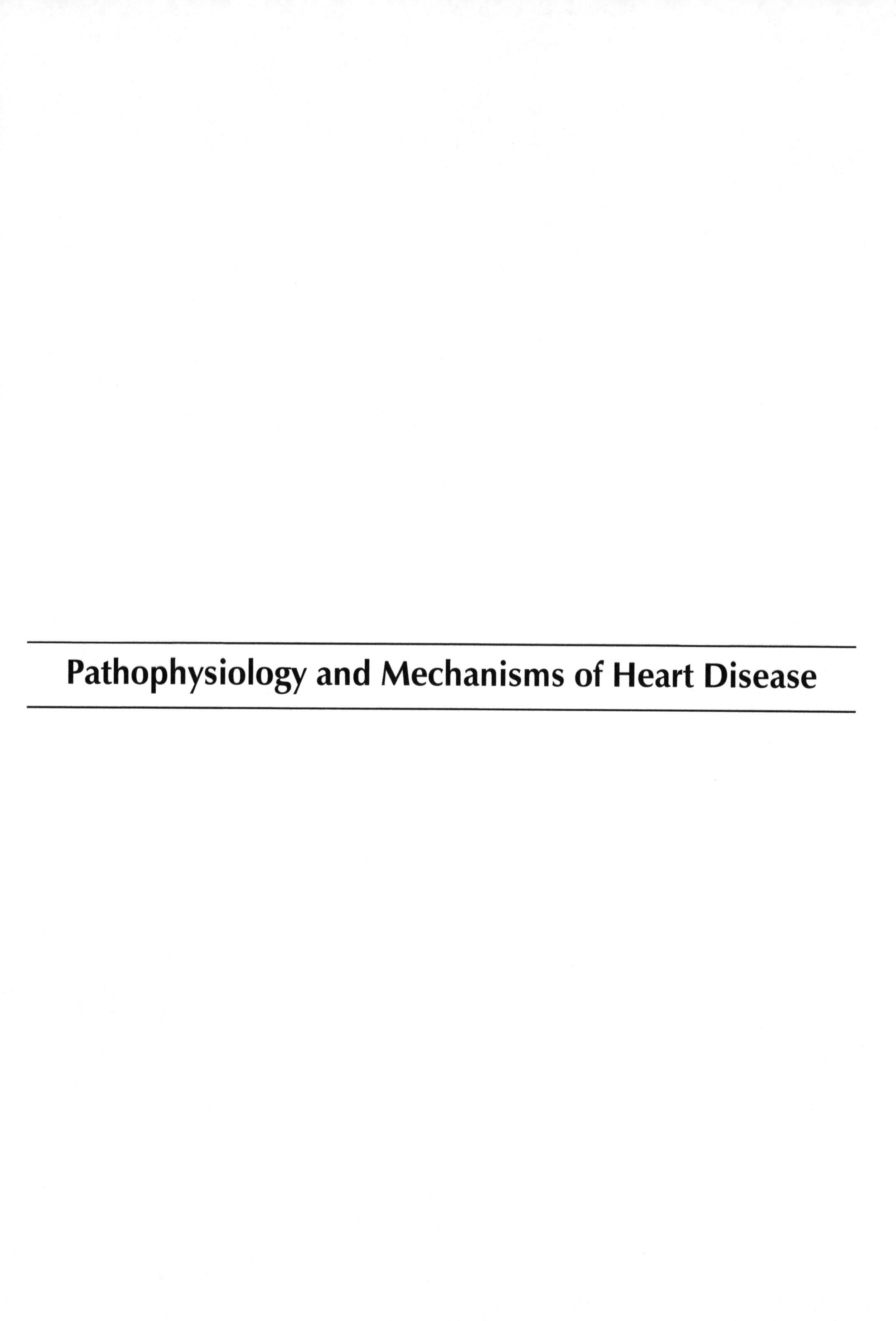

Pathophysiology and Mechanisms of Heart Disease

Pathophysiology and Mechanisms of Heart Disease

Editor: Mia Dunn

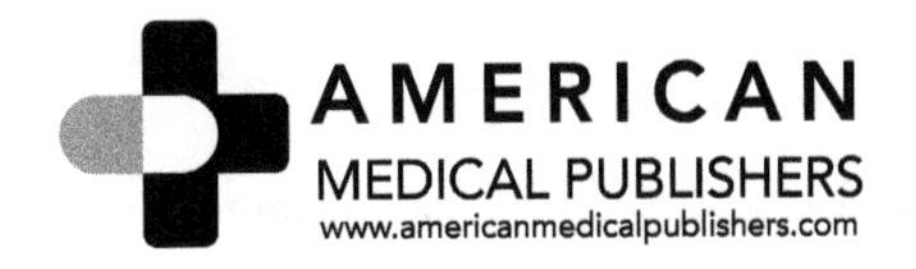

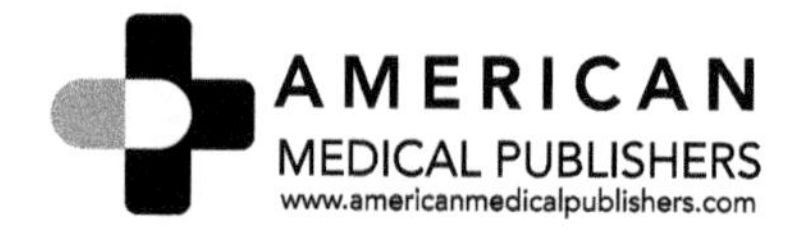

Cataloging-in-Publication Data

Pathophysiology and mechanisms of heart disease / edited by Mia Dunn.
p. cm.
Includes bibliographical references and index.
ISBN 978-1-63927-779-7
1. Heart--Diseases--Pathophysiology. 2. Heart--Pathophysiology. 3. Heart--Diseases.
4. Physiology, Pathological. I. Dunn, Mia.
RC682 .P38 2023
616.12--dc23

American Medical Publishers,
41 Flatbush Avenue,
1st Floor, New York,
NY 11217, USA

ISBN 978-1-63927-779-7 (Hardback)

Contents

Preface

It is often said that books are a boon to mankind. They document every progress and pass on the knowledge from one generation to the other. They play a crucial role in our lives. Thus I was both excited and nervous while editing this book. I was pleased by the thought of being able to make a mark but I was also nervous to do it right because the future of students depends upon it. Hence, I took a few months to research further into the discipline, revise my knowledge and also explore some more aspects. Post this process, I begun with the editing of this book.

Heart diseases refer to various conditions affecting the heart, which include diseases like coronary artery disease, heart arrhythmias, heart failure, heart valve disease, pericardial disease, cardiomyopathy and congenital heart disease. The causal mechanisms vary from disease to disease. In coronary artery disease, fatty plaque builds up in the arteries, which blocks the blood vessels, resulting in stroke, chest pain and heart attack. Deaths due to heart disease are majorly associated with dietary factors. Other risk elements comprise tobacco consumption, age, physical inactivity, sex, family history, obesity, genetic predisposition, increased blood sugar, increased blood pressure, psychological factors and lack of sleep. Majority of the heart diseases are preventable by avoiding the risk factors through exercise, healthy eating, limiting intake of alcohol, and avoiding smoking tobacco. Treatment of risk elements such as blood lipids, diabetes and high blood pressure can also prove beneficial. This book is compiled in such a manner, that it will provide in-depth knowledge about the pathophysiology and mechanisms of heart disease. Those in search of information to further their knowledge will be greatly assisted by it.

I thank my publisher with all my heart for considering me worthy of this unparalleled opportunity and for showing unwavering faith in my skills. I would also like to thank the editorial team who worked closely with me at every step and contributed immensely towards the successful completion of this book. Last but not the least, I wish to thank my friends and colleagues for their support.

Editor

Molecular and Cellular Mechanisms of Electronegative Lipoproteins in Cardiovascular Diseases

Liang-Yin Ke [1,2,3,†], Shi Hui Law [1,†], Vineet Kumar Mishra [1], Farzana Parveen [1], Hua-Chen Chan [3], Ye-Hsu Lu [3,4] and Chih-Sheng Chu [3,4,5,*]

1 Department of Medical Laboratory Science and Biotechnology, College of Health Sciences, Kaohsiung Medical University, Kaohsiung 807378, Taiwan; kly@gap.kmu.edu.tw (L.-Y.K.); shlaw9994@gmail.com (S.H.L.); vineetkmishra.jh@gmail.com (V.K.M.); fparveen.jh@gmail.com (F.P.)
2 Graduate Institute of Medicine, College of Medicine and Drug Development and Value Creation Research Center, Kaohsiung Medical University, Kaohsiung 807378, Taiwan
3 Center for Lipid Biosciences, Kaohsiung Medical University Hospital, Kaohsiung Medical University, Kaohsiung 807377, Taiwan; huachen.chan@gmail.com (H.-C.C.); yehslu@cc.kmu.edu.tw (Y.-H.L.)
4 Division of Cardiology, Department of International Medicine, Kaohsiung Medical University Hospital, Kaohsiung 807377, Taiwan
5 Division of Cardiology, Department of Internal Medicine, Kaohsiung Municipal Ta-Tung Hospital, Kaohsiung 80145, Taiwan
* Correspondence: chucs@kmu.edu.tw
† These authors contributed equally to this work.

Abstract: Dysregulation of glucose and lipid metabolism increases plasma levels of lipoproteins and triglycerides, resulting in vascular endothelial damage. Remarkably, the oxidation of lipid and lipoprotein particles generates electronegative lipoproteins that mediate cellular deterioration of atherosclerosis. In this review, we examined the core of atherosclerotic plaque, which is enriched by byproducts of lipid metabolism and lipoproteins, such as oxidized low-density lipoproteins (oxLDL) and electronegative subfraction of LDL (LDL(−)). We also summarized the chemical properties, receptors, and molecular mechanisms of LDL(−). In combination with other well-known markers of inflammation, namely metabolic diseases, we concluded that LDL(−) can be used as a novel prognostic tool for these lipid disorders. In addition, through understanding the underlying pathophysiological molecular routes for endothelial dysfunction and inflammation, we may reassess current therapeutics and might gain a new direction to treat atherosclerotic cardiovascular diseases, mainly targeting LDL(−) clearance.

Keywords: electronegative LDL; LDL(−); L5 LDL; oxidized LDL; oxLDL; lectin-like oxLDL receptor-1; LOX-1; dyslipidemia; endothelial dysfunction; atherosclerosis; cardiovascular disease

1. Introduction

Approximately 1.9 billion people are obese or overweight worldwide [1]. Obesity is associated with excessive calorific intake and microvasculature damage, resulting in atherosclerosis, diabetes, and cardiovascular diseases (CVDs) [2]. The prevalence of CVDs has significantly increased in the past few decades [3]. Current strategies against CVDs mainly focus on lowering the level of low-density lipoprotein cholesterol (LDL-C) [4,5]. Intensive-dose statin therapy has been endorsed for clinical atherosclerotic vascular disease (ASCVD); however, it also increases statin-related side effects and intolerance [6,7]. To figure out this dilemma and find a balanced solution, here we address the mechanistic players behind these metabolic disturbances through the following disease progression steps: unhealthy lifestyle and unbalanced diet lead to obesity, chronic inflammation, and development of atherosclerosis and CVDs [8–10].

The onset of atherosclerosis initiates vascular lipid deposition, luminal narrowing, and plaque expansion. Unstable plaque deposits further lead to myocardial infarction and stroke [11]. Plaque consists of LDL-C variants, lipids, leukocytes, and inflammasomes in the vascular walls (Figure 1) [11,12]. In addition, several mediators of vasoconstriction, platelet aggregation, inflammatory chemokines, leukocyte adherence, and nitric oxide (NO) disturb the endothelial homeostasis [13]. LDL variants such as oxidized LDL (oxLDL) are essential constituents in the pathogenesis of atherosclerosis and CVDs [14–16]. Differing from the in vitro preparation of oxLDL, electronegative LDL (LDL(−)) is separated from human plasma using fast-protein liquid chromatography equipped with an anion exchange column [17]. According to the physical properties of LDL(−), it can be defined as the minimized oxLDL [18,19].

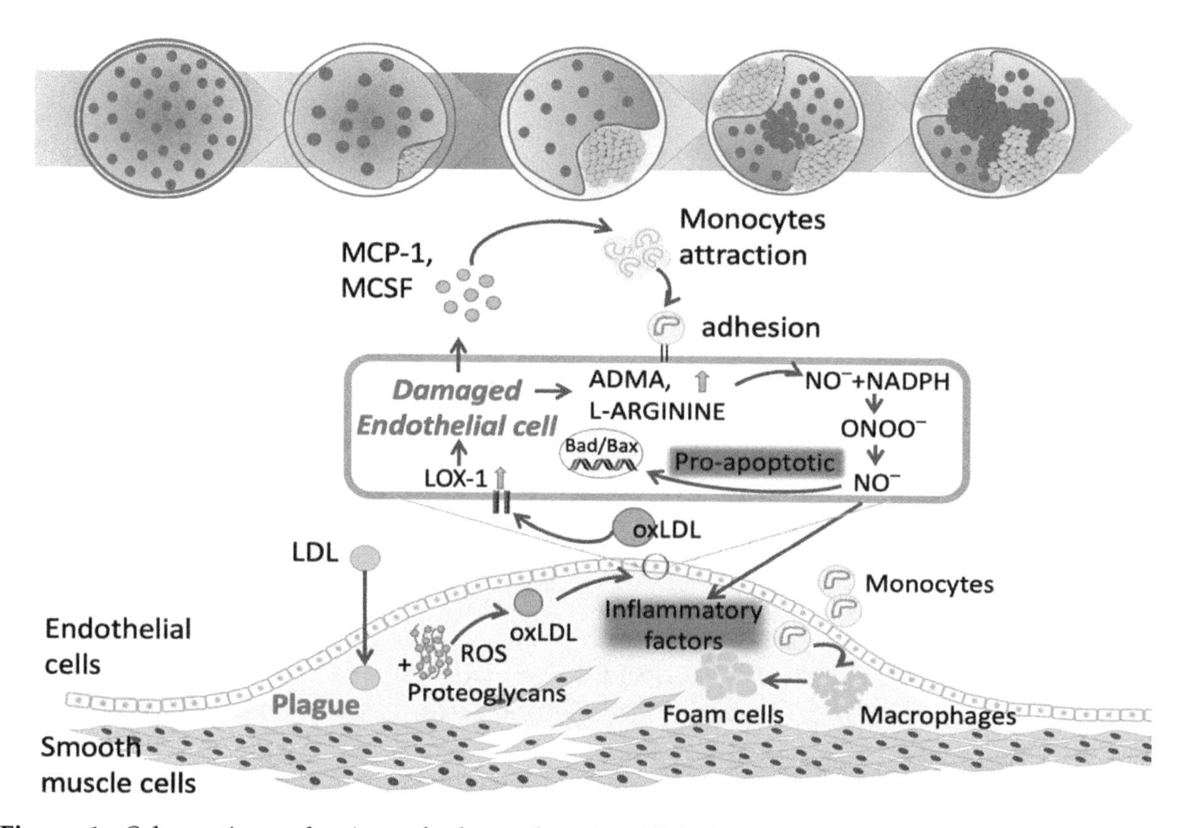

Figure 1. Schematic mechanism of atherosclerosis. LDL: low-density lipoprotein; ROS: reactive oxygen species; oxLDL: oxidized LDL; LOX-1: lectin-like oxidized LDL receptor-1; ADMA: asymmetric dimethylarginine; NO: nitric oxide; NADPH: nicotinamide adenine dinucleotide phosphate; ONOO: peroxynitrite; Bad: BCL2-associated agonist of cell death; Bax: Bcl-2-associated X protein; MCP-1: monocyte chemoattractant protein-1; MCSF: macrophage colony-stimulating factor.

Accumulating evidence shows that LDL(−) could be a novel marker for ASCVD, and levels of LDL(−) are positively correlated with the increasing severity of CVDs [20–22]. LDL(−) serves as a pivotal target for further studies and clinical development strategies beyond statins therapies. By targeting LDL(−), we summarize its pathophysiological links and highlight the molecular mechanisms of atherogenic lipids in the current review.

2. Properties of Electronegative Low-Density Lipoprotein (LDL(−))

2.1. Chemical Properties of LDL(−)

LDL(−) differs from LDL(+) in many aspects [23]. Regarding the lipid components, LDL(−) contains higher concentrations of triglycerides, non-esterified fatty acids (NEFA), lysophosphatidylcholine (LPC), platelet-activating factor (PAF), and ceramide [24–27]. Notably, lipid extracts of LDL(−) contribute to the atherogenic effects on endothelial cells and immune cells [27,28]. Regarding its protein composition, LDL(−) shows additional proteins such as apolipoprotein AI (apoAI), apolipoprotein E (apoE), and apolipoprotein CIII (apoCIII) [29]. Furthermore, the conformation of apoB100 in LDL(−) is altered and has higher competency to bind with proteoglycans [30–32]. Based on the sodium chloride gradient, Chen et al. successfully divided LDL into five subfractions, L1–L5, with increasing electronegativity [29,33,34]. L1 LDL is unmodified; in contrast, L5 LDL is highly *O*-glycosylated on the apoB100 and apoE [28,35]. The terminal glycan of apoE glycosylation (94S, 194T, 289T) in L5 LDL is sialic acid. This sialic-acid-containing glycan increases the electronegativity and hydrophilicity [35]. However, by dividing human plasma LDL into either two subfractions ((+) and (−)) or five (L1–L5), the most electronegative subfractions show similar properties and apoptotic effects on endothelial cells. Thus, we will be using LDL(−) throughout this review.

2.2. Receptors of LDL(−)

LDL(−) is not recognized by the LDL receptor. Instead, it goes through lectin-like oxLDL receptor-1 (LOX-1), which is highly expressed in endothelial cells, immune cells, platelets, and adipocytes [36–39]. Transfection with LOX-1-specific small interfering RNAs (si*LOX-1*) to endothelial cells may attenuate LDL(−)-induced downstream signaling [36]. LOX-1-neutralizing antibodies such as TS20 (for bovine) [40], TS58 (for mouse) [41], and TS92 (for human) [42,43] can inhibit the internalization of LDL(−). Genetic knockout *LOX-1* also protects against the harmful effects of LDL(−) [37,38]. Higher content of PAF on LDL(−) activates the PAF receptor (PAFR) and leads to endothelial cell apoptosis [33]. Incubating PAF acetylhydrolase (PAF-AH) with LDL(−) or pretreatment of WEB-2086 attenuates LDL(−)-induced apoptosis [33]. In addition, ceramide-rich LDL(−) activates toll-like receptor 4 (TLR4) and the cluster of differentiation 14 (CD14) on monocytes that results in cytokine release. Using the TLR4 inhibitor, the viral inhibitory peptide of TLR4 (VIPER), reduces these effects [44,45].

2.3. Structure Modifications and Enzymatic Functions of Electronegative LDL

Electronegativity and apolipoprotein misfolding are two independent features of LDL(−) [46]. The misfolded apoB100 of LDL(−) shows an increased binding affinity to proteoglycans, which may prolong LDL retention in the arterial wall and trigger inflammatory responses [31]. Stabilizing the LDL's structure through the use of 17-β-estradiol (E2) prevents aggregation; however, it cannot prevent the generation of LDL(−) [46,47]. The structural modifications of apoB100 are associated with phospholipolytic activities and exchange of lipid components [28,48,49]. The sphingomyelinase (SMase)-like activity of LDL(−) may hydrolyze sphingomyelin, which produces apoptotic factor, a ceramide [28,48]. The phospholipase D (PLD) activity of LDL(−) degrades phosphorylcholine, LPC, and sphingomyelin, which is associated with self-aggregation and atherogenic properties. Treatment with 400 μM of chlorpromazine may effectively inhibit both the SMase and PLD activities of LDL(−) [48].

2.4. Animal Models Showing Elevated Electronegative LDL

The overproduction of LDL(−) was demonstrated in animal models that consumed a high-fat diet. Lai et al. gave either a standard chow diet or high-fat & high-cholesterol (HFC) diet to each group of 8-week-old male golden Syrian hamsters for six weeks. Plasma LDL-C levels in HFC-diet-fed hamsters were significantly higher than for the control group. Additionally, LDL(−) accounted for 12.5% of all lipoproteins in control hamsters, whereas the value was drastically increased to 42% in HFC-diet-fed hamsters [50]. Recently, Chang et al. distributed an atherogenic diet to sixteen-week-old male New Zealand White rabbits. After six weeks, the LDL(−) from HFC-diet-fed rabbits accounted for about 17.2 ± 5.5% of the LDL fraction. On the other hand, it was almost undetectable in rabbits fed with a control chow diet [51]. Moreover, from the recent publication by Chan et al., LDL(+) and LDL(−) isolated from SLE patients' LDL samples were then injected into eight-week-old apoE knockout mice. Their results showed that only the LDL(−)-injected mice experienced a significant increase in the plasma CX3CL1 level. By observing histological staining results, LDL(−) can trigger endothelial dysfunction and the formation of atherosclerotic lesions in apoE knockout mice [27]. Taken together, we summarized that LDL(−) plays a vital role in atherosclerosis and plaque formation.

3. Mechanisms of Electronegative LDL on Endothelial Cells

The endothelium regulates fluid and molecule trafficking between the bloodstream and tissues for metabolism [52]. In addition, it inhibits platelet aggregation and adhesions by secreting prostacyclin, NO, and exosomes [53,54]. With LDL(−), the atherogenic components lead to endothelial activation and vascular inflammation. Chemokines such as monocyte chemotactic protein-1 (MCP-1) and interleukin-8 (IL-8) are released from the damaged endothelium. The vascular adhesion molecules are highly expressed to promote plaque formation [55]. The mechanisms behind this are listed below.

3.1. Phosphatidylinositol-3 Kinase (PI3K)-Serine/Threonine Kinase (Akt) Signaling

The phosphatidylinositol-3 kinase (PI3K)-serine/threonine kinase (Akt) signaling involves the proliferation and survival of endothelial cells through inhibiting pro-apoptotic proteins [56]. Both fibroblast growth factor 2 (FGF2) and vascular endothelial growth factor (VEGF) activate PI3K/Akt signaling [57,58]; in contrast, LDL(−) disrupts Akt phosphorylation, impairing the FGF2 mRNA expression, as well as induces endothelial cell apoptosis [40,59]. In their study, Lu et al. also demonstrated that the apoptotic effects of LDL(−) on endothelial cells could be attenuated by treatment with FGF2 or constitutively expressing active Akt [59]. LDL(−) inhibits B-cell lymphoma 2 (Bcl-2); in contrast, it triggers the expression of Bad/Bax (Bcl-2-associated agonist cell death) and inflammatory factor tumor necrosis factor-α (TNF-α). These actions result in the release of cytochrome c from mitochondria [36,59].

3.2. Lectin-Like oxLDL Receptor-1 (LOX-1) Signaling

Lectin-like oxLDL receptor-1 (LOX-1) reacts with multiple ligands in response to danger signals [60]. Patients with cerebral stroke and coronary artery diseases exhibited elevated levels of soluble-form LOX-1 (sLOX-1) [61,62]. Furthermore, patients with ST segment elevation myocardial infarction (STEMI) and rheumatoid arthritis (RA) showed increased sLOX-1 expression in the aspirated coronary thrombi [63,64]. Due to earlier release than biochemical markers of myocardial injury, sLOX-1 could be a novel biomarker for plaque instability [65]. In a hypercholesteremic mice model, the LOX-1 knockout reduced the plaque size and atherosclerotic lesions [66–68].

For the detailed mechanisms, LDL(−) leads to the overexpressed changes of LOX-1 on endothelial cells by inducing the expression changes of the pro-inflammatory molecules nuclear factor of kappa light polypeptide gene enhancer in B-cells (NF-κB), vascular cell adhesion molecule (1VCAM-1), and MCP-1 [69,70]. Recently, a similar cohort study was completed to show similar results of LOX-1-mediated inflammation in SLE patients [71]. In addition, the expression of LOX-1 dependents on vasoconstrictors (angiotensin II, endothelin-1) and inflammatory factors such as interferon-γ (IFN-γ), tumor necrosis factor-α (TNF-α), and IL-1β was observed [72]. In vitro, oxidized LDL may enhance the production of angiotensin-converting enzyme (ACE) and endothelin-1 [73,74].

Through LOX-1, LDL(−) downregulates the phosphorylation of Akt and endothelial nitric oxide synthase (eNOS) but increases C-reactive protein (CRP) [11,36,42]. LOX-1 activates Ras homolog family member A (RhoA) and the Ras-related C3 botulinum toxin substrate 1 (Rac1) pathway, leading to the inhibition of intracellular endothelial NO synthesis and overproduction of ROS [75]. Recently, NOS was reported to influence miR-122 expression in hypertension cases, leading to endothelial dysfunction;

however, the expression changes of miR-122-mediating endothelial dysfunction remains unanswered. We, therefore, predict LOX-1 signaling of LDL(−) in such cases [76]. Similarly, ROS overproduction leads to p66shc protein phosphorylation, which further deteriorates mitochondrial DNA and contributes to plaque formation [77–79]. The phenomenon mentioned above can be attenuated by knocking out the *LOX-1* gene [80,81].

3.3. Mitochondria Damage

The basal physiological mechanism of mitochondrial ROS formation is dependent on several factors such as NO, cytosolic Ca2+, and fatty acids [82]. NADPH oxidase 4 (NOX4) in vascular cells inhibits mitochondrial complex I and promotes ROS generation [83]. During the pro-apoptotic conditions, ROS formation is also boosted by growth factor adaptor protein p66Shc, which facilitates the cytochrome c oxidation. Moreover, ROS formation can be further increased by the expression and activation of p66Shc during hyperglycemic conditions [84,85]. LDL(−) inhibits endothelial nitric oxide synthase (eNOS) expression via the Akt signaling pathway, resulting in decreased NO production and leading to endothelial cell apoptosis [86]. Recently, Chen et al. demonstrated that apoE in LDL(−) is responsible for LDL-induced mitochondrial dysfunction. After LDL(−) internalization, apoE translocates from the lysosome to the mitochondria, leading to mitochondrial permeability transition pore (mPTP) opening, dynamin-related protein 1 (DRP1) phosphorylation, and mitochondrial fission [41].

3.4. Endoplasmic Reticulum Stress

The intraluminal oxidation in the endoplasmic reticulum (ER) plays a critical role in maintaining calcium concentration and proper folding of transmembrane proteins. The increased amount of lipoprotein promotes a condition known as ER stress, defined by the accumulation of unfolded protein in the ER lumen [87,88]. The molecular mechanism between LDL oxidation and UPR (unfolded protein response)-mediated expression of IL-8, IL-6, and MCP-1 in endothelial cells, which contributes to endothelial dysfunction, is poorly explained [89,90]. Apart from oxidation, glycation of LDL is also found to be a potent marker for dyslipidemia. Studies showed that glycated LDL could initiate nicotinamide adenine dinucleotide phosphate (NADPH) oxidation via ROS production and could induce apoptosis in endothelial cells [91,92]. Therefore, the LDL oxidation and glycation are involved in amplifying endothelial dysfunction and contributing to atherosclerosis.

4. Mechanisms of Electronegative LDL on Immune Cells

Alongside endothelial cells, immune cells play a significant role in the pathogenesis of atherosclerosis. Monocytes and T lymphocytes create an inflammatory milieu by releasing several cytokines and growth factors. As LDL(−) concentration is elevated in the blood plasma, it tend to interacts with these monocytes and lymphocytes via cytokines and growth factors [93,94]. LDL(−) impregnates the process of oxidation via the feedback loop mechanism shown in Figure 2 and enhances inflammation. The NEFA and ceramide in LDL(−) also show atherogenic properties [93,95–97]. The detailed mechanisms behind this are listed below.

4.1. Monocytes

Numerous studies have described the effects of LDL(−) on inducing cytokine release from monocytes, which may be important in atherosclerosis [25,98]. Remodeling of the vascular extracellular matrix (ECM) seemed to be an important landmark of atherosclerosis. LDL(−) induces the release of matrix metalloproteinase (MMP)-9 and tissue inhibitors of metalloproteinase (TIMP)-1 from monocytes through the TLR4/CD14 inflammatory pathway [45]. Additionally, the downstream signal cascade of TLR4/CD14 will then trigger PI3K/Akt signaling and promote p38 mitogen-activated protein kinase (p38 MAPK) phosphorylation, leading to LDL(−)-induced cytokine release from monocytes [99]. The elevated levels of those cytokines may regulate and contribute to vascular plaque formation.

4.2. Macrophages

Macrophages play a crucial role in the early stage pathogenesis of atherosclerosis [100]. Circulating monocytes undergo differentiation into macrophages and further polarization into classically activated (M1) or alternatively activated (M2) states in order to withstand environmental stimuli. M1 macrophages are responsible for pro-inflammatory properties, whereas M2 macrophages exert opposing anti-inflammatory properties [101].

According to Yang et al., LDL(+) and LDL(−) isolated from patients with ST segment elevation myocardial infarction (STEMI) were treated with THP-1 macrophages. Their results indicated that only LDL(−) could induce the overproduction of interleukin (IL)-1β [102], granulocyte colony-stimulating factor (G-CSF), and granulocyte–macrophage colony-stimulating factor (GM-CSF) in macrophages through LOX-1-, extracellular signal-regulated kinase (ERK)1/2-, and NF-κB-dependent pathways. Inhibition of ERK1/2 and NF-κB activation can prevent G-CSF and GM-CSF production induced by LDL(−) [103].

In 2020, Chang et al. treated THP-1 with LDL(−), which resulted in increased pro-inflammatory cytokines such as IL-1β, IL-6, IL-8, and TNF-α, as well as M1 surface marker CD86; however, M2-related cytokines and surface marker CD206 were not changed by LDL(−) [39]. Additionally, the expression of CD11c, a marker of M1 macrophages, can also be induced by LDL(−) [104]. LDL(−) can induce M1 polarization of human macrophages responsible for secreting pro-inflammatory cytokines, resulting in foam cell formation and vascular plaque formation.

In addition to human macrophages, in treating LDL(+) and LDL(−) with RAW264.7 cell, the results showed that only LDL(−) can induce the expression of CD95 death receptor (Fas), its ligand CD95 L (FasL), and tumor necrosis factor ligand member 10 (Tnfsf10), which stimulate the activation of the caspases, resulting in cell apoptosis [105].

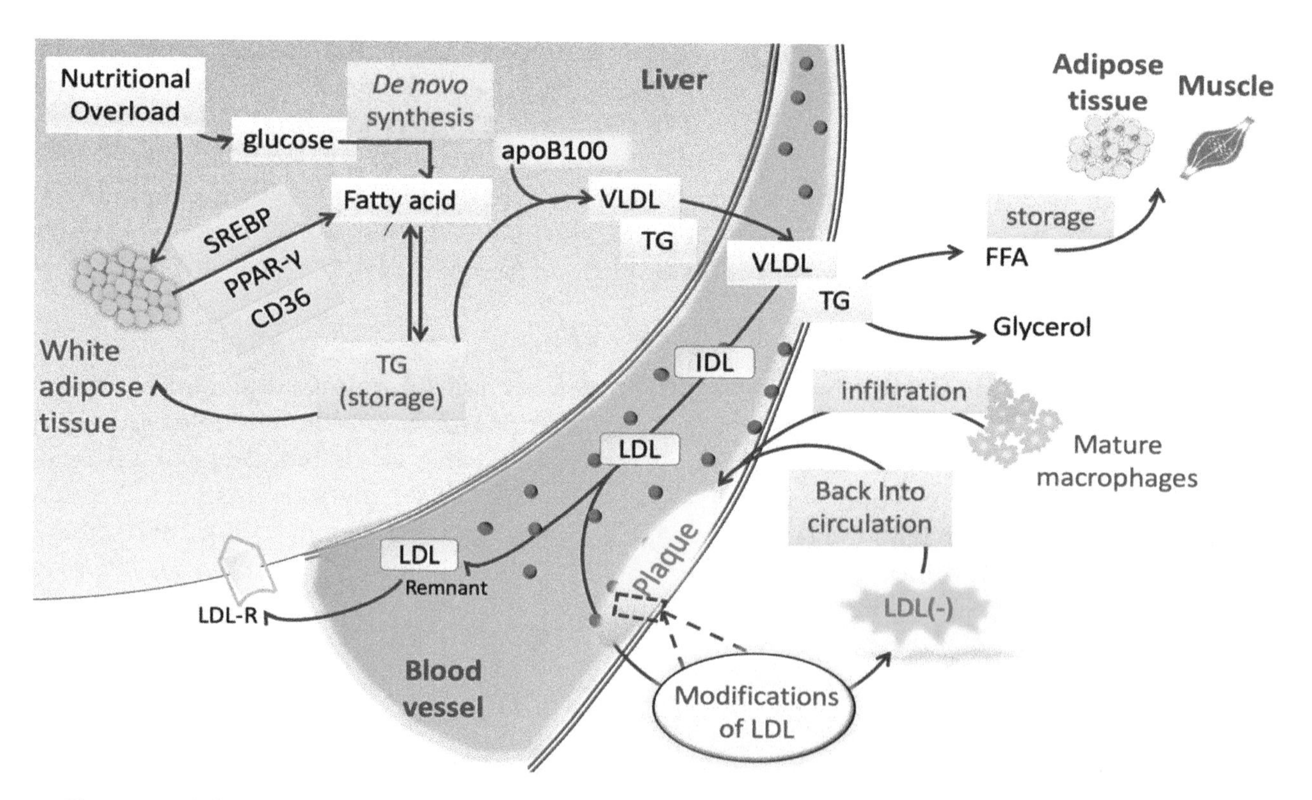

Figure 2. Schematic procedures of lipoprotein metabolism and LDL(−) formation. SREBP: sterol regulatory element-binding protein; PPAR-γ: peroxisome proliferator-activated receptor; CD36: cluster of differentiation 36; TG: triglycerides; apoB100: apolipoprotein B100; VLDL: very low-density lipoprotein; IDL: intermediate-density lipoprotein; LDL: low-density lipoprotein; LDLR: LDL receptor; FFA: free fatty acid.

4.3. *Platelets*

Apart from monocytes and macrophages, accumulating evidence has shown that LDL(−) may trigger platelet activation and aggregation. Platelet hyperreactivity is the most direct evidence contributing to thrombosis in the leading causes of cardiovascular diseases, such as STEMI [106] and stroke [43,107]. As above, Chan et al. separated LDL(+) and LDL(−) from patients with STEMI, with the results illustrating that only LDL(−) was augmented in patients compared to healthy controls. Treating LDL(−) to platelets enhanced their aggregation and adhesion to damaged human aortic endothelial cells (HAECs), which was through LOX-1 and PAFR activation [37]. Furthermore, LDL(−)-induced amyloid β (Aβ) release via IκB kinase 2 (IKK2) in human platelets was reported by Shen et al. in 2016. Besides, LDL(−) works synergistically with Aβ to induce glycoprotein IIb/IIIa receptor activation and phosphorylation of IKK2, IkBa, p65, and c-Jun N-terminal kinase 1 in order to enhance platelet aggregation. These results can be attenuated by inhibiting IKK2, LOX-1, or NF-kB with their inhibitors BMS-345541, TS92, and Bay 117-82, respectively [43]. To conclude, high levels of LDL(−) in patients can trigger platelet activation and aggregation through LOX-1 and PAFR receptors.

5. Electronegative LDL in Vascular Diseases

Figure 2 demonstrates the lipid and lipoprotein metabolism in the liver, blood, and peripheral tissues. Nutritional overload increases fatty acids via the overexpression of cluster of differentiation 36 (CD36) and peroxisome proliferator-activated receptor (PPAR-γ) [108–110]. This phenomenon is highly contrasted to the de novo synthesis pathway, although FFAs from either source in the liver are indistinguishable. The elevated level of free fatty acids ultimately increases triglyceride through esterification. Combined with apoB100 and triglyceride, the efflux of VLDL into circulation promotes the pro-atherogenic metabolic state. VLDL particles deliver lipids hydrolyzed by lipoprotein lipase (LPL) and release FFAs in plasma [111–113].

With the increasing incidence of LDL retention in endothelial cells [114–118], the LDL particles reportedly undergo oxidative modifications by macrophages and endothelial cells within arterial walls (Figure 2) [119–124]. The accumulation of oxLDL further boosts the electronegativity, ultimately generating LDL(−) in circulation [33]. LDL(−) is highly atherogenic and pro-apoptotic to the vascular system, including the endothelium of the blood–brain barrier (BBB). Wang et al. in 2017 explored the role of LDL(−) in pheochromocytoma-derived cell line (PC12) cells, where deliberate dosages of LDL(−) induced neurotoxic stress in a LOX-1-dependent manner [125].

The presence of LDL(−) in circulation correlates with atherosclerosis progression and endothelial dysfunction-mediated cardiovascular diseases. LDL(−) levels are significantly higher in frequent smokers, diabetic patients, and hypercholesterolemia patients [33,34,40,59]. In addition, LDL(−) levels were 10-times higher in STEMI and stroke patients, even though the LDL-C levels were similar to healthy controls [37,43].

6. Current Treatment Strategies Targeting Electronegative LDL

The diagnosis and treatment for endothelial damage are dependent on the ankle–brachial index, vascular imaging, surgery, and revascularization [126–128]. Currently, treatment for dyslipidemia and the prevention of microvasculature damage mainly revolve around reducing LDL-C levels [129–131]. A plethora of studies have demonstrated that excessive levels of lipids lead to endothelial damage; however, only a few studies have outlined strong mechanistic interactions between lipid alterations and endothelial dysfunction (Table 1).

Table 1. Primary dyslipidemia markers and pathways involved in different diseases.

Diseases	Dyslipidemia Markers	Drug Treatment	Effect on ED	Pathway/Phenomenon Involved	Studied on	References
Hypertension	NOS, ROS	α-Linolenic acid	Yes	SIRT-3	Mice	[132]
Hypertension	NOS, ROS	——	Yes	miR-122, CAT-1	Human	[76]
Hypertension, Angina	NOS, CRP, Hyperglycemia	Carvedilol	Yes	β-adrenergic mediate Vasodilation	Human	[133–136]
Heart failure	oxLDL, LDL	Rosuvastatin	Yes	Inflammatory markers	Human	[137,138]
ACS	oxLDL, LDL-C and cardiac fibrosis	perindopril	Yes	-	Human	[139,140]
CKD, CHF	Cardiac fibrosis	carvedilol	Yes	β-adrenergic mediate Vasodilation	Human	[141]
LVF, CKD	oxLDL, LDL and Cardiac fibrosis	Renal and heart transplant	——	——	Human	[142]
STEMI	——	Enoxaparin, Clopidogrel and β-blocker	No	Case study	Human	[143]
STEMI	Atherosclerotic Plaques	Statins, Aspirins, β-blocker, ACE-inhibitor	Yes	——	Human	[144,145]
STEMI	CRP and Atherosclerotic plaques	Vit B, B6, and B12	No	Homocysteine	Human	[146]
STEMI	LDL-C, Ox-LDL and L5	——	——	PKC/AKT pathway	Mice	[37]
CAD, Diabetes	NOS, Hyperinsulinemia, Hyperglycemia	Pioglitazone	Yes	Anti-inflammation, Vasodialation	Human	[147,148]
T1DM	Cardiac fibrosis	Fingolimod (FTY720)	Yes	Rag-1	Mice	[149]
T2DM	Hyperglycemia and Cardiac Fibrosis	H2/H3- RLX	Yes	α-SMA, MMP, TIMP and NLRP3	Rat	[150,151]
T2DM	NOS and Hyperglycemia	Berberine	Yes	AMPK and eNOS Phosphorylation	In-vitro, Ex-vivo	[152–154]
T2DM	Hyperglycemia, oxLDL, LDL, TG	Fenofibrate	Yes	PPAR-α/γ	Rat	[155,156]
RA	CRP, LDL, TG	MTX and Glucocorticoid	Yes	Hemodynamics	Human	[157]
RA	NOS, Myeloperoxidase, LDL	Tocilizimab	Yes	JAK/STAT and mTOR	Human	[158]
Stroke SLE	Atherosclerotic plaques	Glucocorticoids, Immunosuppressant	Yes	——	Human	[159,160]
SLE	Atherosclerotic plaques	Anifrolumab and tsDMARDs	Yes	JAK/BTK	Human Phase III	[161]

RP: C-reactive protein; LDL-C: Low-density lipoprotein cholesterol; TG: Triglyceride; MTX: Methotrexate; RA: Rheumatoid arthritis; NHC: Normal healthy control; T1DM: Type 1 diabetes mellitus; Rag-1: Recombination-activating gene 1; NOS: Nitric oxide synthase; JAK/STAT: Janus kinase/signal transducer activator of transcription protein; T2DM: Type 2 diabetes mellitus; H2/H3-RLX: Relaxin-1 and Relaxin3; mTOR: mammalian target of rapamycin; α-SMA: Alpha smooth muscle actin; MMP: Matrix metallopeptidase; TIMP: Tissue inhibitor of metalloproteinase; NLRP3: NOD-LRR and pyrin-domain-containing protein 3; Ox-LDL: oxidized low-density lipoprotein, CHF: Chronic heart failure; CVD: Cardiovascular disease; AMPK: AMP (Adenosine monophosphate)-activated protein kinase; eNOS: endothelial NOS; PPAR-γ/α: Peroxisome proliferator-activated receptor alpha/gamma; CKD: Chorionic kidney disease; LVF: Left ventricular failure; SLE: Systemic lupus erythematosus; tsDMARDs: Targeted synthetic disease-modifying antirheumatic drugs; JAK/BTK: JAK/Bruton's tyrosine kinase (inhibitor); STEMI: St-elevation myocardial infarction; ACE: Angiotensin-converting enzyme; ROS: Reactive oxygen species; SIRT-3: Nicotinamide adenosine diphosphate (NAD)-dependent deacetylase sirtuin-3; miR122: MicroRNA 122; CAT-1: Cationic amino acid transporter 1; PKC/AKT: Protein kinase C/protein kinase B.

Statins, the inhibitors of β-hydroxy β-methylglutaryl-CoA (HMG-CoA), are successful in lowering cholesterol loadings and expression of LOX-1; they also inhibit atherosclerotic progression and acute atherothrombosis [162–164]. Additionally, statins effectively reduce the proportion of LDL(−) [165–168]; discontinuation leads to LDL(−) approaching baseline levels [42]. However, the mechanisms of LDL(−) reduction are still not clear. Ezetimibe inhibits the Niemann–Pick C1-like 1 transporter (NPC1L1), which leads to decreased cholesterol absorption [169]. Proprotein convertase subtilisin kexin type 9 (PCSK9) is an enzyme for the degradation of LDL receptor (LDLR); blocking PCSK9 may increase LDLR, therefore lowering blood LDL-C concentrations. PCSK9 inhibitors such as alirocumab and evolocumab aggressively reduce the degradation of LDL receptors and increase the clearance of LDL cholesterol in hepatic cells [170]. They increase plaque stability but decrease the necrotic lipid core, as shown in Figure 1 [171–175]. However, other than statins, whether these drugs can decrease LDL(−) or not is currently unclear.

Several anti-inflammatory approaches were taken here to study the management of dyslipidemia, such as cell therapy using mesenchymal stem cells [176], leukotriene inhibitors [177], chemokine ligands (CC motif ligand), MCP-1, IL-1, and TNF-α blockers for the prevention of atherosclerotic plaque formation [178–184]. The currently used drugs significantly decrease LDL-C levels, stabilize vascular plaque, and slowdown atherosclerotic progression; however, new therapeutic strategies for LDL(−) and biomarkers are still needed.

7. Perspective

LDL(−) plays a critical role in the pathophysiology of atherogenesis. It triggers the dysfunction of endothelium by macrophage differentiation, monocyte migration, and platelet aggregation. Moreover, LDL(−) impairs endothelial cells by superoxide overproduction and platelet activation [185–187]. In combination with other well-known markers of inflammation, namely metabolic diseases, we concluded that LDL(−) can be a novel prognostic tool for these lipid disorders. Regarding treatment for the prevention of ASCVD, even though statins can partially reduce the concentration, finding a way to clear LDL(−) remains of utmost importance [22]. In particular, a method involving hydrolyzing atherogenic lipids in LDL(−) and producing harmless metabolites might be a novel therapeutic approach in the future.

Author Contributions: Conceptualization, C.-S.C.; validation, L.-Y.K.; resources, Y.-H.L.; data curation, H.-C.C.; writing—original draft preparation, S.H.L., V.K.M., F.P.; writing—review and editing, S.H.L., L.-Y.K.; visualization, F.P., H.-C.C.; supervision, C.-S.C., Y.-H.L.; project administration, L.-Y.K.; funding acquisition, C.-S.C., H.-C.C., L.-Y.K. All authors have read and agreed to the published version of the manuscript.

Abbreviations

Aβ	Amyloid β
ACE	Angiotensin-converting enzyme
ADP	Adenosine diphosphate
ADPase	Ecto-Adenosine diphosphate
ApoB100	Apolipoprotein B100
ApoCIII	Apolipoprotein CIII
ApoE	Apolipoprotein E
ASCVD	Atherosclerotic cardiovascular diseases
Bad/Bax	BCL2-associated agonist of cell death
Bcl-2	B-cell lymphoma 2
BBB	Blood–brain barrier
BP	Blood pressure
CAD	Coronary artery disease
CCL	Chemokine ligand
CD	Cluster of differentiation
CER	Ceramide
cIMTPWV	Carotid intermedia thickness and pulse wave velocity
COX	Cyclooxygenase
CD36	Cluster of differentiation 36
CRP	C-reactive protein
CVD	Cardiovascular disease
EC	Endothelial cell

ECM	Extracellular matrix
ED	Endothelial dysfunction
ERK	Extracellular signal-regulated kinase
eNOS	Endothelial nitric oxide synthase
ER	Endoplasmic reticulum
Fas	CD95 death receptor
FasL	Ligand CD95 L
FFA	Free fatty acids
FGF2	Fibroblast growth factor 2
FPLC	Fast-protein liquid chromatography
G-CSF	Granulocyte colony-stimulating factor
GDF	Growth differentiation factor
GM-CSF	Granulocyte–macrophage colony-stimulating factor
HDL	High-density lipoprotein
HFC	High-fat, high-cholesterol
HIF-1α	Hypoxia-inducible factor-1α
HMGCoA	β-hydroxy β-methylglutaryl-CoA
HUVECs	Human umbilical vein endothelial cells
ICAM	Intracellular adhesion molecule 1
IDL	Intermediate-density lipoprotein
IFN-γ	Interferon- γ
IKK2	IκB kinase 2
IL	Interleukin
iNOS	Inducible NO synthase
IR	Insulin resistance
IRAK2	Interleukin-1 receptor-associated kinase-2
IRE-1	Inositol requiring enzyme-1
Lp(a)	Lipoprotein (a)
LDL	Low-density lipoprotein
LDL(−)	Electronegative LDL
LDL-C	LDL cholesterol
LPC	Lysophosphatidylcholine
LPL	Lipoprotein lipase
LOX-1	Lectin-like oxidized low-density lipoprotein receptor-1
MAPK	Mitogen-activated protein kinase
MCP-1	Monocyte chemotactic protein-1
MetS	Metabolic syndrome
MMP	Metalloproteinase
MSC	Mesenchymal stem cell
NADPH	Nicotinamide adenine dinucleotide phosphate
NEFA	Non-esterified fatty acids
NF-κB	Nuclear factor kappa light-chain enhancer of activated B cells
NO	Nitric oxide
Nox	NADPH oxidase
NPC1L1	Niemann–pick C1-like
oxLDL	Oxidized LDL
PAFR	Platelet activating factor
PAFR	Platelet activating factor receptor
PC12	Pheochromocytoma cell-derived cell line
PGI2	Prostacyclin 2
PI3K	Phosphatidylinositol-3 kinase
PLD	Phospholipase D
PSCK9	Proprotein convertase subtilisin kexin type 9
RhoA	Ras homology family member A

Rac1	Ras-related C3 botulinum toxin substrate 1
Smase	Sphingomyelinase
STEMI	ST segment elevation myocardial infarction
TGF-β	Transforming growth factor- β
TIMP	Tissue inhibitors of metalloproteinase
TLR4	Toll-like receptor 4
TNF-α	Tumor necrosis factor-α
Tnfsf10	Tumor necrosis factor ligand, member 10
UCP 2	Uncoupling protein 2
UPR	Unfolded protein response
VCAM-1	Vascular cell adhesion molecule-1
VEGF	Vascular endothelial growth factor
VIPER	Viral inhibitory peptide of TLR4
VLDL	Very low-density lipoprotein
VSMCs	Vascular smooth muscle cells

References

1. Saltiel, A.R.; Olefsky, J.M. Inflammatory mechanisms linking obesity and metabolic disease. *J. Clin. Investig.* **2017**, *127*, 1–4. [CrossRef] [PubMed]
2. Benjamin, E.J.; Virani, S.S.; Callaway, C.W.; Chamberlain, A.M.; Chang, A.R.; Cheng, S.; Chiuve, S.E.; Cushman, M.; Delling, F.N.; Deo, R.; et al. Heart Disease and Stroke Statistics-2018 Update: A Report From the American Heart Association. *Circulation* **2018**, *137*, e67–e492. [CrossRef] [PubMed]
3. Hinton, W.; McGovern, A.; Coyle, R.; Han, T.S.; Sharma, P.; Correa, A.; Ferreira, F.; de Lusignan, S. Incidence and prevalence of cardiovascular disease in English primary care: A cross-sectional and follow-up study of the Royal College of General Practitioners (RCGP) Research and Surveillance Centre (RSC). *BMJ Open* **2018**, *8*, e020282. [CrossRef]
4. Goff, D.C., Jr.; Lloyd-Jones, D.M.; Bennett, G.; Coady, S.; D'Agostino, R.B.; Gibbons, R.; Greenland, P.; Lackland, D.T.; Levy, D.; O'Donnell, C.J.; et al. 2013 ACC/AHA guideline on the assessment of cardiovascular risk: A report of the American College of Cardiology/American Heart Association Task Force on Practice Guidelines. *Circulation* **2014**, *129*, S49–S73. [CrossRef] [PubMed]
5. Stone, N.J.; Robinson, J.G.; Lichtenstein, A.H.; Bairey Merz, C.N.; Blum, C.B.; Eckel, R.H.; Goldberg, A.C.; Gordon, D.; Levy, D.; Lloyd-Jones, D.M.; et al. 2013 ACC/AHA guideline on the treatment of blood cholesterol to reduce atherosclerotic cardiovascular risk in adults: A report of the American College of Cardiology/American Heart Association Task Force on Practice Guidelines. *Circulation* **2014**, *129*, S1–S45. [CrossRef] [PubMed]
6. Fernandez-Friera, L.; Fuster, V.; Lopez-Melgar, B.; Oliva, B.; Garcia-Ruiz, J.M.; Mendiguren, J.; Bueno, H.; Pocock, S.; Ibanez, B.; Fernandez-Ortiz, A.; et al. Normal LDL-Cholesterol Levels Are Associated With Subclinical Atherosclerosis in the Absence of Risk Factors. *J. Am. Coll. Cardiol.* **2017**, *70*, 2979–2991. [CrossRef] [PubMed]
7. Toth, P.P.; Patti, A.M.; Giglio, R.V.; Nikolic, D.; Castellino, G.; Rizzo, M.; Banach, M. Management of Statin Intolerance in 2018: Still More Questions Than Answers. *Am. J. Cardiovasc. Drugs* **2018**, *18*, 157–173. [CrossRef]
8. Schwandt, P.; Liepold, E.; Bertsch, T.; Haas, G.M. Lifestyle, Cardiovascular Drugs and Risk Factors in Younger and Elder Adults: The PEP Family Heart Study. *Int. J. Prev. Med.* **2010**, *1*, 56–61.
9. Yasue, H.; Hirai, N.; Mizuno, Y.; Harada, E.; Itoh, T.; Yoshimura, M.; Kugiyama, K.; Ogawa, H. Low-grade inflammation, thrombogenicity, and atherogenic lipid profile in cigarette smokers. *Circ. J.* **2006**, *70*, 8–13. [CrossRef]
10. Hansson, G.K. Inflammation, atherosclerosis, and coronary artery disease. *N. Engl. J. Med.* **2005**, *352*, 1685–1695. [CrossRef]
11. Stancel, N.; Chen, C.C.; Ke, L.Y.; Chu, C.S.; Lu, J.; Sawamura, T.; Chen, C.H. Interplay between CRP, Atherogenic LDL, and LOX-1 and Its Potential Role in the Pathogenesis of Atherosclerosis. *Clin. Chem.* **2016**, *62*, 320–327. [CrossRef] [PubMed]
12. Ross, R. Atherosclerosis—An inflammatory disease. *N. Engl. J. Med.* **1999**, *340*, 115–126. [CrossRef] [PubMed]

13. Mudau, M.; Genis, A.; Lochner, A.; Strijdom, H. Endothelial dysfunction: The early predictor of atherosclerosis. *Cardiovasc. J. Afr.* **2012**, *23*, 222–231. [CrossRef] [PubMed]
14. Carmena, R.; Duriez, P.; Fruchart, J.C. Atherogenic lipoprotein particles in atherosclerosis. *Circulation* **2004**, *109*, III-2–III-7. [CrossRef] [PubMed]
15. Libby, P. Inflammation in atherosclerosis. *Nature* **2002**, *420*, 868–874. [CrossRef]
16. Witztum, J.L.; Steinberg, D. The oxidative modification hypothesis of atherosclerosis: Does it hold for humans? *Trends Cardiovasc. Med.* **2001**, *11*, 93–102. [CrossRef]
17. Estruch, M.; Sanchez-Quesada, J.L.; Ordonez Llanos, J.; Benitez, S. Electronegative LDL: A circulating modified LDL with a role in inflammation. *Mediators Inflamm.* **2013**, *2013*, 181324. [CrossRef]
18. Nyyssonen, K.; Kaikkonen, J.; Salonen, J.T. Characterization and determinants of an electronegatively charged low-density lipoprotein in human plasma. *Scand. J. Clin. Lab. Investig.* **1996**, *56*, 681–689. [CrossRef]
19. Barros, M.R.; Bertolami, M.C.; Abdalla, D.S.; Ferreira, W.P. Identification of mildly oxidized low-density lipoprotein (electronegative LDL) and its auto-antibodies IgG in children and adolescents hypercholesterolemic offsprings. *Atherosclerosis* **2006**, *184*, 103–107. [CrossRef]
20. Ivanova, E.A.; Bobryshev, Y.V.; Orekhov, A.N. LDL electronegativity index: A potential novel index for predicting cardiovascular disease. *Vasc. Health Risk Manag.* **2015**, *11*, 525–532. [CrossRef]
21. Chu, C.S.; Chan, H.C.; Tsai, M.H.; Stancel, N.; Lee, H.C.; Cheng, K.H.; Tung, Y.C.; Chan, H.C.; Wang, C.Y.; Shin, S.J.; et al. Range of L5 LDL levels in healthy adults and L5's predictive power in patients with hyperlipidemia or coronary artery disease. *Sci. Rep.* **2018**, *8*, 11866. [CrossRef] [PubMed]
22. Chu, C.S.; Law, S.H.; Lenzen, D.; Tan, Y.H.; Weng, S.F.; Ito, E.; Wu, J.C.; Chen, C.H.; Chan, H.C.; Ke, L.Y. Clinical Significance of Electronegative Low-Density Lipoprotein Cholesterol in Atherothrombosis. *Biomedicines* **2020**, *8*, 254. [CrossRef]
23. Sanchez-Quesada, J.L.; Benitez, S.; Ordonez-Llanos, J. Electronegative low-density lipoprotein. *Curr. Opin. Lipidol.* **2004**, *15*, 329–335. [CrossRef] [PubMed]
24. Benitez, S.; Camacho, M.; Arcelus, R.; Vila, L.; Bancells, C.; Ordonez-Llanos, J.; Sanchez-Quesada, J.L. Increased lysophosphatidylcholine and non-esterified fatty acid content in LDL induces chemokine release in endothelial cells. Relationship with electronegative LDL. *Atherosclerosis* **2004**, *177*, 299–305. [CrossRef] [PubMed]
25. Estruch, M.; Sanchez-Quesada, J.L.; Beloki, L.; Ordonez-Llanos, J.; Benitez, S. The Induction of Cytokine Release in Monocytes by Electronegative Low-Density Lipoprotein (LDL) Is Related to Its Higher Ceramide Content than Native LDL. *Int. J. Mol. Sci.* **2013**, *14*, 2601–2616. [CrossRef] [PubMed]
26. Ke, L.Y.; Stancel, N.; Bair, H.; Chen, C.H. The underlying chemistry of electronegative LDL's atherogenicity. *Curr. Atheroscler. Rep.* **2014**, *16*, 428. [CrossRef]
27. Chan, H.C.; Chan, H.C.; Liang, C.J.; Lee, H.C.; Su, H.; Lee, A.S.; Shiea, J.; Tsai, W.C.; Ou, T.T.; Wu, C.C.; et al. Role of Low-Density Lipoprotein in Early Vascular Aging Associated With Systemic Lupus Erythematosus. *Arthritis Rheumatol.* **2020**, *72*, 972–984. [CrossRef]
28. Ke, L.Y.; Chan, H.C.; Chen, C.C.; Lu, J.; Marathe, G.K.; Chu, C.S.; Chan, H.C.; Wang, C.Y.; Tung, Y.C.; McIntyre, T.M.; et al. Enhanced Sphingomyelinase Activity Contributes to the Apoptotic Capacity of Electronegative Low-Density Lipoprotein. *J. Med. Chem.* **2016**, *59*, 1032–1040. [CrossRef]
29. Ke, L.Y.; Engler, D.A.; Lu, J.; Matsunami, R.K.; Chan, H.C.; Wang, G.J.; Yang, C.Y.; Chang, J.G.; Chen, C.H. Chemical composition-oriented receptor selectivity of L5, a naturally occurring atherogenic low-density lipoprotein. *Pure Appl. Chem.* **2011**, *83*. [CrossRef]
30. Jayaraman, S.; Chavez, O.R.; Perez, A.; Minambres, I.; Sanchez-Quesada, J.L.; Gursky, O. Binding to heparin triggers deleterious structural and biochemical changes in human low-density lipoprotein, which are amplified in hyperglycemia. *Biochim. Biophys. Acta Mol. Cell Biol. Lipids* **2020**, *1865*, 158712. [CrossRef]
31. Bancells, C.; Benitez, S.; Ordonez-Llanos, J.; Oorni, K.; Kovanen, P.T.; Milne, R.W.; Sanchez-Quesada, J.L. Immunochemical analysis of the electronegative LDL subfraction shows that abnormal N-terminal apolipoprotein B conformation is involved in increased binding to proteoglycans. *J. Biol. Chem.* **2011**, *286*, 1125–1133. [CrossRef] [PubMed]
32. Blanco, F.J.; Villegas, S.; Benitez, S.; Bancells, C.; Diercks, T.; Ordonez-Llanos, J.; Sanchez-Quesada, J.L. 2D-NMR reveals different populations of exposed lysine residues in the apoB-100 protein of electronegative and electropositive fractions of LDL particles. *J. Lipid Res.* **2010**, *51*, 1560–1565. [CrossRef] [PubMed]

33. Chen, C.H.; Jiang, T.; Yang, J.H.; Jiang, W.; Lu, J.; Marathe, G.K.; Pownall, H.J.; Ballantyne, C.M.; McIntyre, T.M.; Henry, P.D.; et al. Low-density lipoprotein in hypercholesterolemic human plasma induces vascular endothelial cell apoptosis by inhibiting fibroblast growth factor 2 transcription. *Circulation* **2003**, *107*, 2102–2108. [CrossRef] [PubMed]
34. Yang, C.Y.; Raya, J.L.; Chen, H.H.; Chen, C.H.; Abe, Y.; Pownall, H.J.; Taylor, A.A.; Smith, C.V. Isolation, characterization, and functional assessment of oxidatively modified subfractions of circulating low-density lipoproteins. *Arterioscler. Thromb. Vasc. Biol.* **2003**, *23*, 1083–1090. [CrossRef] [PubMed]
35. Ke, L.Y.; Chan, H.C.; Chen, C.C.; Chang, C.F.; Lu, P.L.; Chu, C.S.; Lai, W.T.; Shin, S.J.; Liu, F.T.; Chen, C.H. Increased APOE glycosylation plays a key role in the atherogenicity of L5 low-density lipoprotein. *FASEB J.* **2020**, *34*, 9802–9813. [CrossRef]
36. Lu, J.; Yang, J.H.; Burns, A.R.; Chen, H.H.; Tang, D.; Walterscheid, J.P.; Suzuki, S.; Yang, C.Y.; Sawamura, T.; Chen, C.H. Mediation of electronegative low-density lipoprotein signaling by LOX-1: A possible mechanism of endothelial apoptosis. *Circ. Res.* **2009**, *104*, 619–627. [CrossRef]
37. Chan, H.C.; Ke, L.Y.; Chu, C.S.; Lee, A.S.; Shen, M.Y.; Cruz, M.A.; Hsu, J.F.; Cheng, K.H.; Chan, H.C.; Lu, J.; et al. Highly electronegative LDL from patients with ST-elevation myocardial infarction triggers platelet activation and aggregation. *Blood* **2013**, *122*, 3632–3641. [CrossRef]
38. Ke, L.Y.; Chan, H.C.; Chan, H.C.; Kalu, F.C.U.; Lee, H.C.; Lin, I.L.; Jhuo, S.J.; Lai, W.T.; Tsao, C.R.; Sawamura, T.; et al. Electronegative Low-Density Lipoprotein L5 Induces Adipose Tissue Inflammation Associated With Metabolic Syndrome. *J. Clin. Endocrinol. Metab.* **2017**, *102*, 4615–4625. [CrossRef]
39. Chang, S.F.; Chang, P.Y.; Chou, Y.C.; Lu, S.C. Electronegative LDL Induces M1 Polarization of Human Macrophages Through a LOX-1-Dependent Pathway. *Inflammation* **2020**, *43*, 1524–1535. [CrossRef]
40. Tang, D.; Lu, J.; Walterscheid, J.P.; Chen, H.H.; Engler, D.A.; Sawamura, T.; Chang, P.Y.; Safi, H.J.; Yang, C.Y.; Chen, C.H. Electronegative LDL circulating in smokers impairs endothelial progenitor cell differentiation by inhibiting Akt phosphorylation via LOX-1. *J. Lipid Res.* **2008**, *49*, 33–47. [CrossRef]
41. Chen, W.Y.; Chen, Y.F.; Chan, H.C.; Chung, C.H.; Peng, H.Y.; Ho, Y.C.; Chen, C.H.; Chang, K.C.; Tang, C.H.; Lee, A.S. Role of apolipoprotein E in electronegative low-density lipoprotein-induced mitochondrial dysfunction in cardiomyocytes. *Metab. Clin. Exp.* **2020**, *107*, 154227. [CrossRef] [PubMed]
42. Chu, C.S.; Wang, Y.C.; Lu, L.S.; Walton, B.; Yilmaz, H.R.; Huang, R.Y.; Sawamura, T.; Dixon, R.A.; Lai, W.T.; Chen, C.H.; et al. Electronegative low-density lipoprotein increases C-reactive protein expression in vascular endothelial cells through the LOX-1 receptor. *PLoS ONE* **2013**, *8*, e70533. [CrossRef] [PubMed]
43. Shen, M.Y.; Chen, F.Y.; Hsu, J.F.; Fu, R.H.; Chang, C.M.; Chang, C.T.; Liu, C.H.; Wu, J.R.; Lee, A.S.; Chan, H.C.; et al. Plasma L5 levels are elevated in ischemic stroke patients and enhance platelet aggregation. *Blood* **2016**, *127*, 1336–1345. [CrossRef] [PubMed]
44. Estruch, M.; Sanchez-Quesada, J.L.; Ordonez-Llanos, J.; Benitez, S. Ceramide-enriched LDL induces cytokine release through TLR4 and CD14 in monocytes. Similarities with electronegative LDL. *Clin. Investig. Arterioscler.* **2014**, *26*, 131–137. [CrossRef] [PubMed]
45. Ligi, D.; Benitez, S.; Croce, L.; Rivas-Urbina, A.; Puig, N.; Ordonez-Llanos, J.; Mannello, F.; Sanchez-Quesada, J.L. Electronegative LDL induces MMP-9 and TIMP-1 release in monocytes through CD14 activation: Inhibitory effect of glycosaminoglycan sulodexide. *Biochim. Biophys. Acta Mol. Basis Dis.* **2018**, *1864*, 3559–3567. [CrossRef] [PubMed]
46. Brunelli, R.; Balogh, G.; Costa, G.; De Spirito, M.; Greco, G.; Mei, G.; Nicolai, E.; Vigh, L.; Ursini, F.; Parasassi, T. Estradiol binding prevents ApoB-100 misfolding in electronegative LDL(−). *Biochemistry* **2010**, *49*, 7297–7302. [CrossRef]
47. Brunelli, R.; De Spirito, M.; Mei, G.; Papi, M.; Perrone, G.; Stefanutti, C.; Parasassi, T. Misfolding of apoprotein B-100, LDL aggregation and 17-beta -estradiol in atherogenesis. *Curr. Med. Chem.* **2014**, *21*, 2276–2283. [CrossRef]
48. Bancells, C.; Benitez, S.; Villegas, S.; Jorba, O.; Ordonez-Llanos, J.; Sanchez-Quesada, J.L. Novel phospholipolytic activities associated with electronegative low-density lipoprotein are involved in increased self-aggregation. *Biochemistry* **2008**, *47*, 8186–8194. [CrossRef]
49. Sanchez-Quesada, J.L.; Villegas, S.; Ordonez-Llanos, J. Electronegative low-density lipoprotein. A link between apolipoprotein B misfolding, lipoprotein aggregation and proteoglycan binding. *Curr. Opin. Lipidol.* **2012**, *23*, 479–486. [CrossRef]

50. Lai, Y.S.; Yang, T.C.; Chang, P.Y.; Chang, S.F.; Ho, S.L.; Chen, H.L.; Lu, S.C. Electronegative LDL is linked to high-fat, high-cholesterol diet-induced nonalcoholic steatohepatitis in hamsters. *J. Nutr. Biochem.* **2016**, *30*, 44–52. [CrossRef]
51. Chang, P.Y.; Pai, J.H.; Lai, Y.S.; Lu, S.C. Electronegative LDL from Rabbits Fed with Atherogenic Diet Is Highly Proinflammatory. *Mediators Inflamm.* **2019**, *2019*, 6163130. [CrossRef] [PubMed]
52. Kruger-Genge, A.; Blocki, A.; Franke, R.P.; Jung, F. Vascular Endothelial Cell Biology: An Update. *Int. J. Mol. Sci.* **2019**, *20*, 4411. [CrossRef] [PubMed]
53. Yau, J.W.; Teoh, H.; Verma, S. Endothelial cell control of thrombosis. *BMC Cardiovasc. Disord.* **2015**, *15*, 130. [CrossRef] [PubMed]
54. Hamilos, M.; Petousis, S.; Parthenakis, F. Interaction between platelets and endothelium: From pathophysiology to new therapeutic options. *Cardiovasc. Diagn. Ther.* **2018**, *8*, 568–580. [CrossRef]
55. Ziouzenkova, O.; Asatryan, L.; Sahady, D.; Orasanu, G.; Perrey, S.; Cutak, B.; Hassell, T.; Akiyama, T.E.; Berger, J.P.; Sevanian, A.; et al. Dual roles for lipolysis and oxidation in peroxisome proliferation-activator receptor responses to electronegative low density lipoprotein. *J. Biol. Chem.* **2003**, *278*, 39874–39881. [CrossRef]
56. Rommel, C.; Clarke, B.A.; Zimmermann, S.; Nunez, L.; Rossman, R.; Reid, K.; Moelling, K.; Yancopoulos, G.D.; Glass, D.J. Differentiation stage-specific inhibition of the Raf-MEK-ERK pathway by Akt. *Science* **1999**, *286*, 1738–1741. [CrossRef]
57. Kanda, S.; Hodgkin, M.N.; Woodfield, R.J.; Wakelam, M.J.; Thomas, G.; Claesson-Welsh, L. Phosphatidylinositol 3′-kinase-independent p70 S6 kinase activation by fibroblast growth factor receptor-1 is important for proliferation but not differentiation of endothelial cells. *J. Biol. Chem.* **1997**, *272*, 23347–23353. [CrossRef]
58. Abid, M.R.; Guo, S.; Minami, T.; Spokes, K.C.; Ueki, K.; Skurk, C.; Walsh, K.; Aird, W.C. Vascular endothelial growth factor activates PI3K/Akt/forkhead signaling in endothelial cells. *Arterioscler. Thromb. Vasc. Biol.* **2004**, *24*, 294–300. [CrossRef]
59. Lu, J.; Jiang, W.; Yang, J.H.; Chang, P.Y.; Walterscheid, J.P.; Chen, H.H.; Marcelli, M.; Tang, D.; Lee, Y.T.; Liao, W.S.; et al. Electronegative LDL impairs vascular endothelial cell integrity in diabetes by disrupting fibroblast growth factor 2 (FGF2) autoregulation. *Diabetes* **2008**, *57*, 158–166. [CrossRef]
60. Sawamura, T.; Kakino, A.; Fujita, Y. LOX-1: A multiligand receptor at the crossroads of response to danger signals. *Curr. Opin. Lipidol.* **2012**, *23*, 439–445. [CrossRef]
61. Inoue, T.; Ishida, T.; Inoue, T.; Saito, A.; Ezura, M.; Uenohara, H.; Fujimura, M.; Sato, K.; Endo, T.; Omodaka, S.; et al. Lectin-Like Oxidized Low-Density Lipoprotein Receptor-1 Levels as a Biomarker of Acute Intracerebral Hemorrhage. *J. Stroke Cerebrovasc. Dis.* **2019**, *28*, 490–494. [CrossRef] [PubMed]
62. Lubrano, V.; Pingitore, A.; Traghella, I.; Storti, S.; Parri, S.; Berti, S.; Ndreu, R.; Andrenelli, A.; Palmieri, C.; Iervasi, G.; et al. Emerging Biomarkers of Oxidative Stress in Acute and Stable Coronary Artery Disease: Levels and Determinants. *Antioxidants* **2019**, *8*, 115. [CrossRef] [PubMed]
63. Lee, A.S.; Wang, Y.C.; Chang, S.S.; Lo, P.H.; Chang, C.M.; Lu, J.; Burns, A.R.; Chen, C.H.; Kakino, A.; Sawamura, T.; et al. Detection of a High Ratio of Soluble to Membrane-Bound LOX-1 in Aspirated Coronary Thrombi From Patients With ST-Segment-Elevation Myocardial Infarction. *J. Am. Heart Assoc.* **2020**, *9*, e014008. [CrossRef] [PubMed]
64. Ishikawa, M.; Ito, H.; Akiyoshi, M.; Kume, N.; Yoshitomi, H.; Mitsuoka, H.; Tanida, S.; Murata, K.; Shibuya, H.; Kasahara, T.; et al. Lectin-like oxidized low-density lipoprotein receptor 1 signal is a potent biomarker and therapeutic target for human rheumatoid arthritis. *Arthritis Rheum.* **2012**, *64*, 1024–1034. [CrossRef] [PubMed]
65. Hofmann, A.; Brunssen, C.; Wolk, S.; Reeps, C.; Morawietz, H. Soluble LOX-1: A Novel Biomarker in Patients With Coronary Artery Disease, Stroke, and Acute Aortic Dissection? *J. Am. Heart Assoc.* **2020**, *9*, e013803. [CrossRef] [PubMed]
66. Inoue, K.; Arai, Y.; Kurihara, H.; Kita, T.; Sawamura, T. Overexpression of lectin-like oxidized low-density lipoprotein receptor-1 induces intramyocardial vasculopathy in apolipoprotein E-null mice. *Circ. Res.* **2005**, *97*, 176–184. [CrossRef]
67. Mehta, J.L.; Sanada, N.; Hu, C.P.; Chen, J.; Dandapat, A.; Sugawara, F.; Satoh, H.; Inoue, K.; Kawase, Y.; Jishage, K.; et al. Deletion of LOX-1 reduces atherogenesis in LDLR knockout mice fed high cholesterol diet. *Circ. Res.* **2007**, *100*, 1634–1642. [CrossRef]

68. Kataoka, H.; Kume, N.; Miyamoto, S.; Minami, M.; Moriwaki, H.; Murase, T.; Sawamura, T.; Masaki, T.; Hashimoto, N.; Kita, T. Expression of lectinlike oxidized low-density lipoprotein receptor-1 in human atherosclerotic lesions. *Circulation* **1999**, *99*, 3110–3117. [CrossRef]
69. Mattaliano, M.D.; Huard, C.; Cao, W.; Hill, A.A.; Zhong, W.; Martinez, R.V.; Harnish, D.C.; Paulsen, J.E.; Shih, H.H. LOX-1-dependent transcriptional regulation in response to oxidized LDL treatment of human aortic endothelial cells. *Am. J. Physiol. Cell Physiol.* **2009**, *296*, C1329–C1337. [CrossRef]
70. Kattoor, A.J.; Goel, A.; Mehta, J.L. LOX-1: Regulation, Signaling and Its Role in Atherosclerosis. *Antioxidants* **2019**, *8*, 218. [CrossRef]
71. Sagar, D.; Gaddipati, R.; Ongstad, E.L.; Bhagroo, N.; An, L.L.; Wang, J.; Belkhodja, M.; Rahman, S.; Manna, Z.; Davis, M.A.; et al. LOX-1: A potential driver of cardiovascular risk in SLE patients. *PLoS ONE* **2020**, *15*, e0229184. [CrossRef] [PubMed]
72. Xu, S.; Ogura, S.; Chen, J.; Little, P.J.; Moss, J.; Liu, P. LOX-1 in atherosclerosis: Biological functions and pharmacological modifiers. *Cell Mol. Life Sci.* **2013**, *70*, 2859–2872. [CrossRef] [PubMed]
73. Li, D.; Singh, R.M.; Liu, L.; Chen, H.; Singh, B.M.; Kazzaz, N.; Mehta, J.L. Oxidized-LDL through LOX-1 increases the expression of angiotensin converting enzyme in human coronary artery endothelial cells. *Cardiovasc. Res.* **2003**, *57*, 238–243. [CrossRef]
74. Li, D.; Mehta, J.L. Upregulation of endothelial receptor for oxidized LDL (LOX-1) by oxidized LDL and implications in apoptosis of human coronary artery endothelial cells: Evidence from use of antisense LOX-1 mRNA and chemical inhibitors. *Arterioscler. Thromb. Vasc. Biol.* **2000**, *20*, 1116–1122. [CrossRef] [PubMed]
75. Sugimoto, K.; Ishibashi, T.; Sawamura, T.; Inoue, N.; Kamioka, M.; Uekita, H.; Ohkawara, H.; Sakamoto, T.; Sakamoto, N.; Okamoto, Y.; et al. LOX-1-MT1-MMP axis is crucial for RhoA and Rac1 activation induced by oxidized low-density lipoprotein in endothelial cells. *Cardiovasc. Res.* **2009**, *84*, 127–136. [CrossRef] [PubMed]
76. Zhang, H.G.; Zhang, Q.J.; Li, B.W.; Li, L.H.; Song, X.H.; Xiong, C.M.; Zou, Y.B.; Liu, B.Y.; Han, J.Q.; Xiu, R.J. The circulating level of miR-122 is a potential risk factor for endothelial dysfunction in young patients with essential hypertension. *Hypertens. Res.* **2020**. [CrossRef] [PubMed]
77. Shi, Y.; Cosentino, F.; Camici, G.G.; Akhmedov, A.; Vanhoutte, P.M.; Tanner, F.C.; Luscher, T.F. Oxidized low-density lipoprotein activates p66Shc via lectin-like oxidized low-density lipoprotein receptor-1, protein kinase C-beta, and c-Jun N-terminal kinase kinase in human endothelial cells. *Arterioscler. Thromb. Vasc. Biol.* **2011**, *31*, 2090–2097. [CrossRef]
78. Ma, S.C.; Hao, Y.J.; Jiao, Y.; Wang, Y.H.; Xu, L.B.; Mao, C.Y.; Yang, X.L.; Yang, A.N.; Tian, J.; Zhang, M.H.; et al. Homocysteineinduced oxidative stress through TLR4/NFkappaB/DNMT1mediated LOX1 DNA methylation in endothelial cells. *Mol. Med. Rep.* **2017**, *16*, 9181–9188. [CrossRef]
79. Yu, E.P.; Bennett, M.R. The role of mitochondrial DNA damage in the development of atherosclerosis. *Free Radic. Biol. Med.* **2016**, *100*, 223–230. [CrossRef]
80. Hu, C.; Dandapat, A.; Sun, L.; Chen, J.; Marwali, M.R.; Romeo, F.; Sawamura, T.; Mehta, J.L. LOX-1 deletion decreases collagen accumulation in atherosclerotic plaque in low-density lipoprotein receptor knockout mice fed a high-cholesterol diet. *Cardiovasc. Res.* **2008**, *79*, 287–293. [CrossRef]
81. Lu, J.; Mitra, S.; Wang, X.; Khaidakov, M.; Mehta, J.L. Oxidative stress and lectin-like ox-LDL-receptor LOX-1 in atherogenesis and tumorigenesis. *Antioxid. Redox. Signal.* **2011**, *15*, 2301–2333. [CrossRef]
82. Murphy, M.P. How mitochondria produce reactive oxygen species. *Biochem. J.* **2009**, *417*, 1–13. [CrossRef]
83. Koziel, R.; Pircher, H.; Kratochwil, M.; Lener, B.; Hermann, M.; Dencher, N.A.; Jansen-Durr, P. Mitochondrial respiratory chain complex I is inactivated by NADPH oxidase Nox4. *Biochem. J.* **2013**, *452*, 231–239. [CrossRef] [PubMed]
84. Giorgio, M.; Migliaccio, E.; Orsini, F.; Paolucci, D.; Moroni, M.; Contursi, C.; Pelliccia, G.; Luzi, L.; Minucci, S.; Marcaccio, M.; et al. Electron transfer between cytochrome c and p66Shc generates reactive oxygen species that trigger mitochondrial apoptosis. *Cell* **2005**, *122*, 221–233. [CrossRef] [PubMed]
85. Trinei, M.; Berniakovich, I.; Beltrami, E.; Migliaccio, E.; Fassina, A.; Pelicci, P.; Giorgio, M. P66Shc signals to age. *Aging (Albany N.Y.)* **2009**, *1*, 503–510. [CrossRef] [PubMed]
86. Chang, C.T.; Wang, G.J.; Kuo, C.C.; Hsieh, J.Y.; Lee, A.S.; Chang, C.M.; Wang, C.C.; Shen, M.Y.; Huang, C.C.; Sawamura, T.; et al. Electronegative Low-density Lipoprotein Increases Coronary Artery Disease Risk in Uremia Patients on Maintenance Hemodialysis. *Medicine* **2016**, *95*, e2265. [CrossRef] [PubMed]

87. Ron, D.; Walter, P. Signal integration in the endoplasmic reticulum unfolded protein response. *Nat. Rev. Mol. Cell Biol.* **2007**, *8*, 519–529. [CrossRef]
88. Sanson, M.; Auge, N.; Vindis, C.; Muller, C.; Bando, Y.; Thiers, J.C.; Marachet, M.A.; Zarkovic, K.; Sawa, Y.; Salvayre, R.; et al. Oxidized low-density lipoproteins trigger endoplasmic reticulum stress in vascular cells: Prevention by oxygen-regulated protein 150 expression. *Circ. Res.* **2009**, *104*, 328–336. [CrossRef]
89. Gora, S.; Maouche, S.; Atout, R.; Wanherdrick, K.; Lambeau, G.; Cambien, F.; Ninio, E.; Karabina, S.A. Phospholipolyzed LDL induces an inflammatory response in endothelial cells through endoplasmic reticulum stress signaling. *FASEB J.* **2010**, *24*, 3284–3297. [CrossRef]
90. Gargalovic, P.S.; Gharavi, N.M.; Clark, M.J.; Pagnon, J.; Yang, W.P.; He, A.; Truong, A.; Baruch-Oren, T.; Berliner, J.A.; Kirchgessner, T.G.; et al. The unfolded protein response is an important regulator of inflammatory genes in endothelial cells. *Arterioscler. Thromb. Vasc. Biol.* **2006**, *26*, 2490–2496. [CrossRef]
91. Xie, X.; Zhao, R.; Shen, G.X. Impact of cyanidin-3-glucoside on glycated LDL-induced NADPH oxidase activation, mitochondrial dysfunction and cell viability in cultured vascular endothelial cells. *Int. J. Mol. Sci.* **2012**, *13*, 15867–15880. [CrossRef] [PubMed]
92. Zhao, R.; Xie, X.; Le, K.; Li, W.; Moghadasian, M.H.; Beta, T.; Shen, G.X. Endoplasmic reticulum stress in diabetic mouse or glycated LDL-treated endothelial cells: Protective effect of Saskatoon berry powder and cyanidin glycans. *J. Nutr. Biochem.* **2015**, *26*, 1248–1253. [CrossRef]
93. Benitez, S.; Bancells, C.; Ordonez-Llanos, J.; Sanchez-Quesada, J.L. Pro-inflammatory action of LDL(−) on mononuclear cells is counteracted by increased IL10 production. *Biochim. Biophys. Acta* **2007**, *1771*, 613–622. [CrossRef]
94. Benitez, S.; Camacho, M.; Bancells, C.; Vila, L.; Sanchez-Quesada, J.L.; Ordonez-Llanos, J. Wide proinflammatory effect of electronegative low-density lipoprotein on human endothelial cells assayed by a protein array. *Biochim. Biophys. Acta* **2006**, *1761*, 1014–1021. [CrossRef] [PubMed]
95. De Castellarnau, C.; Sanchez-Quesada, J.L.; Benitez, S.; Rosa, R.; Caveda, L.; Vila, L.; Ordonez-Llanos, J. Electronegative LDL from normolipemic subjects induces IL-8 and monocyte chemotactic protein secretion by human endothelial cells. *Arterioscler. Thromb. Vasc. Biol.* **2000**, *20*, 2281–2287. [CrossRef] [PubMed]
96. Demuth, K.; Myara, I.; Chappey, B.; Vedie, B.; Pech-Amsellem, M.A.; Haberland, M.E.; Moatti, N. A cytotoxic electronegative LDL subfraction is present in human plasma. *Arterioscler. Thromb. Vasc. Biol.* **1996**, *16*, 773–783. [CrossRef] [PubMed]
97. Hodis, H.N.; Kramsch, D.M.; Avogaro, P.; Bittolo-Bon, G.; Cazzolato, G.; Hwang, J.; Peterson, H.; Sevanian, A. Biochemical and cytotoxic characteristics of an in vivo circulating oxidized low density lipoprotein (LDL-). *J. Lipid Res.* **1994**, *35*, 669–677.
98. Estruch, M.; Rajamaki, K.; Sanchez-Quesada, J.L.; Kovanen, P.T.; Oorni, K.; Benitez, S.; Ordonez-Llanos, J. Electronegative LDL induces priming and inflammasome activation leading to IL-1beta release in human monocytes and macrophages. *Biochim. Biophys. Acta* **2015**, *1851*, 1442–1449. [CrossRef]
99. Estruch, M.; Sanchez-Quesada, J.L.; Ordonez-Llanos, J.; Benitez, S. Inflammatory intracellular pathways activated by electronegative LDL in monocytes. *Biochim. Biophys. Acta* **2016**, *1861 Pt A*, 963–969. [CrossRef]
100. Glass, C.K.; Witztum, J.L. Atherosclerosis. the road ahead. *Cell* **2001**, *104*, 503–516. [CrossRef]
101. Gordon, S.; Martinez, F.O. Alternative activation of macrophages: Mechanism and functions. *Immunity* **2010**, *32*, 593–604. [CrossRef] [PubMed]
102. Yang, T.C.; Chang, P.Y.; Lu, S.C. L5-LDL from ST-elevation myocardial infarction patients induces IL-1beta production via LOX-1 and NLRP3 inflammasome activation in macrophages. *Am. J. Physiol. Heart Circ. Physiol.* **2017**, *312*, H265–H274. [CrossRef] [PubMed]
103. Yang, T.C.; Chang, P.Y.; Kuo, T.L.; Lu, S.C. Electronegative L5-LDL induces the production of G-CSF and GM-CSF in human macrophages through LOX-1 involving NF-kappaB and ERK2 activation. *Atherosclerosis* **2017**, *267*, 1–9. [CrossRef] [PubMed]
104. Chang, C.K.; Chen, P.K.; Lan, J.L.; Chang, S.H.; Hsieh, T.Y.; Liao, P.J.; Chen, C.H.; Chen, D.Y. Association of Electronegative LDL with Macrophage Foam Cell Formation and CD11c Expression in Rheumatoid Arthritis Patients. *Int. J. Mol. Sci.* **2020**, *21*, 5883. [CrossRef] [PubMed]
105. Pedrosa, A.M.; Faine, L.A.; Grosso, D.M.; de Las Heras, B.; Bosca, L.; Abdalla, D.S. Electronegative LDL induction of apoptosis in macrophages: Involvement of Nrf2. *Biochim. Biophys. Acta* **2010**, *1801*, 430–437. [CrossRef] [PubMed]

106. Parguina, A.F.; Grigorian-Shamagian, L.; Agra, R.M.; Lopez-Otero, D.; Rosa, I.; Alonso, J.; Teijeira-Fernandez, E.; Gonzalez-Juanatey, J.R.; Garcia, A. Variations in platelet proteins associated with ST-elevation myocardial infarction: Novel clues on pathways underlying platelet activation in acute coronary syndromes. *Arterioscler. Thromb. Vasc. Biol.* **2011**, *31*, 2957–2964. [CrossRef]
107. Podrez, E.A.; Byzova, T.V. Prothrombotic lipoprotein patterns in stroke. *Blood* **2016**, *127*, 1221–1222. [CrossRef]
108. Hou, X.; Summer, R.; Chen, Z.; Tian, Y.; Ma, J.; Cui, J.; Hao, X.; Guo, L.; Xu, H.; Wang, H.; et al. Lipid Uptake by Alveolar Macrophages Drives Fibrotic Responses to Silica Dust. *Sci. Rep.* **2019**, *9*, 399. [CrossRef]
109. Yoshida, H.; Quehenberger, O.; Kondratenko, N.; Green, S.; Steinberg, D. Minimally oxidized low-density lipoprotein increases expression of scavenger receptor A, CD36, and macrosialin in resident mouse peritoneal macrophages. *Arterioscler. Thromb. Vasc. Biol.* **1998**, *18*, 794–802. [CrossRef]
110. Nagy, L.; Tontonoz, P.; Alvarez, J.G.; Chen, H.; Evans, R.M. Oxidized LDL regulates macrophage gene expression through ligand activation of PPARgamma. *Cell* **1998**, *93*, 229–240. [CrossRef]
111. Rahalkar, A.R.; Hegele, R.A. Monogenic pediatric dyslipidemias: Classification, genetics and clinical spectrum. *Mol. Genet. Metab.* **2008**, *93*, 282–294. [CrossRef] [PubMed]
112. Tall, A.R. Protease variants, LDL, and coronary heart disease. *N. Engl. J. Med.* **2006**, *354*, 1310–1312. [CrossRef] [PubMed]
113. Sisman, G.; Erzin, Y.; Hatemi, I.; Caglar, E.; Boga, S.; Singh, V.; Senturk, H. Familial chylomicronemia syndrome related chronic pancreatitis: A single-center study. *Hepatobiliary Pancreat. Dis. Int.* **2014**, *13*, 209–214. [CrossRef]
114. Steinberg, D. Atherogenesis in perspective: Hypercholesterolemia and inflammation as partners in crime. *Nat. Med.* **2002**, *8*, 1211–1217. [CrossRef]
115. Brown, M.S.; Goldstein, J.L. A receptor-mediated pathway for cholesterol homeostasis. *Science* **1986**, *232*, 34–47. [CrossRef]
116. Stalenhoef, A.F.; van 't Laar, A. Clinical significance of current perspectives in cholesterol metabolism. *Ned. Tijdschr. Geneeskd.* **1986**, *130*, 951–955.
117. Goldstein, J.L.; Brown, M.S. Molecular medicine. The cholesterol quartet. *Science* **2001**, *292*, 1310–1312. [CrossRef]
118. Horton, J.D.; Goldstein, J.L.; Brown, M.S. SREBPs: Activators of the complete program of cholesterol and fatty acid synthesis in the liver. *J. Clin. Investig.* **2002**, *109*, 1125–1131. [CrossRef]
119. Steinberg, D. The LDL modification hypothesis of atherogenesis: An update. *J. Lipid Res.* **2009**, *50*, S376–S381. [CrossRef]
120. Parthasarathy, S.; Wieland, E.; Steinberg, D. A role for endothelial cell lipoxygenase in the oxidative modification of low density lipoprotein. *Proc. Natl. Acad. Sci. USA* **1989**, *86*, 1046–1050. [CrossRef]
121. Benz, D.J.; Mol, M.; Ezaki, M.; Mori-Ito, N.; Zelan, I.; Miyanohara, A.; Friedmann, T.; Parthasarathy, S.; Steinberg, D.; Witztum, J.L. Enhanced levels of lipoperoxides in low density lipoprotein incubated with murine fibroblast expressing high levels of human 15-lipoxygenase. *J. Biol. Chem.* **1995**, *270*, 5191–5197. [CrossRef] [PubMed]
122. Steinberg, D. Low density lipoprotein oxidation and its pathobiological significance. *J. Biol. Chem.* **1997**, *272*, 20963–20966. [CrossRef] [PubMed]
123. Yoshida, H.; Ishikawa, T.; Hosoai, H.; Suzukawa, M.; Ayaori, M.; Hisada, T.; Sawada, S.; Yonemura, A.; Higashi, K.; Ito, T.; et al. Inhibitory effect of tea flavonoids on the ability of cells to oxidize low density lipoprotein. *Biochem. Pharmacol.* **1999**, *58*, 1695–1703. [CrossRef]
124. Yoshida, H.; Sasaki, K.; Namiki, Y.; Sato, N.; Tada, N. Edaravone, a novel radical scavenger, inhibits oxidative modification of low-density lipoprotein (LDL) and reverses oxidized LDL-mediated reduction in the expression of endothelial nitric oxide synthase. *Atherosclerosis* **2005**, *179*, 97–102. [CrossRef] [PubMed]
125. Wang, J.Y.; Lai, C.L.; Lee, C.T.; Lin, C.Y. Electronegative Low-Density Lipoprotein L5 Impairs Viability and NGF-Induced Neuronal Differentiation of PC12 Cells via LOX-1. *Int. J. Mol. Sci.* **2017**, *18*, 1744. [CrossRef]
126. Gerhard-Herman, M.D.; Gornik, H.L.; Barrett, C.; Barshes, N.R.; Corriere, M.A.; Drachman, D.E.; Fleisher, L.A.; Fowkes, F.G.R.; Hamburg, N.M.; Kinlay, S.; et al. 2016 AHA/ACC Guideline on the Management of Patients With Lower Extremity Peripheral Artery Disease: A Report of the American College of Cardiology/American Heart Association Task Force on Clinical Practice Guidelines. *J. Am. Coll. Cardiol.* **2017**, *69*, e71–e126. [CrossRef]

127. Pollak, A.W.; Norton, P.T.; Kramer, C.M. Multimodality imaging of lower extremity peripheral arterial disease: Current role and future directions. *Circ. Cardiovasc. Imaging* **2012**, *5*, 797–807. [CrossRef]
128. Shishehbor, M.H.; White, C.J.; Gray, B.H.; Menard, M.T.; Lookstein, R.; Rosenfield, K.; Jaff, M.R. Critical Limb Ischemia: An Expert Statement. *J. Am. Coll. Cardiol.* **2016**, *68*, 2002–2015. [CrossRef]
129. Grundy, S.M.; Stone, N.J.; Bailey, A.L.; Beam, C.; Birtcher, K.K.; Blumenthal, R.S.; Braun, L.T.; de Ferranti, S.; Faiella-Tommasino, J.; Forman, D.E.; et al. 2018 AHA/ACC/AACVPR/AAPA/ABC/ACPM/ADA/AGS/APhA/ASPC/NLA/PCNA Guideline on the Management of Blood Cholesterol: A Report of the American College of Cardiology/American Heart Association Task Force on Clinical Practice Guidelines. *J. Am. Coll. Cardiol.* **2019**, *73*, e285–e350. [CrossRef]
130. Wadhera, R.K.; Steen, D.L.; Khan, I.; Giugliano, R.P.; Foody, J.M. A review of low-density lipoprotein cholesterol, treatment strategies, and its impact on cardiovascular disease morbidity and mortality. *J. Clin. Lipidol.* **2016**, *10*, 472–489. [CrossRef]
131. Koskinas, K.C.; Siontis, G.C.M.; Piccolo, R.; Mavridis, D.; Raber, L.; Mach, F.; Windecker, S. Effect of statins and non-statin LDL-lowering medications on cardiovascular outcomes in secondary prevention: A meta-analysis of randomized trials. *Eur. Heart J.* **2018**, *39*, 1172–1180. [CrossRef] [PubMed]
132. Li, G.; Wang, X.; Yang, H.; Zhang, P.; Wu, F.; Li, Y.; Zhou, Y.; Zhang, X.; Ma, H.; Zhang, W.; et al. alpha-Linolenic acid but not linolenic acid protects against hypertension: Critical role of SIRT3 and autophagic flux. *Cell Death Dis.* **2020**, *11*, 83. [CrossRef] [PubMed]
133. Stafylas, P.C.; Sarafidis, P.A. Carvedilol in hypertension treatment. *Vasc. Health Risk Manag.* **2008**, *4*, 23–30. [CrossRef] [PubMed]
134. Leonetti, G.; Egan, C.G. Use of carvedilol in hypertension: An update. *Vasc. Health Risk Manag.* **2012**, *8*, 307–322. [CrossRef] [PubMed]
135. Sy, R.G.; Nevado, J.B., Jr.; Llanes, E.J.B.; Magno, J.D.A.; Ona, D.I.D.; Punzalan, F.E.R.; Reganit, P.F.M.; Santos, L.E.G.; Tiongco, R.H.P., 2nd; Aherrera, J.A.M.; et al. The Klotho Variant rs36217263 Is Associated With Poor Response to Cardioselective Beta-Blocker Therapy Among Filipinos. *Clin. Pharmacol. Ther.* **2020**, *107*, 221–226. [CrossRef]
136. Silva, I.V.G.; de Figueiredo, R.C.; Rios, D.R.A. Effect of Different Classes of Antihypertensive Drugs on Endothelial Function and Inflammation. *Int. J. Mol. Sci.* **2019**, *20*, 3548. [CrossRef] [PubMed]
137. Erbs, S.; Beck, E.B.; Linke, A.; Adams, V.; Gielen, S.; Krankel, N.; Mobius-Winkler, S.; Hollriegel, R.; Thiele, H.; Hambrecht, R.; et al. High-dose rosuvastatin in chronic heart failure promotes vasculogenesis, corrects endothelial function, and improves cardiac remodeling—Results from a randomized, double-blind, and placebo-controlled study. *Int. J. Cardiol.* **2011**, *146*, 56–63. [CrossRef]
138. Szygula-Jurkiewicz, B.; Szczurek, W.; Krol, B.; Zembala, M. The role of statins in chronic heart failure. *Kardiochir Torakochirurgia Pol.* **2014**, *11*, 301–305. [CrossRef]
139. Cangiano, E.; Marchesini, J.; Campo, G.; Francolini, G.; Fortini, C.; Carra, G.; Miccoli, M.; Ceconi, C.; Tavazzi, L.; Ferrari, R. ACE inhibition modulates endothelial apoptosis and renewal via endothelial progenitor cells in patients with acute coronary syndromes. *Am. J. Cardiovasc. Drugs* **2011**, *11*, 189–198. [CrossRef]
140. Brugts, J.J.; Bertrand, M.; Remme, W.; Ferrari, R.; Fox, K.; MacMahon, S.; Chalmers, J.; Simoons, M.L.; Boersma, E. The Treatment Effect of an ACE-Inhibitor Based Regimen with Perindopril in Relation to Beta-Blocker use in 29,463 Patients with Vascular Disease: A Combined Analysis of Individual Data of ADVANCE, EUROPA and PROGRESS Trials. *Cardiovasc. Drugs Ther.* **2017**, *31*, 391–400. [CrossRef]
141. Rangaswami, J.; McCullough, P.A. Heart Failure in End-Stage Kidney Disease: Pathophysiology, Diagnosis, and Therapeutic Strategies. *Semin. Nephrol.* **2018**, *38*, 600–617. [CrossRef] [PubMed]
142. Weaver, D.J.; Mitsnefes, M. Cardiovascular Disease in Children and Adolescents With Chronic Kidney Disease. *Semin. Nephrol.* **2018**, *38*, 559–569. [CrossRef] [PubMed]
143. Kern, A.; Gil, R.; Gorny, J.; Sienkiewicz, E.; Bojko, K.; Wasilewski, G. Patient with ST-elevation myocardial infarction, coronary artery embolism and no signs of coronary atherosclerosis in angiography. *Postepy Kardiol. Interwencyjnej* **2015**, *11*, 334–336. [CrossRef] [PubMed]
144. Vernon, S.T.; Coffey, S.; D'Souza, M.; Chow, C.K.; Kilian, J.; Hyun, K.; Shaw, J.A.; Adams, M.; Roberts-Thomson, P.; Brieger, D.; et al. ST-Segment-Elevation Myocardial Infarction (STEMI) Patients Without Standard Modifiable Cardiovascular Risk Factors-How Common Are They, and What Are Their Outcomes? *J. Am. Heart Assoc.* **2019**, *8*, e013296. [CrossRef]

145. Corretti, M.C.; Anderson, T.J.; Benjamin, E.J.; Celermajer, D.; Charbonneau, F.; Creager, M.A.; Deanfield, J.; Drexler, H.; Gerhard-Herman, M.; Herrington, D.; et al. Guidelines for the ultrasound assessment of endothelial-dependent flow-mediated vasodilation of the brachial artery: A report of the International Brachial Artery Reactivity Task Force. *J. Am. Coll. Cardiol.* **2002**, *39*, 257–265. [CrossRef]
146. Chen, C.J.; Yang, T.C.; Chang, C.; Lu, S.C.; Chang, P.Y. Homocysteine is a bystander for ST-segment elevation myocardial infarction: A case-control study. *BMC Cardiovasc. Disord.* **2018**, *18*, 33. [CrossRef]
147. Zou, C.; Hu, H. Use of pioglitazone in the treatment of diabetes: Effect on cardiovascular risk. *Vasc. Health Risk Manag.* **2013**, *9*, 429–433. [CrossRef]
148. Yu, X.; Chen, P.; Wang, H.; Zhu, T. Pioglitazone ameliorates endothelial dysfunction in those with impaired glucose regulation among the first-degree relatives of type 2 diabetes mellitus patients. *Med. Princ. Pract.* **2013**, *22*, 156–160. [CrossRef]
149. Abdullah, C.S.; Li, Z.; Wang, X.; Jin, Z.Q. Depletion of T lymphocytes ameliorates cardiac fibrosis in streptozotocin-induced diabetic cardiomyopathy. *Int. Immunopharmacol.* **2016**, *39*, 251–264. [CrossRef]
150. Samuel, C.S.; Hewitson, T.D.; Zhang, Y.; Kelly, D.J. Relaxin ameliorates fibrosis in experimental diabetic cardiomyopathy. *Endocrinology* **2008**, *149*, 3286–3293. [CrossRef]
151. Zhang, X.; Pan, L.; Yang, K.; Fu, Y.; Liu, Y.; Chi, J.; Zhang, X.; Hong, S.; Ma, X.; Yin, X. H3 Relaxin Protects Against Myocardial Injury in Experimental Diabetic Cardiomyopathy by Inhibiting Myocardial Apoptosis, Fibrosis and Inflammation. *Cell Physiol. Biochem.* **2017**, *43*, 1311–1324. [CrossRef] [PubMed]
152. Zhang, M.; Wang, C.M.; Li, J.; Meng, Z.J.; Wei, S.N.; Li, J.; Bucala, R.; Li, Y.L.; Chen, L. Berberine protects against palmitate-induced endothelial dysfunction: Involvements of upregulation of AMPK and eNOS and downregulation of NOX4. *Mediators Inflamm.* **2013**, *2013*, 260464. [CrossRef] [PubMed]
153. Wang, Y.; Huang, Y.; Lam, K.S.; Li, Y.; Wong, W.T.; Ye, H.; Lau, C.W.; Vanhoutte, P.M.; Xu, A. Berberine prevents hyperglycemia-induced endothelial injury and enhances vasodilatation via adenosine monophosphate-activated protein kinase and endothelial nitric oxide synthase. *Cardiovasc. Res.* **2009**, *82*, 484–492. [CrossRef] [PubMed]
154. Suganya, N.; Bhakkiyalakshmi, E.; Sarada, D.V.; Ramkumar, K.M. Reversibility of endothelial dysfunction in diabetes: Role of polyphenols. *Br. J. Nutr.* **2016**, *116*, 223–246. [CrossRef]
155. Forcheron, F.; Basset, A.; Abdallah, P.; Del Carmine, P.; Gadot, N.; Beylot, M. Diabetic cardiomyopathy: Effects of fenofibrate and metformin in an experimental model—The Zucker diabetic rat. *Cardiovasc. Diabetol.* **2009**, *8*, 16. [CrossRef]
156. Baraka, A.; AbdelGawad, H. Targeting apoptosis in the heart of streptozotocin-induced diabetic rats. *J. Cardiovasc. Pharmacol. Ther.* **2010**, *15*, 175–181. [CrossRef]
157. Arosio, E.; De Marchi, S.; Rigoni, A.; Prior, M.; Delva, P.; Lechi, A. Forearm haemodynamics, arterial stiffness and microcirculatory reactivity in rheumatoid arthritis. *J. Hypertens.* **2007**, *25*, 1273–1278. [CrossRef] [PubMed]
158. Ruiz-Limon, P.; Ortega, R.; Arias de la Rosa, I.; Abalos-Aguilera, M.D.C.; Perez-Sanchez, C.; Jimenez-Gomez, Y.; Peralbo-Santaella, E.; Font, P.; Ruiz-Vilches, D.; Ferrin, G.; et al. Tocilizumab improves the proatherothrombotic profile of rheumatoid arthritis patients modulating endothelial dysfunction, NETosis, and inflammation. *Transl. Res.* **2017**, *183*, 87–103. [CrossRef] [PubMed]
159. Fanouriakis, A.; Pamfil, C.; Rednic, S.; Sidiropoulos, P.; Bertsias, G.; Boumpas, D.T. Is it primary neuropsychiatric systemic lupus erythematosus? Performance of existing attribution models using physician judgment as the gold standard. *Clin. Exp. Rheumatol.* **2016**, *34*, 910–917. [PubMed]
160. Nikolopoulos, D.; Fanouriakis, A.; Boumpas, D.T. Cerebrovascular Events in Systemic Lupus Erythematosus: Diagnosis and Management. *Mediterr. J. Rheumatol.* **2019**, *30*, 7–15. [CrossRef] [PubMed]
161. Aringer, M.; Leuchten, N.; Dorner, T. Biologicals and small molecules for systemic lupus erythematosus. *Z. Rheumatol.* **2020**, *79*, 232–240. [CrossRef] [PubMed]
162. Lee, S.E.; Chang, H.J.; Sung, J.M.; Park, H.B.; Heo, R.; Rizvi, A.; Lin, F.Y.; Kumar, A.; Hadamitzky, M.; Kim, Y.J.; et al. Effects of Statins on Coronary Atherosclerotic Plaques: The PARADIGM Study. *JACC Cardiovasc. Imaging* **2018**, *11*, 1475–1484. [CrossRef]
163. Nicholls, S.J.; Nelson, A.J. Monitoring the Response to Statin Therapy: One Scan at a Time. *JACC Cardiovasc. Imaging* **2018**, *11*, 1485–1486. [CrossRef] [PubMed]

164. Yla-Herttuala, S.; Bentzon, J.F.; Daemen, M.; Falk, E.; Garcia-Garcia, H.M.; Herrmann, J.; Hoefer, I.; Jauhiainen, S.; Jukema, J.W.; Krams, R.; et al. Stabilization of atherosclerotic plaques: An update. *Eur. Heart J.* **2013**, *34*, 3251–3258. [CrossRef] [PubMed]
165. Chu, C.S.; Ke, L.Y.; Chan, H.C.; Chan, H.C.; Chen, C.C.; Cheng, K.H.; Lee, H.C.; Kuo, H.F.; Chang, C.T.; Chang, K.C.; et al. Four Statin Benefit Groups Defined by The 2013 ACC/AHA New Cholesterol Guideline are Characterized by Increased Plasma Level of Electronegative Low-Density Lipoprotein. *Acta Cardiol. Sin.* **2016**, *32*, 667–675. [CrossRef] [PubMed]
166. Zhang, B.; Miura, S.; Yanagi, D.; Noda, K.; Nishikawa, H.; Matsunaga, A.; Shirai, K.; Iwata, A.; Yoshinaga, K.; Adachi, H.; et al. Reduction of charge-modified LDL by statin therapy in patients with CHD or CHD risk factors and elevated LDL-C levels: The SPECIAL Study. *Atherosclerosis* **2008**, *201*, 353–359. [CrossRef]
167. Zhang, B.; Matsunaga, A.; Rainwater, D.L.; Miura, S.; Noda, K.; Nishikawa, H.; Uehara, Y.; Shirai, K.; Ogawa, M.; Saku, K. Effects of rosuvastatin on electronegative LDL as characterized by capillary isotachophoresis: The ROSARY Study. *J. Lipid Res.* **2009**, *50*, 1832–1841. [CrossRef]
168. Sena-Evangelista, K.C.; Pedrosa, L.F.; Paiva, M.S.; Dias, P.C.; Ferreira, D.Q.; Cozzolino, S.M.; Faulin, T.E.; Abdalla, D.S. The hypolipidemic and pleiotropic effects of rosuvastatin are not enhanced by its association with zinc and selenium supplementation in coronary artery disease patients: A double blind randomized controlled study. *PLoS ONE* **2015**, *10*, e0119830. [CrossRef]
169. Vavlukis, M.; Vavlukis, A. Adding ezetimibe to statin therapy: Latest evidence and clinical implications. *Drugs Context* **2018**, *7*, 212534. [CrossRef]
170. Page, M.M.; Watts, G.F. PCSK9 inhibitors—Mechanisms of action. *Aust. Prescr.* **2016**, *39*, 164–167. [CrossRef]
171. Ikegami, Y.; Inoue, I.; Inoue, K.; Shinoda, Y.; Iida, S.; Goto, S.; Nakano, T.; Shimada, A.; Noda, M. The annual rate of coronary artery calcification with combination therapy with a PCSK9 inhibitor and a statin is lower than that with statin monotherapy. *NPJ Aging Mech. Dis.* **2018**, *4*, 7. [CrossRef] [PubMed]
172. Alonso, R.; Mata, P.; Muniz, O.; Fuentes-Jimenez, F.; Diaz, J.L.; Zambon, D.; Tomas, M.; Martin, C.; Moyon, T.; Croyal, M.; et al. PCSK9 and lipoprotein (a) levels are two predictors of coronary artery calcification in asymptomatic patients with familial hypercholesterolemia. *Atherosclerosis* **2016**, *254*, 249–253. [CrossRef] [PubMed]
173. Kuhnast, S.; van der Hoorn, J.W.; Pieterman, E.J.; van den Hoek, A.M.; Sasiela, W.J.; Gusarova, V.; Peyman, A.; Schafer, H.L.; Schwahn, U.; Jukema, J.W.; et al. Alirocumab inhibits atherosclerosis, improves the plaque morphology, and enhances the effects of a statin. *J. Lipid Res.* **2014**, *55*, 2103–2112. [CrossRef]
174. Pouwer, M.G.; Pieterman, E.J.; Worms, N.; Keijzer, N.; Jukema, J.W.; Gromada, J.; Gusarova, V.; Princen, H.M.G. Alirocumab, evinacumab, and atorvastatin triple therapy regresses plaque lesions and improves lesion composition in mice. *J. Lipid Res.* **2020**, *61*, 365–375. [CrossRef] [PubMed]
175. Berbee, J.F.; Wong, M.C.; Wang, Y.; van der Hoorn, J.W.; Khedoe, P.P.; van Klinken, J.B.; Mol, I.M.; Hiemstra, P.S.; Tsikas, D.; Romijn, J.A.; et al. Resveratrol protects against atherosclerosis, but does not add to the antiatherogenic effect of atorvastatin, in APOE*3-Leiden.CETP mice. *J. Nutr. Biochem.* **2013**, *24*, 1423–1430. [CrossRef] [PubMed]
176. Mishra, V.K.; Shih, H.H.; Parveen, F.; Lenzen, D.; Ito, E.; Chan, T.F.; Ke, L.Y. Identifying the Therapeutic Significance of Mesenchymal Stem Cells. *Cells* **2020**, *9*, 1145. [CrossRef]
177. Back, M. Leukotriene signaling in atherosclerosis and ischemia. *Cardiovasc. Drugs Ther.* **2009**, *23*, 41–48. [CrossRef]
178. Charo, I.F.; Taub, R. Anti-inflammatory therapeutics for the treatment of atherosclerosis. *Nat. Rev. Drug Discov.* **2011**, *10*, 365–376. [CrossRef]
179. Bertrand, M.J.; Tardif, J.C. Inflammation and beyond: New directions and emerging drugs for treating atherosclerosis. *Expert Opin. Emerg. Drugs* **2017**, *22*, 1–26. [CrossRef]
180. Tuttolomondo, A. Editorial: Treatment of atherosclerosis as an inflammatory disease. *Curr. Pharm. Des.* **2012**, *18*, 4265. [CrossRef]
181. Raggi, P.; Genest, J.; Giles, J.T.; Rayner, K.J.; Dwivedi, G.; Beanlands, R.S.; Gupta, M. Role of inflammation in the pathogenesis of atherosclerosis and therapeutic interventions. *Atherosclerosis* **2018**, *276*, 98–108. [CrossRef] [PubMed]
182. Riccioni, G.; Zanasi, A.; Vitulano, N.; Mancini, B.; D'Orazio, N. Leukotrienes in atherosclerosis: New target insights and future therapy perspectives. *Mediators Inflamm.* **2009**, *2009*, 737282. [CrossRef] [PubMed]

183. Lin, J.; Kakkar, V.; Lu, X. Impact of MCP-1 in atherosclerosis. *Curr. Pharm. Des.* **2014**, *20*, 4580–4588. [CrossRef] [PubMed]
184. Tousoulis, D.; Oikonomou, E.; Economou, E.K.; Crea, F.; Kaski, J.C. Inflammatory cytokines in atherosclerosis: Current therapeutic approaches. *Eur. Heart J.* **2016**, *37*, 1723–1732. [CrossRef] [PubMed]
185. Pieper, G.M. Enhanced, unaltered and impaired nitric oxide-mediated endothelium-dependent relaxation in experimental diabetes mellitus: Importance of disease duration. *Diabetologia* **1999**, *42*, 204–213. [CrossRef] [PubMed]
186. Li, H.; Forstermann, U. Nitric oxide in the pathogenesis of vascular disease. *J. Pathol.* **2000**, *190*, 244–254. [CrossRef]
187. McLeod, D.S.; Lefer, D.J.; Merges, C.; Lutty, G.A. Enhanced expression of intracellular adhesion molecule-1 and P-selectin in the diabetic human retina and choroid. *Am. J. Pathol.* **1995**, *147*, 642–653.

2

Prediction of Major Depressive Disorder Following Beta-Blocker Therapy in Patients with Cardiovascular Diseases

Suho Jin [1], Kristin Kostka [2], Jose D. Posada [3], Yeesuk Kim [4], Seung In Seo [5], Dong Yun Lee [6], Nigam H. Shah [3], Sungwon Roh [7], Young-Hyo Lim [8], Sun Geu Chae [9], Uram Jin [10], Sang Joon Son [6], Christian Reich [2], Peter R. Rijnbeek [11], Rae Woong Park [1,12,*] and Seng Chan You [1,*]

1 Department of Biomedical Informatics, Ajou University School of Medicine, Suwon 16499, Korea; jshsh7553@ajou.ac.kr
2 Real World Solutions, IQVIA, Cambridge, MA 02139, USA; kristin.kostka@iqvia.com (K.K.); christian.reich@iqvia.com (C.R.)
3 Department of Medicine, School of Medicine, Stanford University, Stanford, CA 94305, USA; jdposada@stanford.edu (J.D.P.); nigam@stanford.edu (N.H.S.)
4 Department of Orthopaedic Surgery, College of Medicine, Hanyang University, Seoul 04763, Korea; estone96@gmail.com
5 Department of Internal Medicine, Kangdong Sacred Heart Hospital, Hallym University College of Medicine, Seoul 05355, Korea; doctorssi@kdh.or.kr
6 Department of Psychiatry, Ajou University School of Medicine, Suwon 16499, Korea; dongyun909@gmail.com (D.Y.L.); sjsonpsy@ajou.ac.kr (S.J.S.)
7 Department of Psychiatry, College of Medicine, Hanyang University, Seoul 04763, Korea; swroh@hanyang.ac.kr
8 Division of Cardiology, Department of Internal Medicine, College of Medicine, Hanyang University, Seoul 04763, Korea; mdoim@hanyang.ac.kr
9 Department of Industrial Engineering, Hanyang University, Seoul 04763, Korea; sgchae@psm.hanyang.ac.kr
10 Department of Cardiology, Ajou University School of Medicine, Suwon 16499, Korea; statery@aumc.ac.kr
11 Department of Medical Informatics, Erasmus Medical Center, 3015 GD Rotterdam, The Netherlands; p.rijnbeek@erasmusmc.nl
12 Department of Biomedical Sciences, Ajou University Graduate School of Medicine, Suwon 16499, Korea
* Correspondence: veritas@ajou.ac.kr (R.W.P.); seng.chan.you@ohdsi.org (S.C.Y.)

Abstract: Incident depression has been reported to be associated with poor prognosis in patients with cardiovascular disease (CVD), which might be associated with beta-blocker therapy. Because early detection and intervention can alleviate the severity of depression, we aimed to develop a machine learning (ML) model predicting the onset of major depressive disorder (MDD). A model based on $L1$ regularized logistic regression was trained against the South Korean nationwide administrative claims database to identify risk factors for the incident MDD after beta-blocker therapy in patients with CVD. We identified 50,397 patients initiating beta-blockers for CVD, with 774 patients developing MDD within 365 days after initiating beta-blocker therapy. An area under the receiver operating characteristic curve (AUC) of 0.74 was achieved. A history of non-selective beta-blockers and factors related to anxiety disorder, sleeping problems, and other chronic diseases were the most strong predictors. AUCs of 0.62–0.71 were achieved in the external validation conducted on six independent electronic health records and claims databases in the USA and South Korea. In conclusion, an ML model that identifies patients at high-risk for incident MDD was developed. Application of ML to identify susceptible patients for adverse events of treatment may serve as an important approach for personalized medicine.

Keywords: adrenergic beta-antagonists; depressive disorder; machine learning; cardiovascular diseases

1. Introduction

Incidence of depression in patients with cardiovascular disease (CVD) is higher than that in healthy individuals [1]. Depression following CVD has been reported to be associated with mortality and new cardiovascular events [2,3]. The severity of depression and poor prognosis have a directly proportional relationship [1]. Furthermore, early diagnosis and intervention for depression in patients with CVD alleviate the disease severity and eventually benefit treatment outcome [4,5]. However, clinical predictors of incident depression following CVD are not well established [6].

Studies have suggested that subsequent depression or mood disturbance after CVD might be associated with beta-blocker therapy [7–9]. Beta-blockers are a widely prescribed drug for CVDs, including hypertension, myocardial infarction, coronary arteriosclerosis, angina pectoris, cardiac arrhythmia, and heart failure [10]. Nonetheless, the use of beta-blockers in patients with stable coronary artery disease, myocardial infarction, heart failure with preserved ejection fraction, or hypertension has been challenged due to paucity of evidence about the benefit of beta-blockers in these patients [11–14]. Unnecessary prescription of medications to susceptible patients may violate the so-called 'First, do no harm' injunction [15]. Risk stratification of patients with beta-blockers for subsequent depression may reduce drug-related morbidity, which is in line with personalized medicine [16].

Machine learning (ML) is widely used to solve prediction problems in medicine. Existing depression prediction models have mostly focused on limited socio-psychological factors and medical histories [17,18]. By contrast, ML can handle a large number of variables through a data-driven approach [19], so that developing reproducible machine-learning algorithms and validating the developed algorithms using heterogeneous external data sets has been demanding. Reps et al. proposed a standardized machine-learning framework to generate and evaluate a clinical prediction model that leverages standardized clinical databases to overcome this daunting challenge [20].

Therefore, we aimed to develop a robust prediction model that stratifies patients at risk of incident major depressive disorder (MDD) after using beta-blockers for CVD based on the standardized framework.

2. Materials and Methods

2.1. Data Source

We developed a prediction model using the National Health Insurance Service-National Sample Cohort (NHIS-NSC) database, South Korea [21]. This database is generated from claims of South Korea's national health insurance. It is designed to represent the general population of South Korea by systematical sampling from all eligible insured individuals. In 2002, approximately one million individuals, which is equivalent to 2.2% of the South Korean population, were sampled and followed up for 11 years. The database covers information about age, sex, diagnosis, drugs, and procedures.

External validation was conducted on six electronic health records (EHR) and claims databases from the USA and South Korea. The databases from the USA include two EHR databases called IQVIA US Ambulatory Electronic Medical Record (EMR) and the STAnford medicine Research data Repository (STARR)—Observational Medical Outcomes Partnership (OMOP), and one claims database called IQVIA OpenClaims. The databases from South Korea include EHR databases from three tertiary teaching hospitals, Ajou University Hospital, Hanyang University Hospital, and Kangdong Sacred Heart Hospital.

The IQVIA US Ambulatory EMR database is composed of longitudinal, de-identified EHR originating from ambulatory clients spanning from 2006 to 2020. The database covers more than 40 million patients. IQVIA Open Claims database consists of open, pre-adjudicated medical (inpatient and outpatient) and pharmacy claims from 2013 to 2020. These data cover more than 200 million unique patients. The STARR, a clinical data warehouse, contains live Epic data from various hospitals.

STARR-OMOP contains EHR data for more than 3 million patients from 2008 to 2020 [22]. More detailed information about the databases from the USA is available in Supplementary Table S1.

Ajou University Hospital database contains medical records of approximately 3 million inpatients and outpatients who visited between 1994 and 2018. Hanyang University Hospital database includes approximately 1.7 million inpatients and outpatients who visited between 2001 and 2018. Kangdong Sacred Heart Hospital database includes approximately 1.1 million inpatients and outpatients who visited between 1986 and 2019.

All databases had been converted to a standardized format called the OMOP common data model (CDM) [23]. Regional of institutional drug and diagnosis codes were converted to standardized OMOP vocabulary to provide interoperability between databases using different code systems, which has been developed and maintained by an international collaborative initiative, Observational Health Data Sciences and Informatics (OHDSI) [24].

2.2. *Design*

2.2.1. Study Population and Outcome

Patients who were prescribed beta-blockers for a continuous exposure period of 30 days or more, were enrolled in the cohort. If the prescription interval for a particular drug is less than 30 days, it was regarded as continuous exposure. The first prescription date during a continuous exposure period is considered as the index date of a subject enters the cohort. Only beta-blockers used for CVD were included. We required patients to have a diagnosis record of hypertension, myocardial infarction, coronary arteriosclerosis, angina pectoris, or heart failure, within 3 days before and after the index date. Patients with a prescription history of antidepressants, or a diagnosis history of schizophrenia or depressive disorder, at any time before the index date were excluded. The patient's age had to be 18 years or older on the index date. In addition, patients without 365 days of observable period prior to the index date were excluded to ensure that the index event was the first beta-blocker prescription longer than 30 days.

We defined outcome event as the onset of MDD within 365 days after the index date. Only the first MDD diagnosis within the follow up period was used as an outcome event. Patients without an observable period of 365 days after the index date were excluded to ensure that patients with non-occurrence of the outcome event are event-free.

Target cohort and outcome events were extracted using clinical data from claims and EHR databases converted to OMOP-CDM. The list of concepts and logics utilized to define the target cohort and outcome events are provided in Supplementary Table S2.

2.2.2. Variables and Analysis

Variables to train the prediction model were generated from clinical data for 365 days of observable time prior to the index date. Clinical data include sex, age, diagnosis, prescription, and procedure. Furthermore, diagnosis covers various categories of disease such as cardiovascular diseases, mental disorders, and common chronic diseases. Clinical data were converted to binary format (yes or no), which has high usability for training the ML model. Variables were coded "no" for non-occurrence of a particular record. Exceptionally, age is used as continuous variable. Through this process, a total of 10,004 variables were generated.

The baseline characteristics of the study population with outcome, and without outcome, were compared. Mean age was calculated based on the index date, and age was also grouped by 10-year interval. Beta-blocker indication was derived from the records of CVD for three days before and after the index date. Other baseline characteristics of diagnoses and drugs were extracted from the history of 365 days prior to the index date. History of common chronic diseases, mental disorders, nutritional disorders, and medications associated with CVD and immunosuppressive therapy in the year prior to the index date, were compared. Differences of categorical variables between outcome and non-outcome groups were evaluated using the chi-squared test. When the frequency of categorical variables is less than 5, the Fisher's exact test was used. The t-test was used to compare continuous variables. Statistical significance was defined as a p-value of <0.05 in a two-tailed test.

We investigated $L1$ regularized logistic regression, random forest, and gradient boosting machine as candidate algorithms to be used in the prediction model. These algorithms are widely used and are suitable for solving classification problems, such as the prediction of clinical outcomes [25]. Using default settings in each algorithm, we built three models using the NHIS-NSC claims database, for the comparison of performance. We found that the performances of three models were similar (area under the receiver operating characteristic curve (AUC) range, 0.67–0.69). However, the $L1$ regularized logistic regression algorithm significantly reduced the number of variables compared to other methods (58 versus 121–2597). The details of default algorithm settings and the results are provided in Supplementary Table S3. Considering that the need for more data in the clinical field is directly associated with increased cost, the prediction model is desirable for using fewer variables. Also, previous studies have demonstrated the usefulness of regression-based algorithms in clinical prediction compared with other modern ML algorithms [25,26].

Thus, the prediction model was developed based on the logistic regression method with $L1$ regularization. Logistic regression was used, because the variables used to train the model were binary. $L1$ regularization is a data-driven algorithm selecting the most predictive variables from numerous variables converted from clinical data. This enabled regression to be applied to extremely high-dimensional data, which have variables larger than sample size. Moreover, regularization reduces overfitting induced by including the training data-specific association in the model.

The model was trained against the NHIS-NSC database. The study population who met the inclusion and exclusion criteria was randomly split into 80% of the training set and 20% of the validation set. The training set was again randomly split into five groups, and the optimal parameters were derived for each group. Among them, the parameter of the best performed model was chosen. Then, the model was fitted using whole training set with the chosen parameters. This helps in suppressing the overfitting and retaining the generality across the databases. For the evaluation of model performance, AUC, sensitivity, and specificity were calculated. Furthermore, external validation of the developed model was conducted against six EHR and claims databases to demonstrate generalizability and to identify the possibility of overfitting.

Two additional analyses were conducted to improve understanding of the development data and the model. First, we investigated the distribution of beta-blockers in the development database by molecular type and year. The prescriptions were counted by year, from 2003 to 2012. Also, the numbers of beta-blocker prescriptions were counted by selectivity and lipophilicity. Furthermore, we calculated the incidence of MDD among patients with and without strong predictors.

This study followed the Transparent Reporting of a Multivariable Prediction Model for Individual Prognosis or Diagnosis (TRIPOD) reporting guideline for prediction algorithm validation [27]. All development of the prediction model and statistical analysis were carried out with R 3.6, and the framework including packages followed the patient-level prediction from the OHDSI community [20]. A dedicated R package to validate and apply the developed prediction model has been published in GitHub (https://github.com/ohdsi-studies/MddAfterBbValidation). The institutional review board (IRB) at Ajou University Hospital, Suwon, Korea, approved this study (IRB approval number: AJIRB-MED-MDB-20-382, AJIRB-MED-EXP-20-390).

3. Results

3.1. Baseline Characteristics

There were a total of 50,397 beta-blocker users who met the inclusion and exclusion criteria in the training database. Among them, 774 patients developed MDD within the following 365 days from the index date. Incident rate was 1.5%. Basic characteristics of the study population with outcome, and non-outcome are listed in Table 1.

Table 1. Basic characteristics of study population with outcome, and non-outcome.

Characteristics	Outcome (n = 774)	Non-Outcome (n = 49,623)	p-Value
Age (years, mean ± standard deviation (SD))	61.2 ± 12.9	58.7 ± 13.1	0.510
Male [1]	298 (38.5)	25,527 (51.4)	<0.001
Beta-blocker indication [2]			
Hypertensive disorder	726 (93.8)	47,321 (95.4)	0.050
Myocardial infarction	46 (5.9)	2456 (4.9)	0.238
Angina pectoris	205 (26.5)	8899 (17.9)	<0.001
Coronary arteriosclerosis	13 (1.7)	1592 (3.2)	0.021
Heart failure	98 (12.7)	4688 (9.4)	0.003
Chronic disease [3]			
Cancer	24 (3.1)	1056 (2.1)	0.084
Chronic lung disease	98 (12.7)	4621 (9.3)	0.002
Stroke	45 (5.8)	1441 (2.9)	<0.001
Alzheimer's disease	7 (0.9)	114 (0.2)	<0.001
Diabetes	135 (17.4)	9691 (19.5)	0.159
Chronic kidney disease	12 (1.6)	490 (1.0)	0.167
Mental disorder			
Anxiety disorder	150 (14.9)	3911 (7.9)	<0.001
Neurosis	62 (8.0)	1731 (3.5)	<0.001
Organic mental disorder	30 (3.9)	603 (1.2)	<0.001
Adjustment disorder	6 (0.8)	116 (0.2)	0.012
Personality disorder	0 (0.0)	60 (0.1)	1.000
Delusional disorder	1 (0.1)	14 (0.0)	0.207
Nutritional disorder			
Vitamin deficiency	9 (1.2)	301 (0.6)	0.08
Undernutrition	16 (2.1)	371 (0.7)	<0.001
Medication [3]			
VKA	13 (1.7)	599 (1.2)	0.305
Aspirin	304 (39.3)	10,990 (22.1)	<0.001
Antiplatelet agents	66 (8.5)	2604 (5.2)	<0.001
ACEi	165 (21.5)	4795 (9.7)	<0.001
Angiotensin II receptor blocker	233 (30.1)	14,926 (30.1)	1.000
Selective beta-blocker	556 (71.8)	37,234 (75.0)	0.046
Non-selective beta-blocker	375 (48.4)	17,768 (35.8)	<0.001
Hydrophilic beta-blocker	543 (71.8)	36,302 (73.2)	0.068
Lipophilic beta-blocker	388 (50.1)	18,700 (37.7)	<0.001
Diuretic	400 (51.7)	25,985 (52.4)	0.732
Calcium channel antagonist	415 (53.6)	28,057 (56.5)	0.112
Cardiac glycoside	26 (3.4)	1575 (3.2)	0.851
Aldosterone antagonist	52 (6.7)	2846 (5.7)	0.277
Verapamil/diltiazem	80 (10.3)	3204 (6.5)	<0.001
Antiarrhythmics	14 (1.8)	517 (1.0)	0.058
Other immunosuppressants [4]	1 (0.1)	153 (0.3)	0.735
Calcineurin inhibitors	4 (0.5)	132 (0.3)	0.157
Selective immunosuppressants	1 (0.1)	78 (0.2)	1.000
Tumor necrosis factor alpha -inhibitor	0 (0.0)	2 (0.0)	1.000

Number of persons were presented as number (percent in outcome or non-outcome group), except age. The chi-squared test was used for comparison between categorical variables, and the Fisher's exact test was used for the categorical variables with frequency less than 5. The t-test was used for continuous variables. Statistical significance was defined as a p-value of <0.05 in a two-tailed test. [1] Mean of continuous variables were presented as mean (standard deviation). [2] Diagnosis record of cardiovascular disease at the time of beta-blocker prescription were counted and each diagnosis is not exclusive. [3] Diagnosis or drug exposure history in one year prior to index date were counted. VKA, vitamin K antagonist; ACEi, angiotensin converting enzyme inhibitors. [4] Other immunosuppressants include methotrexate, azathioprine, and thalidomide.

Mean age of the outcome group and non-outcome group was 61.2 (standard deviation = 12.9) and 58.7 (standard deviation = 13.1) respectively, with no statistical significance. When the patients were grouped by age at 10-year intervals, we observed that patients in their 20s have a high incidence of outcome, especially in males. Thereafter, the incidence rate fell sharply and again gradually increased with age. The number of patients and their outcome incidence by age groups are presented in Supplementary Table S4. The proportion of males in the outcome group was 38.5%, which is significantly lower than 51.4% in the non-outcome group. The most frequent CVD in both outcome and non-outcome group was hypertensive disorder, 93.8% and 95.4% respectively ($p = 0.050$). Among CVD that showed statistical significance, angina pectoris and heart failure showed a higher proportion in the outcome group ($p < 0.001$, $p = 0.003$) and coronary arteriosclerosis was higher in non-outcome group ($p = 0.021$). Prevalence of chronic lung disease, stroke, and Alzheimer's disease was higher in the outcome group with statistical significance ($p = 0.002$, $p < 0.001$, and $p < 0.001$, respectively). Among the mental disorders, anxiety disorder, neurosis, organic mental disorder, and adjustment disorder were more frequent in the outcome group with statistical significance ($p < 0.001$, $p < 0.001$, $p < 0.001$, and $p = 0.012$, respectively). In the case of nutritional disorder, undernutrition was more prevalent in the outcome group with statistical significance ($p < 0.001$). Among cardiovascular medication history, aspirin, antiplatelet agent, angiotensin-converting enzyme inhibitors, non-selective beta-blocker, and verapamil/diltiazem were more frequent in the outcome group with statistical significance (all $p < 0.001$). The selective beta-blocker was significantly lower in the outcome group ($p < 0.001$).

3.2. Variables

To train the *L*1 regularized logistic regression model, the NHIS-NSC database was converted to a total of 10,004 variables including clinical information about age, sex, diagnosis, drug, and procedure from about one million individuals. Among them, 74 variables were selected by *L*1 regularization and were included in the final model. Some of these variables are listed in Figure 1.

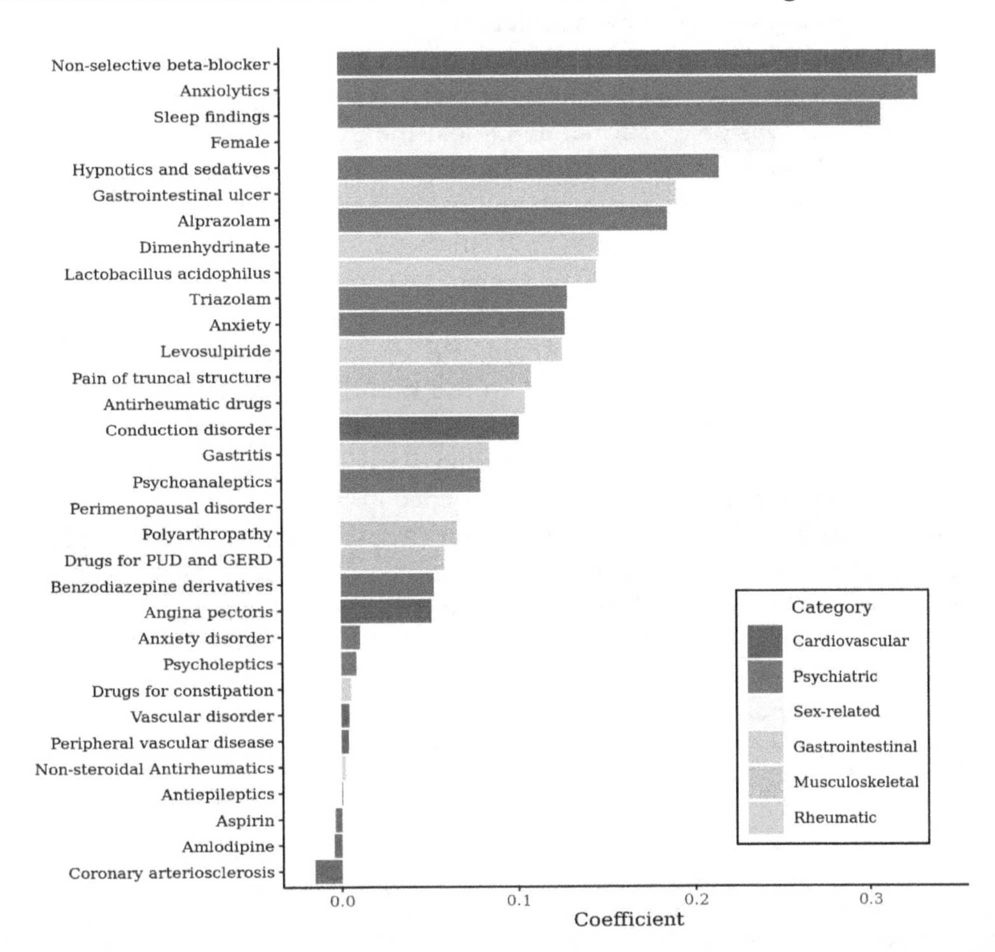

Figure 1. Coefficients of variables included in the developed model, as predictors for incident major depressive disorder. The higher coefficient means more predictive. PUD: peptic ulcer disease; GERD: gastro-esophageal reflux disease.

Among 74 variables finally selected in the model, the non-selective beta-blocker was the predictor with the highest coefficient (coefficient = 0.34). The following high coefficient predictors were anxiolytics, sleep findings, and female sex. Conditions and drugs associated with psychiatric disorders were included in the model such as sedatives, alprazolam, triazolam, anxiety, and benzodiazepines. Also, factors related to chronic disease such as gastrointestinal, musculoskeletal, and rheumatic chronic disorders were also predictors with high coefficients. Among CVDs used as the indication of a beta-blocker, angina pectoris was most predictive to MDD development and coronary arteriosclerosis was most predictive to not developing MDD. A full list of 74 variables selected as predictors of the model and their standardized mean difference is shown in Supplementary Table S5.

3.3. Model Performance

A total of 154 (1.53%) MDD outcome events from 10,078 beta-blockers users in internal validation were obtained, with an AUC value of 0.74. Sensitivity and specificity were 83.1% and 49.5%, respectively. The performance of the model in internal and external validations is listed in Table 2. In six external validations, the number of outcomes was 19, 15, 26, 439, 59045, and 3342, respectively. AUCs were 0.71, 0.66, 0.70, 0.62, 0.62, and 0.62, each. Incidence ranged from 0.22% to 1.67%, some are much lower than internal validation data. Sensitivity and specificity were 78.9% and 49.0% in External 1, 86.7% and 49.4% in External 2, 80.8% and 49.9% in External 3, 77.2% and 40.4% in External 4, 75.1% and 40.2% in External 5, and 75.4% and 40.1% in External 6. The receiver operating characteristic (ROC) curve plot and calibration plot of each validation set are listed in Figure 2. Some of the ROC curves are rough due to the small number of outcomes causing a decrease of AUC. However, sensitivity and specificity were relatively retained comparing with internal validation.

Calibration plots depict the proportion between predicted probability calculated by the prediction model and the fraction of true observed outcome. In internal validation, we found that predicted risk and real observed outcome was proportional in a linear manner. In three external validations using the database from South Korea, the confidence interval was wide due to low frequency of outcome. However, a proportional tendency between predicted risk and fraction of outcome was still comparable. In three external validations using the databases from the USA, the proportion of observed outcome and predicted probability were proportional with a narrow confidence interval.

Furthermore, comparison of the standardized mean difference of the predictors, across internal and South Korean validation sets, was conducted and is shown in Figure 3. The following were consistently higher in the outcome group than in the non-outcome group across validation sets: female sex, non-selective beta-blocker, anxiolytics, triazolam, and drugs for peptic ulcer disease or gastro-esophageal reflux disease (GERD). Among variables showing a consistent difference, anxiolytics had the highest standardized mean difference in internal and external 1 validation sets (0.38, 0.69) and female sex had the highest standardized mean difference in external 2 and external 3 (0.20, 0.59). However, the incidence of angina pectoris and coronary arteriosclerosis were inconsistent across databases, although they were selected to be predictive in the model.

Table 2. Performance of the model in internal and external validations.

Validation Set	Name	*n*	Outcome	Incidence (%)	AUC	Sensitivity	Specificity
Internal	NHIS	10,078	154	1.53	0.74	83.1%	49.5%
External 1	Ajou	8511	19	0.22	0.71	78.9%	49.0%
External 2	Hanyang	5112	15	0.29	0.66	86.7%	49.4%
External 3	Kandong	5097	26	0.51	0.70	80.8%	49.9%
External 4	STARR	26,258	439	1.67	0.62	77.2%	40.4%
External 5	OpenClaims	4,295,013	59,045	1.38	0.62	75.1%	40.2%
External 6	AmbEMR	883,198	3342	0.38	0.62	75.4%	40.1%

AUC, area under the receiver operating characteristic curve.

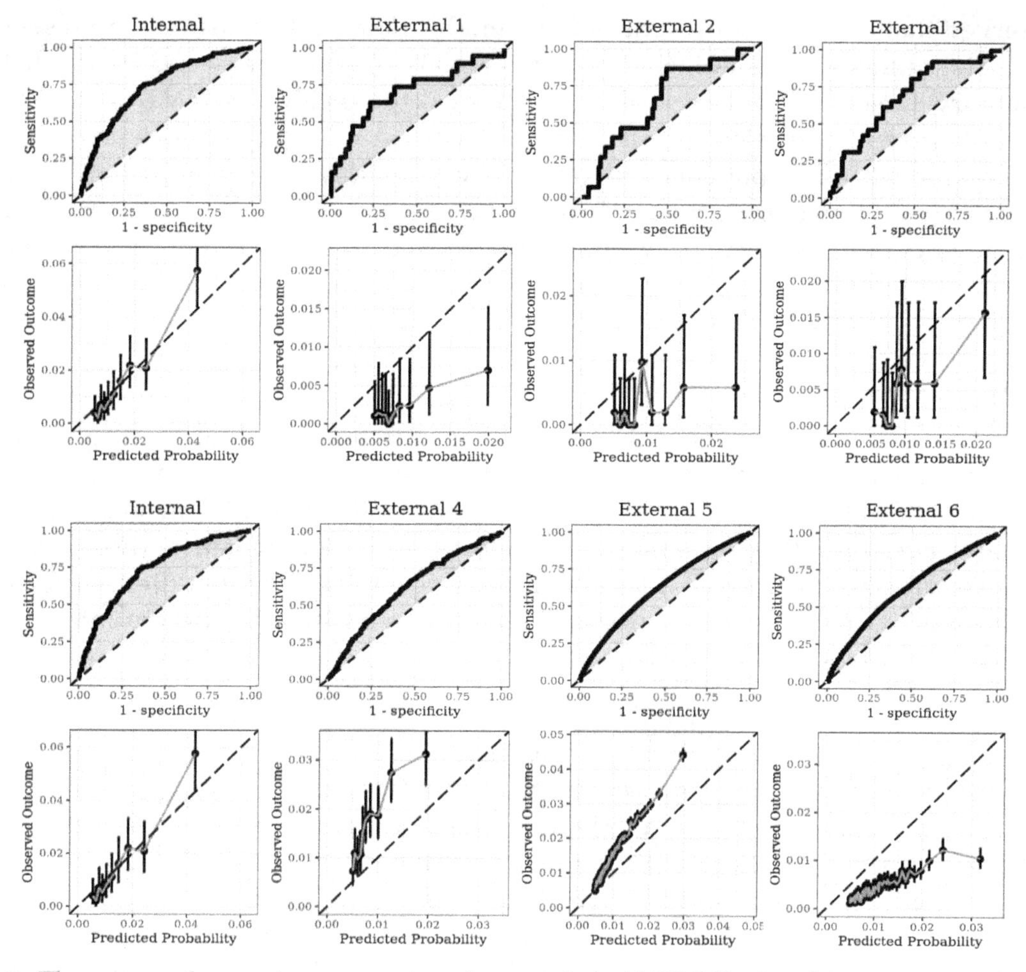

Figure 2. The area under receiver operating characteristic (AUROC) plot showing the performance of the $L1$ regularized logistic regression model and calibration plot comparing predicted probability calculated by the prediction model with the fraction of observed outcome.

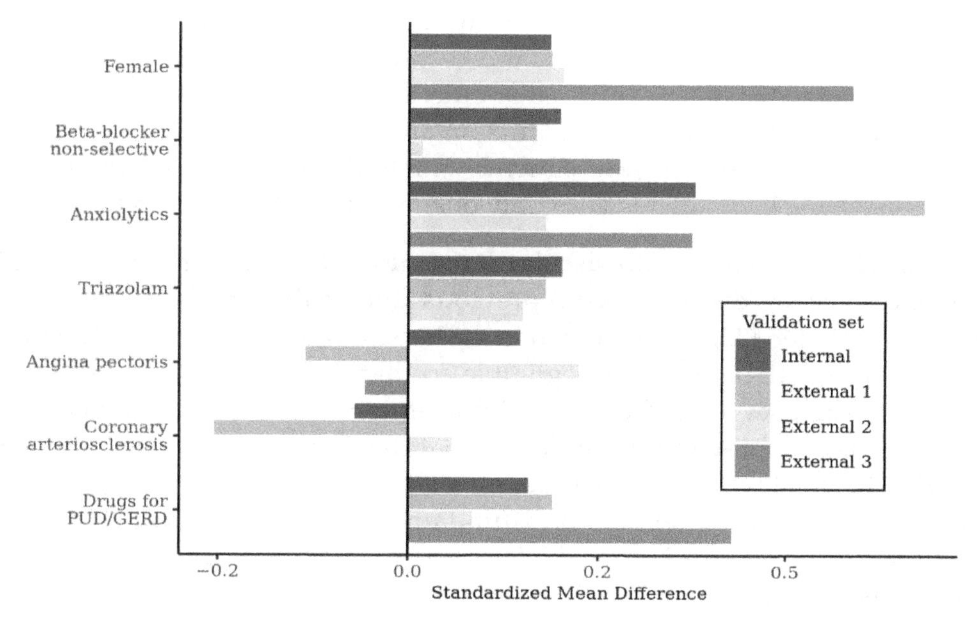

Figure 3. The comparison of the standardized mean differences of the predictors of major depressive disorder across databases in which validation is done. Positive number of standardized mean difference means that the variable is more frequent in outcome group than non-outcome group. PUD, peptic ulcer disease, GERD, gastro-esophageal reflux disease.

We observed that the general prescription of beta-blockers is decreasing in both selectivity and lipophilicity. The number of beta-blocker prescriptions by its selectivity and lipophilicity is listed in Supplementary Table S6. Furthermore, we calculated the incidence of MDD in patients with a history of anxiolytics and non-selective beta-blockers, which are the predictors with a high coefficient in the prediction model. While patients with no history of anxiolytics and no history of non-selective beta-blockers had only 0.8% of incident MDD, incidence increased to 2.5% and 3.4% in patients with a history of anxiolytics or non-selective beta-blockers, respectively. For patients with a history of both anxiolytics and non-selective beta-blockers, the incidence rate was 4.3%. The number of patients with a different history is listed in Supplementary Table S7.

4. Discussion

An ML model predicting incident MDD in patients initiating beta-blocker therapy for CVD was developed on the nationwide longitudinal claims database. The robustness of model performance was validated on multiple independent EHR and claims databases from South Korea and the USA. To the best of our knowledge, this is the first research utilizing extensive clinical data for discovering predictors of incident MDD in cardiovascular patients with beta-blockers. We identified various predictors including non-selective beta-blockers, anxiety disorder, sleep disorder, and chronic cardiovascular, musculoskeletal, and rheumatoid diseases.

Although we do not argue that there is independent causal relationship between use of non-selective beta-blockers and the risk of incident MDD in patients with CVD, the exposure of non-selective beta-blocker was the predictor with the highest coefficient value in our model. This aligns with a previous study that reported non-selective beta-blockers induce more depressive symptoms than other hypertensives [28]. There is still controversy as to whether beta-blocker induce depression in cardiovascular patients [29,30]. Mostly, old papers appear to be relevant, and relatively new ones are not [31]. This inconsistency might be due to the dilution of the effects of non-selective beta-blockers by various types of beta-blocker developed over time. Since the newer beta-blockers are mostly moderately lipophilic or hydrophilic, there is a possibility that overall association between beta-blockers and depression became weak.

Variables related to anxiety disorder were also strong predictors. Anxiety was often comorbid with depression [32], and there is a previous study that presented anxiety is a risk factor of depression [33]. Since anxiety is associated with poor cardiovascular outcome in patients with acute coronary syndrome, more vigilance is needed about comorbid depression and anxiety disorder [34]. We found that the incidence of MDD is numerically higher in patients with both a history of anxiolytics and the use of non-selective beta-blockers than patients with only one or none of these predictors.

Variables related to chronic cardiovascular, musculoskeletal, and rheumatoid diseases were selected as predictors. This is consistent with previous studies that showed a relationship between these diseases and depression [35,36]. As shown in the baseline characteristics of the study population, the prevalence of chronic diseases is not negligible so that the chance of a cardiovascular patient having other chronic diseases should be carefully examined. In addition, female sex was also a strong predictor of MDD. A previous study found that the lifetime prevalence of major depressive episodes was higher in females than in males and the onset was earlier in females [37]. This difference may arise from behavioral characteristics and fundamental genetic reasons [38,39]. In addition, perimenopausal disorder may contribute to the female sex being predictive of MDD, as shown in our model and a previous study [40].

This study has several limitations. First, the use of non-selective and lipophilic beta-blockers might decrease over time, although it was not evident in our development database. Second, outcomes reflecting depression severity were not included in the model due to limitation of the datasets.

Not only onset, but also disease severity prediction is important regarding the proportional relationship between depression severity and poor prognosis [1]. However, this model predicted the onset of depression with only existing clinical data, unlike other studies that used variables that need to be newly measured or assessed [17,18]. Third, using only a diagnosis code for defining outcome event is another limitation. Nonetheless, this study used clearly specified standardized codes which is compatible with various code systems worldwide, and a previous study that showed the validity of defining depression using a code system in NHIS-NSC [41].

5. Conclusions

We developed a prediction model for incident MDD following long-term beta-blocker use in patients with CVDs. Variables including use of non-selective beta-blockers, female sex, history of anxiety, and common chronic diseases, such as gastrointestinal and musculoskeletal diseases, were predictive.

Table S1: Description of the USA databases used in validation, Table S2: The concepts and logics used to define the target cohort and outcome event, Table S3: The settings and results of experimental models, Table S4: Number of patients and outcome incidence by age group, Table S5: Full list of variables selected in the final model, Table S6: The number of beta-blocker prescriptions by its selectivity and lipophilicity, Table S7: Number of patients and outcome incidence by history records.

Author Contributions: Conceptualization, S.J., Y.K., S.I.S., D.Y.L., U.J., S.J.S., R.W.P., S.C.Y.; data curation, S.J.; formal analysis, S.J., S.G.C., S.C.Y.; funding acquisition, R.W.P.; investigation, S.J., S.C.Y.; methodology, S.J.; project administration, R.W.P., S.C.Y.; resources, R.W.P.; supervision, Y.K., R.W.P., S.C.Y.; validation, Y.K., S.I.S., K.K., C.R., N.H.S., J.D.P., S.R., Y.-H.L., S.G.C.; writing–original draft, S.J., S.C.Y.; writing–review and editing S.J., Y.K., S.I.S., D.Y.L., U.J., S.J.S., K.K., J.D.P., S.R., Y.-H.L., P.R.R., N.H.S., C.R., R.W.P., S.C.Y. All authors have read and agreed to the published version of the manuscript.

References

1. Hare, D.L.; Toukhsati, S.R.; Johansson, P.; Jaarsma, T. Depression and cardiovascular disease: A clinical review. *Eur. Heart J.* **2014**, *35*, 1365–1372. [CrossRef]
2. Strik, J.J.; Denollet, J.; Lousberg, R.; Honig, A. Comparing symptoms of depression and anxiety as predictors of cardiac events and increased health care consumption after myocardial infarction. *J. Am. Coll. Cardiol.* **2003**, *42*, 1801–1807. [CrossRef]
3. Van Melle, J.P.; De Jonge, P.; Spijkerman, T.A.; Tijssen, J.G.; Ormel, J.; Van Veldhuisen, D.J.; Van Den Brink, R.H.; Van Den Berg, M.P. Prognostic association of depression following myocardial infarction with mortality and cardiovascular events: A meta-analysis. *Psychosom. Med.* **2004**, *66*, 814–822. [CrossRef] [PubMed]
4. Carney, R.M.; Freedland, K.E. Depression and coronary heart disease. *Nat. Rev. Cardiol.* **2017**, *14*, 145. [CrossRef] [PubMed]
5. Kim, J.-M.; Stewart, R.; Lee, Y.-S.; Lee, H.-J.; Kim, M.C.; Kim, J.-W.; Kang, H.-J.; Bae, K.-Y.; Kim, S.-W.; Shin, I.-S. Effect of escitalopram vs placebo treatment for depression on long-term cardiac outcomes in patients with acute coronary syndrome: A randomized clinical trial. *JAMA* **2018**, *320*, 350–357. [CrossRef] [PubMed]
6. Carney, R.M.; Freedland, K.E.; Steinmeyer, B.C.; Rubin, E.H.; Rich, M.W. Clinical predictors of depression treatment outcomes in patients with coronary heart disease. *J. Psychosom. Res.* **2016**, *88*, 36–41. [CrossRef]
7. Avorn, J.; Everitt, D.E.; Weiss, S. Increased Antidepressant Use in Patients Prescribed β-Blockers. *JAMA* **1986**, *255*, 357–360. [CrossRef]
8. Thiessen, B.Q.; Wallace, S.M.; Blackburn, J.L.; Wilson, T.W.; Bergman, U. Increased Prescribing of Antidepressants Subsequent to ß-Blocker Therapy. *Arch. Intern. Med.* **1990**, *150*, 2286–2290. [CrossRef]
9. Boal, A.H.; Smith, D.J.; McCallum, L.; Muir, S.; Touyz, R.M.; Dominiczak, A.F.; Padmanabhan, S. Monotherapy with major antihypertensive drug classes and risk of hospital admissions for mood disorders. *Hypertension* **2016**, *68*, 1132–1138. [CrossRef]
10. Luc, P.; Sheldon, W.T. Contemporary Use of β-Blockers: Clinical Relevance of Subclassification. *Can J. Cardiol.* **2014**, *30*, S9–S15.

11. Bavishi, C.; Chatterjee, S.; Ather, S.; Patel, D.; Messerli, F.H. Beta-blockers in heart failure with preserved ejection fraction: A meta-analysis. *Heart Fail. Rev.* **2015**, *20*, 193–201. [CrossRef] [PubMed]
12. Dondo, T.B.; Hall, M.; West, R.M.; Jernberg, T.; Lindahl, B.; Bueno, H.; Danchin, N.; Deanfield, J.E.; Hemingway, H.; Fox, K.A. β-blockers and mortality after acute myocardial infarction in patients without heart failure or ventricular dysfunction. *J. Am. Coll. Cardiol.* **2017**, *69*, 2710–2720. [CrossRef] [PubMed]
13. Wiysonge, C.S.; Bradley, H.A.; Volmink, J.; Mayosi, B.M.; Opie, L.H. Beta-blockers for hypertension. *Cochrane Database Syst. Rev.* **2017**. [CrossRef]
14. Bangalore, S.; Steg, G.; Deedwania, P.; Crowley, K.; Eagle, K.A.; Goto, S.; Ohman, E.M.; Cannon, C.P.; Smith, S.C.; Zeymer, U. β-Blocker use and clinical outcomes in stable outpatients with and without coronary artery disease. *JAMA* **2012**, *308*, 1340–1349. [CrossRef]
15. Smith, C.M. Origin and uses of primum non nocere—Above all, do no harm! *J. Clin. Pharmacol.* **2005**, *45*, 371–377. [CrossRef] [PubMed]
16. Stevenson, J.M.; Williams, J.L.; Burnham, T.G.; Prevost, A.T.; Schiff, R.; Erskine, S.D.; Davies, J.G. Predicting adverse drug reactions in older adults; a systematic review of the risk prediction models. *Clin. Interv. Aging* **2014**, *9*, 1581. [CrossRef]
17. Liu, R.; Yue, Y.; Jiang, H.; Lu, J.; Wu, A.; Geng, D.; Wang, J.; Lu, J.; Li, S.; Tang, H. A risk prediction model for post-stroke depression in Chinese stroke survivors based on clinical and socio-psychological features. *Oncotarget* **2017**, *8*, 62891. [CrossRef]
18. Cattelani, L.; Murri, M.B.; Chesani, F.; Chiari, L.; Bandinelli, S.; Palumbo, P. Risk prediction model for late life depression: Development and validation on three large European datasets. *IEEE J. Biomed. Health Inform.* **2018**, *23*, 2196–2204. [CrossRef]
19. Chua, W.; Purmah, Y.; Cardoso, V.R.; Gkoutos, G.V.; Tull, S.P.; Neculau, G.; Thomas, M.R.; Kotecha, D.; Lip, G.Y.; Kirchhof, P. Data-driven discovery and validation of circulating blood-based biomarkers associated with prevalent atrial fibrillation. *Eur. Heart J.* **2019**, *40*, 1268–1276. [CrossRef]
20. Reps, J.M.; Schuemie, M.J.; Suchard, M.A.; Ryan, P.B.; Rijnbeek, P.R. Design and implementation of a standardized framework to generate and evaluate patient-level prediction models using observational healthcare data. *J. Am. Med. Inform. Assoc.* **2018**, *25*, 969–975. [CrossRef]
21. Lee, J.; Lee, J.S.; Park, S.-H.; Shin, S.A.; Kim, K. Cohort profile: The national health insurance service–national sample cohort (NHIS-NSC), South Korea. *Int. J. Epidemiol.* **2017**, *46*, e15. [CrossRef] [PubMed]
22. Datta, S.; Posada, J.; Olson, G.; Li, W.; O'Reilly, C.; Balraj, D.; Mesterhazy, J.; Pallas, J.; Desai, P.; Shah, N. A new paradigm for accelerating clinical data science at Stanford Medicine. *arXiv* **2020**, arXiv:2003.10534.
23. FitzHenry, F.; Resnic, F.; Robbins, S.; Denton, J.; Nookala, L.; Meeker, D.; Ohno-Machado, L.; Matheny, M. Creating a common data model for comparative effectiveness with the observational medical outcomes partnership. *Appl. Clin. Inform.* **2015**, *6*, 536. [PubMed]
24. Hripcsak, G.; Duke, J.D.; Shah, N.H.; Reich, C.G.; Huser, V.; Schuemie, M.J.; Suchard, M.A.; Park, R.W.; Wong, I.C.K.; Rijnbeek, P.R. Observational Health Data Sciences and Informatics (OHDSI): Opportunities for observational researchers. *Stud. Health Technol. Inform.* **2015**, *216*, 574.
25. Christodoulou, E.; Ma, J.; Collins, G.S.; Steyerberg, E.W.; Verbakel, J.Y.; Van Calster, B. A systematic review shows no performance benefit of machine learning over logistic regression for clinical prediction models. *J. Clin. Epidemiol.* **2019**, *110*, 12–22. [CrossRef]
26. Sanchez-Pinto, L.N.; Venable, L.R.; Fahrenbach, J.; Churpek, M.M. Comparison of variable selection methods for clinical predictive modeling. *Int. J. Med. Inform.* **2018**, *116*, 10–17. [CrossRef]
27. Collins, G.S.; Reitsma, J.B.; Altman, D.G.; Moons, K.G. Transparent Reporting of a Multivariable Prediction Model for Individual Prognosis or Diagnosis (TRIPOD) The TRIPOD Statement. *Circulation* **2015**, *131*, 211–219. [CrossRef]
28. Agustini, B.; Mohebbi, M.; Woods, R.L.; McNeil, J.J.; Nelson, M.R.; Shah, R.C.; Murray, A.M.; Ernst, M.E.; Reid, C.M.; Tonkin, A. The association of antihypertensive use and depressive symptoms in a large older population with hypertension living in Australia and the United States: A cross-sectional study. *J. Hum. Hypertens.* **2020**, *34*, 787–794. [CrossRef]
29. Kessing, L.V.; Rytgaard, H.C.; Ekstrøm, C.T.; Torp-Pedersen, C.; Berk, M.; Gerds, T.A. Antihypertensive drugs and risk of depression: A nationwide population-based study. *Hypertension* **2020**, *76*, 1263–1279. [CrossRef]
30. Armstrong, C.; Kapolowicz, M.R. A Preliminary Investigation on the Effects of Atenolol for Treating Symptoms of Anxiety. *Mil. Med.* **2020**, usaa170. [CrossRef]

31. Luijendijk, H.J.; Koolman, X. The incentive to publish negative studies: How beta-blockers and depression got stuck in the publication cycle. *J. Clin. Epidemiol.* **2012**, *65*, 488–492. [CrossRef] [PubMed]
32. Haug, T.T.; Mykletun, A.; Dahl, A.A. The association between anxiety, depression, and somatic symptoms in a large population: The HUNT-II study. *Psychosom. Med.* **2004**, *66*, 845–851. [CrossRef] [PubMed]
33. Stein, M.B.; Fuetsch, M.; Müller, N.; Höfler, M.; Lieb, R.; Wittchen, H.-U. Social anxiety disorder and the risk of depression: A prospective community study of adolescents and young adults. *Arch. Gen. Psychiatry* **2001**, *58*, 251–256. [CrossRef] [PubMed]
34. Huffman, J.C.; Celano, C.M.; Januzzi, J.L. The relationship between depression, anxiety, and cardiovascular outcomes in patients with acute coronary syndromes. *Neuropsychiatr. Dis. Treat.* **2010**, *6*, 123. [CrossRef]
35. Edwards, R.R.; Cahalan, C.; Mensing, G.; Smith, M.; Haythornthwaite, J.A. Pain, catastrophizing, and depression in the rheumatic diseases. *Nat. Rev. Rheumatol.* **2011**, *7*, 216. [CrossRef] [PubMed]
36. Magni, G.; Moreschi, C.; Rigatti-Luchini, S.; Merskey, H. Prospective study on the relationship between depressive symptoms and chronic musculoskeletal pain. *Pain* **1994**, *56*, 289–297. [CrossRef]
37. Kessler, R.C.; McGonagle, K.A.; Swartz, M.; Blazer, D.G.; Nelson, C.B. Sex and depression in the National Comorbidity Survey I: Lifetime prevalence, chronicity and recurrence. *J. Affect. Disord.* **1993**, *29*, 85–96. [CrossRef]
38. Nolen-Hoeksema, S. Sex differences in unipolar depression: Evidence and theory. *Psychol. Bull.* **1987**, *101*, 259. [CrossRef] [PubMed]
39. Kang, H.-J.; Park, Y.; Yoo, K.-H.; Kim, K.-T.; Kim, E.-S.; Kim, J.-W.; Kim, S.-W.; Shin, I.-S.; Yoon, J.-S.; Kim, J.H. Sex differences in the genetic architecture of depression. *Sci. Rep.* **2020**, *10*, 9927. [CrossRef]
40. Bromberger, J.T.; Assmann, S.F.; Avis, N.E.; Schocken, M.; Kravitz, H.M.; Cordal, A. Persistent mood symptoms in a multiethnic community cohort of pre-and perimenopausal women. *Am. J. Epidemiol.* **2003**, *158*, 347–356. [CrossRef]
41. Kim, G.E.; Jo, M.-W.; Shin, Y.-W. Increased prevalence of depression in South Korea from 2002 to 2013. *Sci. Rep.* **2020**, *10*, 16979. [CrossRef] [PubMed]

3

Altered Metabolomic Profile in Patients with Peripheral Artery Disease

Ahmed Ismaeel [1], Marco E. Franco [2], Ramon Lavado [2], Evlampia Papoutsi [1], George P. Casale [3], Matthew Fuglestad [3], Constance J. Mietus [3], Gleb R. Haynatzki [4], Robert S. Smith [5], William T. Bohannon [5], Ian Sawicki [5], Iraklis I. Pipinos [3] and Panagiotis Koutakis [1,*]

1 Department of Nutrition, Food and Exercise Sciences, Florida State University, Tallahassee, FL 32306, USA
2 Department of Environmental Science, Baylor University, Waco, TX 76798, USA
3 Department of Surgery, University of Nebraska at Medical Center, Omaha, NE 68198, USA
4 Department of Biostatistics, University of Nebraska Medical Center, Omaha, NE 68198, USA
5 Department of Surgery, Baylor Scott and White Hospital, Temple, TX 76508, USA
* Correspondence: pkoutakis@fsu.edu

Abstract: Peripheral artery disease (PAD) is a common atherosclerotic disease characterized by narrowed or blocked arteries in the lower extremities. Circulating serum biomarkers can provide significant insight regarding the disease progression. Here, we explore the metabolomics signatures associated with different stages of PAD and investigate potential mechanisms of the disease. We compared the serum metabolites of a cohort of 26 PAD patients presenting with claudication and 26 PAD patients presenting with critical limb ischemia (CLI) to those of 26 non-PAD controls. A difference between the metabolite profiles of PAD patients from non-PAD controls was observed for several amino acids, acylcarnitines, ceramides, and cholesteryl esters. Furthermore, our data demonstrate that patients with CLI possess an altered metabolomic signature different from that of both claudicants and non-PAD controls. These findings provide new insight into the pathophysiology of PAD and may help develop future diagnostic procedures and therapies for PAD patients.

Keywords: peripheral artery disease (PAD); metabolomics; claudication; critical limb ischemia (CLI)

---

1. Introduction

Peripheral artery disease (PAD) is an atherosclerotic condition of the arteries supplying the lower extremities. PAD affects over 200 million people around the world, with an estimated prevalence of more than 20% for individuals over 80 years old [1,2]. The most common manifestation of symptomatic PAD is intermittent claudication (IC), a painful discomfort in the leg muscles during walking that produces gait dysfunction and severe functional limitation. A small subset of PAD patients (approximately 1.3%) present with critical limb ischemia (CLI), the more severe form of PAD, manifested by ischemic rest pain and tissue loss/gangrene [3,4]. Work from several groups, including our own, has demonstrated significant degenerative changes in all the tissues of the chronically ischemic legs of patients with PAD, including skin, muscles, nerves, and subcutaneous tissues [5,6]. These changes have been best studied in the skeletal muscle of the affected limbs [7–9] and demonstrate an acquired myopathy with significant metabolic components. The biochemical characteristics of this myopathy include mitochondrial dysfunction, accumulation of metabolic intermediates, increased oxidative damage, and cytokine upregulation [1,5,6,10–14]. These metabolic myopathic changes are present in the legs of both IC and CLI patients, with the myopathy of CLI being more severe than that of IC [15]. Beyond this ischemic myopathy, PAD is also directly associated with conditions like dyslipidemia, obesity or cachexia, diabetes, and insulin resistance, all of which involve dysregulation of metabolism and energy homeostasis [16,17].

Metabolomics, the study of small-molecule metabolites in biological systems [18,19], has been increasingly applied to cardiovascular disease, leading to recent discoveries in disease-specific biomarkers and their mechanistic implications [20]. Metabolomics can detect, quantify, and identify a number of intermediate compounds and end products of cellular metabolism in body fluids, tissues, and cells, thus providing a molecular phenotype that directly reflects biochemical activity [21,22]. This strategy can therefore be useful in identifying the signature profiles of patients at different stages of a disease, and has the potential of improving our understanding of the pathogenesis, diagnosis, risk-stratification, monitoring of disease progression, personalization of treatment [23], and monitoring of the response to different therapies [24].

The clinical application of metabolomics in the study of PAD has been thus far explored with two studies evaluating near-term mortality and arterial stiffness in PAD patients. The first study showed that the ^{1}H NMR metabolomic profiles of plasma lipid molecules are correlated with mortality in PAD patients [25]. Specifically, alterations in lipoprotein and phospholipid structures were the major chemical signals that were distinct between PAD patients who died in the near-term versus those PAD patients who did not. The second study demonstrated that tyrosine and oxidized low-density lipoprotein (oxLDL) are associated with arterial stiffness in PAD patients [26]. These two seminal studies point to the potential of metabolomic profiling for providing significant insight into the pathophysiology of PAD. With this study, we aimed to expand the metabolomic mapping of PAD and to compare the circulating metabolites of patients with IC, patients with CLI, and non-PAD controls.

2. Materials and Methods

2.1. *Study Approval and Subjects*

Twenty-six non-PAD controls, 26 patients with IC, and 26 patients with CLI were recruited by vascular surgeons at the University of Nebraska Medical Center (UNMC, 00707), the Veterans Affairs Nebraska-Western Iowa Medical Center, and Baylor Scott and White Hospital (BSWI, 160390) under approved IRB protocols. IC or CLI diagnoses were made after examination of medical history, a physical examination, measurement of the ankle-brachial index (ABI), and computerized or standard arteriography. All non-PAD controls had normal blood flow to their legs and were undergoing operations for manifestations other than PAD (Table 1). These patients also had no history of PAD symptoms, normal lower limb pulses, normal ABIs at rest and after stress, were sex-matched, and all led sedentary lifestyles.

2.2. *Sample Collection and Preparation*

Blood samples were obtained in the morning after an overnight fast. In total, 30 mL of blood was obtained from each patient and was immediately centrifuged for 10 minutes, 2000× *g* at 4 °C. Serum was aliquoted into separate polypropylene tubes and immediately stored at −80 °C. The Biocrates AbsoluteIDQ p400 HR kit (Biocrates Life Science AG, Innsbruck, Austria) was used to analyze 100 μL of serum from each patient. Compared to manual liquid chromatography-tandem mass spectrometry (LC-MS/MS) (Applied Biosystems/MDS Sciex., Foster City, CA, USA)) analysis and other technologies, the Biocrates kit allows for higher efficiency of separation, better limits of detection, decreased consumption of solvents, and absolute quantification of metabolites [27].

2.3. *Targeted Identification and Quantification*

The Biocrates AbsoluteIDQ p400 HR kit was used to measure more than 400 metabolites, including 21 amino acids, 21 biogenic amines, the sum of hexoses (as one metabolite, primarily glucose), 55 acylcarnitines, 18 diglycerides, 42 triglycerides, 24 lysophosphatidylcholines, 172 phosphatidylcholines, 31 sphingomyelins, 9 ceramides, and 14 cholesteryl esters. The complete list of metabolites assayed are provided in the Supplementary Material. Serum samples, blanks, calibration standards, and quality controls were prepared according to manual instructions. LC-MS/MS was used to analyze the amino acids and biogenic amines, and the remaining metabolites were analyzed by flow injection analysis (FIA) coupled with tandem mass spectrometry. All amino acids and biogenic amines were derivatized with phenylisothiocyanate. Metabolites were quantified using internal standards and multiple reactions monitoring (MRM). The samples were analyzed on a Thermo Scientific UltiMate 3000 Rapid Separation Quaternary HPLC System (Thermo Scientific, Madison, WI, USA), connected to a QExactive™ Focus Hybrid Quadrupole-Orbitrap™ Mass Spectrometer (Thermo Scientific, Waltham, MA, USA). The chromatographic column was obtained from Biocrates. Data first underwent a pre-processing step of peak integration to determine concentration based on calibration curves using Multiquant software (version 3.0, AB Sciex, Darmstadt, Germany). Following, data were uploaded into Biocrates MetIDQ software, and concentrations of FIA-monitored metabolites were calculated in MetIDQ. The experiment was also validated using the Biocrates software (version 5, MetIDQ, Biocrates, Innsbruck, Austria).

2.4. *Phenylalanine/Tyrosine Ratio and Cholesteryl Esters CE (18:1)/CE (18:2)*

We calculated the ratio of phenylalanine to tyrosine as a marker of inflammation [28] and the ratio of cholesteryl esters CE (18:1)/CE (18:2) as an indicator of the ratio of acyl-coenzyme A (CoA) cholesterol acyltransferase (ACAT), a pro-atherogenic enzyme, to serum lecithin cholesterol acyltransferase (LCAT), an anti-atherogenic enzyme that facilitates reverse cholesterol transport [29]. This relationship is based on the observation that CE (18:1) is the preferred fatty acid of ACAT, and CE (18:2) is preferred by LCAT. A higher (18:1) to (18:2) ratio is therefore believed to suggest higher ACAT activity [30,31].

2.5. *Statistical Analyses*

Baseline characteristics between non-PAD control, IC, and CLI subjects were compared using Chi-square and Fisher exact tests for categorical variables and analysis of variance (ANOVA) for continuous variables. One-way analysis of covariance (ANCOVA) was used for the rest of the analyses controlling for age, ABI, and diabetes mellitus. MetaboAnalyst 4.0 (www.metaboanalyst.ca) (version 4, McGill University, Montreal, QC, Canada) was used for statistical analysis of the metabolites' data, processed with normalization, scaling, and filtering [32].

A one-way analysis of covariance was used to identify differences between non-PAD control, IC, and CLI groups for all the metabolites adjusting for any significant covariates, followed by *post-hoc* analyses with Bonferroni correction. Pearson correlations were calculated to evaluate associations between the ABI and the metabolites. Discriminant function models were developed to classify patients as non-PAD control, IC, or CLI. First, discriminant analysis assumptions were verified, and the multivariate data were standardized to remove units and place each variable on the same scale. A stepwise selection procedure was used to analyze variable contribution [33]. This method uses both forward selection and backward elimination procedures to determine the contribution of parameters to the discriminatory power of the model. Further, after derivation of a discriminant model, the model was used to classify new observations. A full cross-validation procedure was executed to evaluate the model performance. Cross-validation is a standard multivariate statistical method used on small data sets, validating the model by assessing stability and determining how well it will perform on other data sets [33]. During training, the cross-validation technique rotates the membership of the metabolite, verifying that the results are not dependent on calibration versus validation group membership, thus ensuring that the model is not overfitting the data. All analyses were performed using SAS statistical software (version 9.3, SAS Institute Inc., Cary, NC, USA).

3. Results

3.1. Patient Demographics

The baseline demographic and clinical characteristics are presented in Table 1. As expected, IC and CLI patients had significantly lower ABI values than non-PAD control subjects (IC: 0.51 ± 0.18 vs. CLI: 0.18 ± 0.10 vs. non-PAD controls: 1.05 ± 0.05, $p < 0.001$). IC patients were younger than CLI patients ($p = 0.044$) and CLI patients had a higher ratio of diabetes mellitus ($p = 0.005$). No other differences were found among the different groups of subjects.

Table 1. Patient demographics at enrollment. Data are shown as mean ± standard deviation.

	Non-PAD Control (n = 26)	IC (n = 26)	CLI (n = 26)	p
Age (years)	63.2 ± 7.4	62.0 ± 7.3	67.6 ± 9.9 †	**0.044**
Male sex (%)	23 (88.50)	24 (92.3)	26 (100)	0.224
Body mass index	29.6 ± 6.5	27.1 ± 9.9	27.8 ± 5.6	0.476
ABI	1.05 ± 0.05	0.51 ± 0.18 *	0.18 ± 0.10 *,†	**<0.001**
Risk factors (%)				
Tobacco use				0.073
Current	10 (38.5)	14 (53.8)	6 (23.1)	
Never	9 (34.6)	3 (11.5)	6 (23.1)	
Former	7 (26.9)	9 (34.6)	14 (53.8)	
Hypertension	17 (65.4)	22 (84.6)	23 (88.5)	0.087
Diabetes mellitus	4 (15.4)	8 (30.8)	15 (57.7) *,†	**0.005**
Coronary Artery Disease	9 (34.6)	13 (50.0)	16 (61.5)	0.150
Obesity	9 (34.6)	7 (26.9)	6 (23.1)	0.642
Dyslipidemia	21 (80.8)	19 (73.1)	16 (61.5)	0.300

Note: The values presented in the column "p-value" represent the overall difference between the three groups; bold font indicates a significant difference between groups ($p < 0.05$); post-hoc differences in comparisons between individual groups are denoted below as: * = significant difference from non-PAD control, $p < 0.05$; † = significant difference from IC, $p < 0.05$.

3.2. Amino Acids

Nineteen amino acids were measured for all subjects, and the phenylalanine/tyrosine ratio was also calculated. The amino acids arginine, glutamine, proline, tryptophan, and tyrosine were significantly lower in CLI patients when compared to both IC patients and non-PAD controls (Table 2). In addition, levels of histidine and ornithine were significantly lower in both CLI and IC patients compared to non-PAD controls. The phenylalanine/tyrosine ratio was significantly higher in both CLI and IC patients compared to non-PAD controls (Table 2). No other differences were observed.

Table 2. Serum amino acids concentrations of the study subjects. Data are shown as mean ± standard error (μmol/L).

	Non-PAD Control (n = 26)	IC (n = 26)	CLI (n = 26)	p
Alanine	291.3 ± 23.1	356.1 ± 22.6 *	258.6 ± 24.0 †	**0.014**
Arginine	109.1 ± 5.3	117.4 ± 5.2	89.1 ± 5.5 *,†	**0.002**
Asparagine	31.7 ± 2.1	34.1 ± 2.0	30.5 ± 2.2	0.482
Citrulline	32.7 ± 3.6	37.5 ± 3.6	34.8 ± 3.8	0.626
Glutamine	580.5 ± 20.2	583.8 ± 19.8	495.3 ± 20.9 *,†	**0.007**
Glutamate	88.0 ± 5.9	65.7 ± 5.8 *	72.7 ± 6.2	**0.029**
Glycine	271.4 ± 20.1	298.6 ± 19.7	275.1 ± 20.9	0.575
Histidine	80.4 ± 2.7	73.0 ± 2.6 *	54.6 ± 2.8 *,†	**<0.001**
Leucine	199.5 ± 12.6	203.5 ± 12.4	177.6 ± 13.1	0.352
Lysine	146.2 ± 9.2	143.3 ± 8.9	121.9 ± 9.1	0.165
Methionine	30.8 ± 7.3	50.8 ± 7.2	30.4 ± 7.6	0.083
Ornithine	70.1 ± 3.9	60.7 ± 3.9 *	53.3 ± 4.2 *	**0.016**

Table 2. *Cont.*

	Non-PAD Control (n = 26)	IC (n = 26)	CLI (n = 26)	p
Phenylalanine	70.1 ± 3.7	69.7 ± 3.6	64.6 ± 3.9	0.567
Proline	207.2 ± 11.3	224.4 ± 11.9	158.9 ± 11.7 *,†	**0.001**
Serine	120.4 ± 4.9	117.7 ± 4.8	105.5 ± 5.1	0.116
Threonine	122.9 ± 8.3	121.6 ± 8.2	108.8 ± 8.6	0.473
Tryptophan	48.9 ± 3.1	53.6 ± 3.1	32.5 ± 3.2 *,†	**<0.001**
Tyrosine	62.7 ± 3.2	58.1 ± 3.2	46.6 ± 3.4 *,†	**0.006**
Valine	72.9 ± 5.1	80.6 ± 5.5	71.1 ± 5.3	0.376
Phenylalanine/Tyrosine	1.05 ± 0.06	1.25 ± 0.06 *	1.45 ± 0.07 *,†	**0.001**

Note: The values presented in the column "p-value" represent the overall difference between the three groups; bold font indicates a significant difference between groups ($p < 0.05$); post-hoc differences in comparisons between individual groups are denoted below as: * = significant difference from non-PAD control, $p < 0.05$; † = significant difference from IC, $p < 0.05$.

Of the amino acids, ABI was significantly correlated with histidine ($r = 0.463, p < 0.001$), ornithine ($r = 0.277, p = 0.017$), tryptophan ($r = 0.451, p < 0.001$), and the phenylalanine/tyrosine ratio ($r = -0.428$, $p < 0.001$).

3.3. *Acylcarnitines, Hexoses, and Biogenic Amines*

Acycarnitine was significantly lower in CLI patients compared to IC patients and non-PAD controls. Acylcarnitne was also associated with the ABI ($r = 0.378$, $p = 0.001$). In contrast, hydroxypropionylcarnitine, propionylcarnitine, and tiglylcarnitine were significantly higher in both the IC and CLI patients compared to non-PAD controls (Table 3). Of the biogenic amines, only putrescine was significantly different, higher in CLI patients compared to both IC patients and non-PAD controls (Table 4). No other differences were observed.

Table 3. Concentrations of serum acylcarnitines and hexoses of the study subjects. Data are shown as mean ± standard error (μmol/L).

	Non-PAD Control (n = 26)	IC (n = 26)	CLI (n = 26)	p
Acylcarnitine	43.5 ± 2.1	40.6 ± 2.1	31.1 ± 2.2 *,†	**0.001**
Acetyl-L-carnitine	8.7 ± 1.0	9.5 ± 1.1	9.6 ± 1.1	0.816
Propionylcarnitine	0.351 ± 0.038	0.391 ± 0.037	0.294 ± 0.039	0.221
Malonylcarnitine	0.006 ± 0.001	0.006 ± 0.001	0.007 ± 0.001	0.452
Hydroxypropionylcarnitine	0.040 ± 0.002	0.046 ± 0.002 *	0.047 ± 0.002 *	**0.003**
Propenoylcarnitine	0.017 ± 0.001	0.019 ± 0.001 *	0.019 ± 0.001 *	**0.050**
Butyrylcarnitine	0.169 ± 0.023	0.168 ± 0.023	0.153 ± 0.024	0.869
Hydroxybutyrylcarnitine	0.055 ± 0.015	0.093 ± 0.015	0.084 ± 0.016	0.189
Butenylcarnitine	0.030 ± 0.001	0.030 ± 0.001	0.029 ± 0.001	0.879
Isovalerylcarnitine	0.086 ± 0.01	0.092 ± 0.01	0.066 ± 0.01	0.189
Tiglylcarnitine	0.023 ± 0.01	0.025 ± 0.01 *	0.026 ± 0.01 *	**0.038**
Hexoses	5266 ± 489	6034 ± 479	5967 ± 508	0.476

Note: The values presented in the column "p-value" represent the overall difference between the three groups; bold font indicates a significant difference between groups ($p < 0.05$); post-hoc differences in comparisons between individual groups are denoted below as * = significant difference from non-PAD control, $p < 0.05$; † = significant difference from IC, $p < 0.05$.

Table 4. Concentrations of serum biogenic amines of the study subjects. Data are shown as mean ± standard error (μmol/L). ADMA: Asymmetric dimethyl arginine. SDMA: Symmetric dimethyl arginine. Met-SO: Methionine sulfoxide. t4-OH-Pro: Trans-4-hydroxyproline.

	Control (n = 26)	IC (n = 24)	CLI (n = 24)	p
ADMA	0.549 ± 0.03	0.543 ± 0.03	0.591 ± 0.03	0.544
SDMA	0.491 ± 0.05	0.530 ± 0.04	0.614 ± 0.05	0.249
Creatinine	92.8 ± 19.6	103.1 ± 19.5	139.1 ± 19.5	0.260
Kynurenine	2.03 ± 0.203	1.90 ± 0.199	2.42 ± 0.211	0.211
Met-SO	1.35 ± 0.847	3.47 ± 0.830	2.35 ± 0.880	0.198
Putrescine	0.011 ± 0.063	0.059 ± 0.062	0.328 ± 0.066 *,†	**0.003**
Serotonin	0.503 ± 0.107	0.793 ± 0.089	0.769 ± 0.114	0.096
Spermide	0.453 ± 0.137	0.312 ± 0.134	0.440 ± 0.142	0.716
t4-OH-Pro	11.0 ± 1.68	10.8 ± 1.65	10.4 ± 1.64	0.938
Taurine	86.7 ± 10.1	88.3 ± 12.3	65.6 ± 12.2	0.370

Note: The values presented in the column "p-value" represent the overall difference between the three groups; bold font indicates a significant difference between groups ($p < 0.05$); post-hoc differences in comparisons between individual groups are denoted below as: * = significant difference from non-PAD control, $p < 0.05$; † = significant difference from IC, $p < 0.05$.

3.4. Ceramides, Cholesteryl Esters, Sphingomyelins, Diglycerides, Triglycerides, and Phosphatidylcholines

Ceramides (Cer) (40:1), (41:1), and (42:1) were significantly lower in CLI patients compared to IC patients and non-PAD controls (Table 5). Cer (43:1) and (44:0) were significantly lower in both CLI and IC patients compared to non-PAD controls. Cholesteryl esters (CE) (16:0), (17:1), (18:2), (19:2), and (20:4) were significantly lower in CLI patients compared to IC patients and non-PAD controls (Table 6). Additionally, CE (17:0) was significantly lower in both CLI and IC patients compared to non-PAD controls, and the ratio of CE (18:1)/CE (18:2) was significantly higher in both CLI and IC patients compared to non-PAD controls. (Table 6). Finally, sphingomyelins, lysophosphatidylcholines, and phosphatidylcholines were all significantly lower in CLI patients compared to both IC patients and non-PAD controls (Table 6).

Table 5. Concentrations of serum ceramides of the study subjects. Data are shown as mean ± standard error (μmol/L).

	Control (n = 26)	IC (n = 24)	CLI (n = 24)	p
Cer (34:0)	0.054 ± 0.002	0.052 ± 0.002	0.045 ± 0.02*	**0.038**
Cer (34:1)	0.174 ± 0.011	0.182 ± 0.011	0.168 ± 0.012	0.664
Cer (38:1)	0.136 ± 0.01	0.129 ± 0.01	0.114± 0.01	0.356
Cer (40:1)	0.702 ± 0.05	0.688 ± 0.04	0.508 ± 0.05 *,†	**0.014**
Cer (41:1)	0.550 ± 0.04	0.530 ± 0.04	0.312 ± 0.04 *,†	**0.001**
Cer (42:1)	2.16 ± 0.151	2.31 ± 0.148	1.35 ± 0.156 *,†	**<0.001**
Cer (42:2)	1.39 ± 0.083	1.46 ± 0.081	1.19 ± 0.086	0.094
Cer (43:1)	0.555 ± 0.030	0.466 ± 0.030 *	0.300 ± 0.032 *,†	**<0.001**
Cer (44:0)	0.286 ± 0.026	0.207 ± 0.025 *	0.202 ± 0.027 *	**0.048**

Note: The values presented in the column "p-value" represent the overall difference between the three groups; bold font indicates a significant difference between groups ($p < 0.05$); post-hoc differences in comparisons between individual groups are denoted below as: * = significant difference from non-PAD control, $p < 0.05$; † = significant difference from IC, $p < 0.05$.

Table 6. Concentrations of serum cholesteryl esters (CE), sphingomyelins, diglycerides, triglycerides, and phosphatidylcholines of the study subjects. Data are shown as mean ± standard error (μmol/L).

	Control (n = 26)	IC (n = 24)	CLI (n = 24)	p
CE (16:0)	168.9 ± 10.3	160.2 ± 10.1	106.8 ± 10.7 *,†	**0.001**
CE (16:1)	96.6 ± 14.9	103.6 ± 14.6	69.4 ± 15.5	0.281
CE (17:0)	10.9 ± 0.56	9.4 ± 0.55 *	7.2 ± 0.58 *,†	**0.001**
CE (17:1)	8.82 ± 0.76	8.45 ± 0.75	5.37 ± 0.79 *,†	**0.007**
CE (17:2)	0.94 ± 0.16	0.85 ± 0.15	0.49 ± 0.16	0.152
CE (18:1)	244 ± 55	422 ± 54	302 ± 58	0.067
CE (18:2)	3,015± 176	2,791 ± 172	1,870 ± 183 *,†	**<0.001**
CE (18:3)	119 ± 12.3	123.2 ± 12.0	83.8 ± 12.7	0.069
CE (19:2)	5.58 ± 0.64	5.82 ± 0.63	2.69 ± 0.66 *,†	**0.001**
CE (19:3)	0.92 ± 0.266	1.86 ± 0.26 *	0.49 ± 0.277 †	**0.002**
CE (20:4)	911 ± 70	892 ± 69	662 ± 73 *,†	**0.041**
CE (20:5)	91.9 ± 7.5	78.5 ± 7.4	59.7 ± 7.8 *	**0.022**
CE (22:5)	43.3 ± 2.5	46.2 ± 2.4	37.6 ± 2.6	0.069
CE (22:6)	91.3 ± 5.9	87.0 ± 5.8	71.4 ± 6.2	0.078
CE (18:1)/CE (18:2)	0.084 ± 0.02	0.169 ± 0.02 *	0.186 ± 0.02 *	**0.008**
Sphingomyelins	11.1 ± 0.49	10.8 ± 0.48	8.80 ± 0.51 *,†	**0.007**
Diglycerides	3.48 ± 0.34	4.47 ± 0.33 *	3.07 ± 0.348 †	**0.014**
Triglycerides	29.1 ± 3.91	40.1 ± 3.83	27.8 ± 4.06	0.055
Lysophosphatidylcholines	4.13 ± 0.24	4.44 ± 0.24	2.66 ± 0.25 *,†	**0.001**
Phosphatidylcholines	10.2 ± 0.65	12.2 ± 0.63 *	8.38 ± 0.67 *,†	**0.001**

Note: The values presented in the column "p-value" represent the overall difference between the three groups; bold font indicates a significant difference between groups ($p < 0.05$); post-hoc differences in comparisons between individual groups are denoted below as: * = significant difference from non-PAD control, $p < 0.05$; † = significant difference from IC, $p < 0.05$.

Of the ceramides, ABI was significantly associated with Cer (40:1) ($r = 0.505$, $p < 0.001$), Cer (41:1) ($r = 0.541$, $p < 0.001$), Cer (42:1) ($r = 0.488$, $p < 0.001$), and Cer (43:1) ($r = 0.638$, $p < 0.001$). Of the CEs, ABI was significantly associated with CE (16:0) ($r = 0.374$, $p = 0.001$), CE(17:0) ($r = 0.482$, $p < 0.001$), CE (17:1) ($r = 0.446$, $p < 0.001$), CE (18:2) ($r = 0.447$, $p < 0.001$), and CE (20:5) ($r = 0.459$, $p < 0.001$) (Table 7).

Table 7. Pearson correlation between ankle brachial index (ABI) and metabolites.

Metabolite/Metabolite Ratio	Pearson Correlation Coefficient (r)	Significance (p)
Acylcarnitine	0.378	0.001
Histidine	0.463	<0.001
Ornithine	0.277	0.017
Trytophan	0.451	<0.001
Phenylalanine/Tyrosine	−0.428	<0.001
Cer (40:1)	0.505	<0.001
Cer (41:1)	0.541	<0.001
Cer (42:1)	0.488	<0.001
Cer (43:1)	0.638	<0.001
CE (16:0)	0.374	0.001
CE (17:0)	0.482	<0.001
CE (17:1)	0.446	<0.001
CE (18:2)	0.447	<0.001
CE (20:5)	0.459	<0.001

3.5. Discriminant Function Analysis: Non-PAD Control vs. PAD and IC vs. CLI

The discriminant function analysis model was able to correctly classify the non-PAD control and PAD patients with a 93.6% accuracy. Using a cross-validation procedure to evaluate the discriminant model performance and stability also yielded an 87.2% accuracy in patient classification. Sensitivity and specificity are two basic quantities for measuring the accuracy of a diagnostic test. The sensitivity of a diagnostic test quantifies its ability to correctly identify non-PAD control subjects without the disease and is a measure of how well the test detects non-PAD control subjects. The sensitivity of the analysis was 73.1%. The specificity refers to the ability of a test to correctly identify subjects with PAD. The specificity of the analysis was 94.2%. Figure 1A represents the plot of the original discriminant function scores, and Equation (1) represents the unstandardized canonical discriminant function coefficients:

$$\begin{aligned} Di = & -2.539 - 0.057(Carnitine) + 243.9(Hydroxypropionylcarnitine) \\ & -449.2(Propionylcarnitine) + 1.36\left(\frac{Phenylalanine}{Tyrosine}\right) \\ & +0.006(Alanine) - 0.020(Glutamate). \end{aligned} \quad (1)$$

The discriminant function analysis model correctly classified the IC and CLI patients with a 90.4% accuracy. Using a cross-validation procedure to evaluate the discriminant model performance and stability also yielded an 84.6% accuracy in patient classification. For this model, the sensitivity (correctly identify IC patients) was 80.8%, and the specificity (correctly identify CLI patients) was 88.5%. Figure 1B represents the plot of the original discriminant function scores, and Equation (2) represents the unstandardized canonical discriminant function coefficients:

$$\begin{aligned} Di = & -3.346 + 0.032(Histidine) + 5.83(Butyrylcarnitine) + 0.051(Tryptophan) \\ & -0.865(Kynurenine). \end{aligned} \quad (2)$$

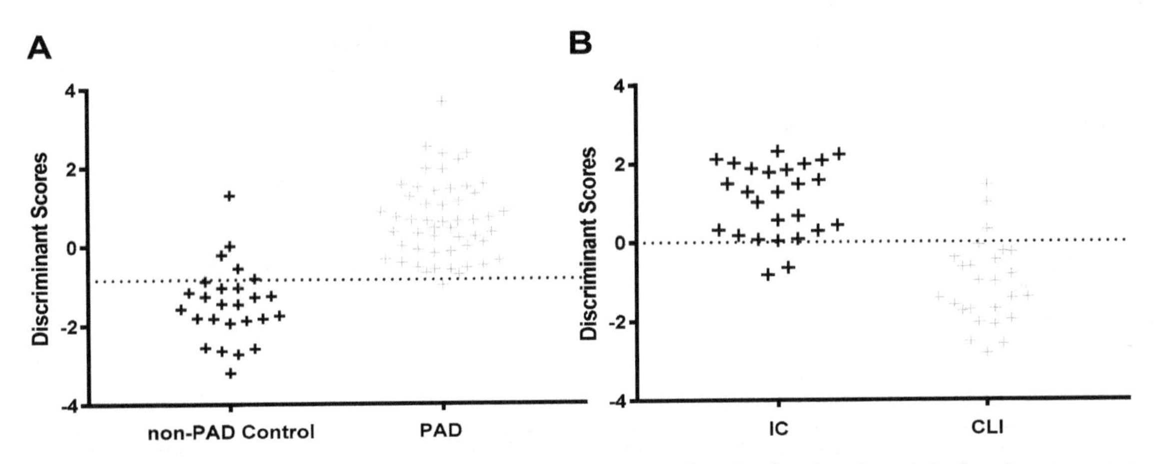

Figure 1. Discriminant function analysis model. Note: On the basis of metabolomic parameters, patient discriminant function scores can separate non-peripheral artery disease (PAD) control from PAD patients (**A**), and intermittent claudication (IC) patients from critical limb ischemia (CLI) patients (**B**).

4. Discussion

We conducted a broad metabolomic profiling of small molecules and lipids and compared metabolites between patients with IC, patients with CLI, and non-PAD controls. To our knowledge, this is the first example of metabolomics applied to evaluate patients in the two symptomatic categories of PAD versus controls. Compared to non-PAD controls, we found significant changes in the circulating levels of multiple metabolites in patients with CLI and patients with IC (Table 8). Our discriminant function analysis was able to correctly classify subjects into symptomatic PAD (both IC and CLI) vs. non-PAD controls, as well as IC vs. CLI groups, with a 93.6% and 87.2% accuracy, respectively. We found that a series of metabolites or metabolite ratios, including histidine, ornithine, phenylalanine/tyrosine, hydroxypropionyl-carnitine, propenoylcarnitine, tiglylcarnitine, Cer (43:1), Cer (44:0), CE (17:0), and CE (18:1)/CE (18:2), are significantly different in symptomatic PAD patients compared to non-PAD controls (Table 8). Several of these metabolites were also significantly correlated with the ABI, a test which may indicate PAD severity. These variables may therefore prove useful as diagnostic markers to identify PAD patients among a large population [34]. The measurement of some or a combination of these metabolites, although not currently common in most clinical laboratories, could become a much-needed, standard test for the early detection of PAD and may be incorporated into routine care cardiovascular risk prediction [35]. Additionally, the levels of a number of metabolites or metabolite ratios, including arginine, glutamine, proline, tryptophan, tyrosine, acylcarnitine, putrescine, Cer (40:1), Cer (41:1), Cer (42:1), CE (16:0), CE (17:1), CE (18:2), CE (19:2), CE (20:4), sphingomyelins, phosphatidylcholines, and lysophosphatidylcholines, were significantly different in CLI patients compared to IC patients and may prove to be valuable biomarkers for indicating which patients with IC are at higher risk of progressing to CLI. The moderate correlations between several of the ceramides and the ABI further support this. Notably, the strongest association between any of the metabolites with the ABI was that for Cer (43:1) ($r = 0.638$). It is possible that these metabolites alone or in combination can be used to produce a high-risk profile for PAD patients, allowing a personalized approach (more aggressive management, earlier intervention, and more frequent follow up for higher risk patients and less aggressive for lower risk patients) to providing care for PAD patients. The utility of such a profile should be tested in the near future as it may be able to direct the general care of PAD patients.

Table 8. List of altered metabolites in PAD.

Metabolite Class	Different in CLI	Higher/Lower	Different in PAD	Higher/Lower
Amino Acids	Arginine	↓	Histidine	↓
	Glutamine	↓	Ornithine	↓
	Proline	↓	Phenylalanine/tyrosine	↑
	Tryptophan	↓		
	Tyrosine	↓		
Acylcarnitines	Acylcarnitine	↓	Hydroxypropionyl-carnitine	↑
			Propenoylcarnitine	↑
			Tigylcarnitine	↑
Biogenic amines	Putrescine	↑		
Ceramides	Cer (40:1)	↓	Cer (43:1)	↓
	Cer (41:1)	↓	Cer (44:0)	↓
	Cer (42:1)	↓		
Cholesteryl esters, Sphingomyelin phosphatidyl-cholines	CE (16:0)	↓	CE (17:0)	↓
	CE (17:1)	↓	CE (18:1)/CE (18:2)	↑
	CE (18:2)	↓		
	CE (19:2)	↓		
	CE (20:4)	↓		
	Sphingomyelins	↓		
	Phosphatidyl-cholines	↓		
	Lysophosphatidyl-cholines	↓		

Note: "Different in CLI" are the metabolites or metabolite ratios that were significantly different between CLI patients and both IC patients and non-PAD controls. "Different in PAD" are the metabolites or metabolite ratios that were significantly different between both CLI and IC patients and non-PAD controls. ↑ represents higher and ↓ represents lower.

Several of the metabolite changes observed in this study in PAD patients are consistent with other reports from different pathologies. For example, serum levels of arginine were significantly reduced in CLI, which is consistent with several disorders linked to nitric oxide (NO) deficiency [36–38]. Likewise, ornithine, a byproduct of arginine, was reduced in both IC and CLI patients. Since NO is synthesized from *L*-arginine, lack of availability of this substrate is believed to be a factor that can lead to decreased plasma NO [36]. Impaired endothelial production of NO has been demonstrated in IC patients, and this may in fact be worse in patients with CLI [39]. Further, the ratio between serum levels of phenylalanine and tyrosine was elevated in PAD patients (both IC and CLI), and the phenylalanine/tyrosine ratio was inversely correlated with the ABI ($r = -0.428$). An elevated phenylalanine/tyrosine ratio has similarly been shown in different conditions associated with oxidative stress and inflammation, including acute brain ischemia [28]. This increased ratio may suggest diminished activity of the phenylalanine hydroxylase (PAH) enzyme by oxidation as well as tetrahydrobiopterin (BH4) deficiency, an essential cofactor of PAH [28]. Since BH4 is also a cofactor of nitric oxide synthase (NOS) and can be depleted by oxidative stress and inflammation, this ratio may also be indicative of NO dysregulation [39,40]

(Figure 2). Notably, oxidative stress and inflammation are hallmarks of PAD [41–44]. Several biomarkers of oxidative stress and inflammation, including malondyaldheide (MDA), 4-hydroxynonenale (4-HNE), isoprostanes, protein carbonyl groups, C-reactive protein (CRP), fibrinogen, tumor necrosis factor alpha (TNF-α), interferon-gamma (IFN-γ), monocyte chemoattractant protein-1 (MCP-1), and interleukin 6 (IL-6), have all been shown to be elevated in PAD patients in both circulation and skeletal muscle, and to increase with increasing disease stage [45].

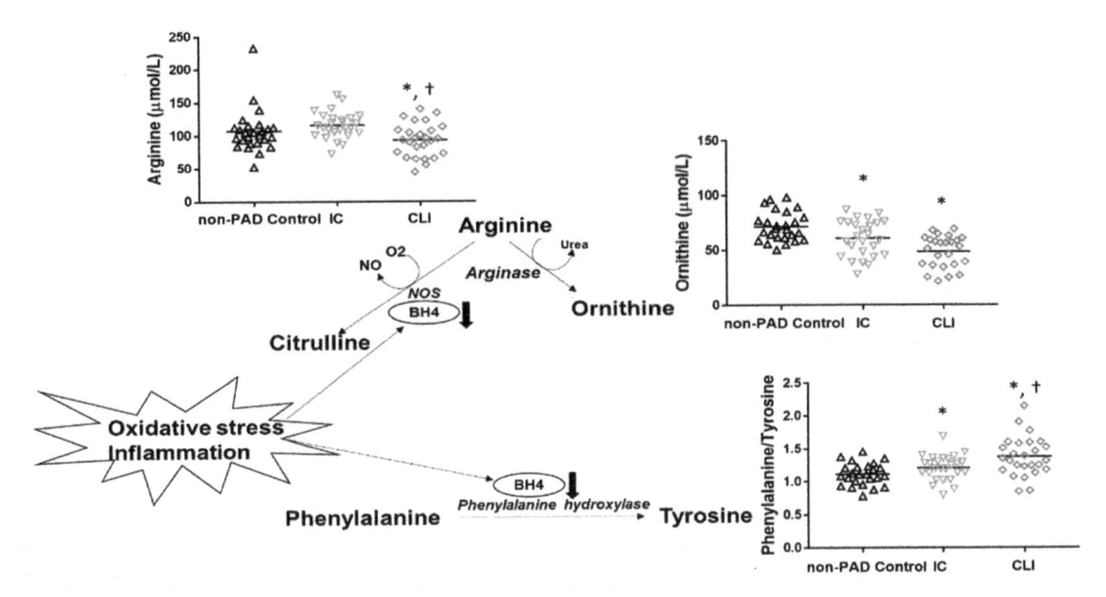

Figure 2. Potential mechanism (oxidative stress and inflammation) operating to produce decreased arginine and ornithine, increased phenylalanine to tyrosine ratio, and decreased nitric oxide bioavailability in PAD. Note: Tetrahydrobiopterin (BH4), an essential cofactor of nitric oxide synthase (NOS) and phenylalanine hydroxylase (PAH), is depleted by oxidative stress and inflammation. Therefore, reduced BH4 may explain the decreased turnover of phenylalanine to tyrosine observed in IC and CLI patients. Reduced BH4, as well as a lack of arginine availability, may play a role in impairing production of NO in PAD patients, leading to endothelial dysfunction. * denotes a significant difference from non-PAD controls and † denotes a significant difference from IC.

PAD patients also demonstrated significantly reduced levels of histidine, an amino acid with antioxidant and anti-inflammatory properties [46]. In vitro, histidine has been shown to blunt pro-inflammatory cytokine expression, and histidine supplementation has been used to control inflammation in obese patients with metabolic syndrome [47]. Patients with different conditions of enhanced oxidative stress, such as chronic kidney disease and coronary heart disease, have also been shown to have reduced levels of histidine [46,48], suggesting that depletion of histidine may indicate elevated oxidative stress, a condition that is well described in patients with IC and CLI [41,49,50].

CLI patients demonstrated further perturbations in amino acids not observed in IC patients that are also consistent with reports from other diseases and disorders. For example, reduced tryptophan levels have been associated with inflammation and immune activation, and have been shown to predict higher mortality in cardiovascular disease [51]. Specifically, reduced tryptophan may be due to accelerated conversion to kynurenine by indoleamine 2,3-dioxygenase (IDO1), which is activated by cytokines, such as tumor necrosis factor-alpha (TNF-α) and interferon gamma (IFN-γ) (Figure 3) [52]. Levels of kynurenine were also higher in CLI patients compared to both ICs and non-PAD controls, although differences were not significant statistically. In addition, glutamine levels were significantly lower in CLI patients. Reduced levels of glutamine are thought to be indicative of skeletal muscle catabolism [53]. Interestingly, CLI patients exhibit a severe myopathy that is characterized by myofiber degeneration, fibrosis, and muscle atrophy [49].

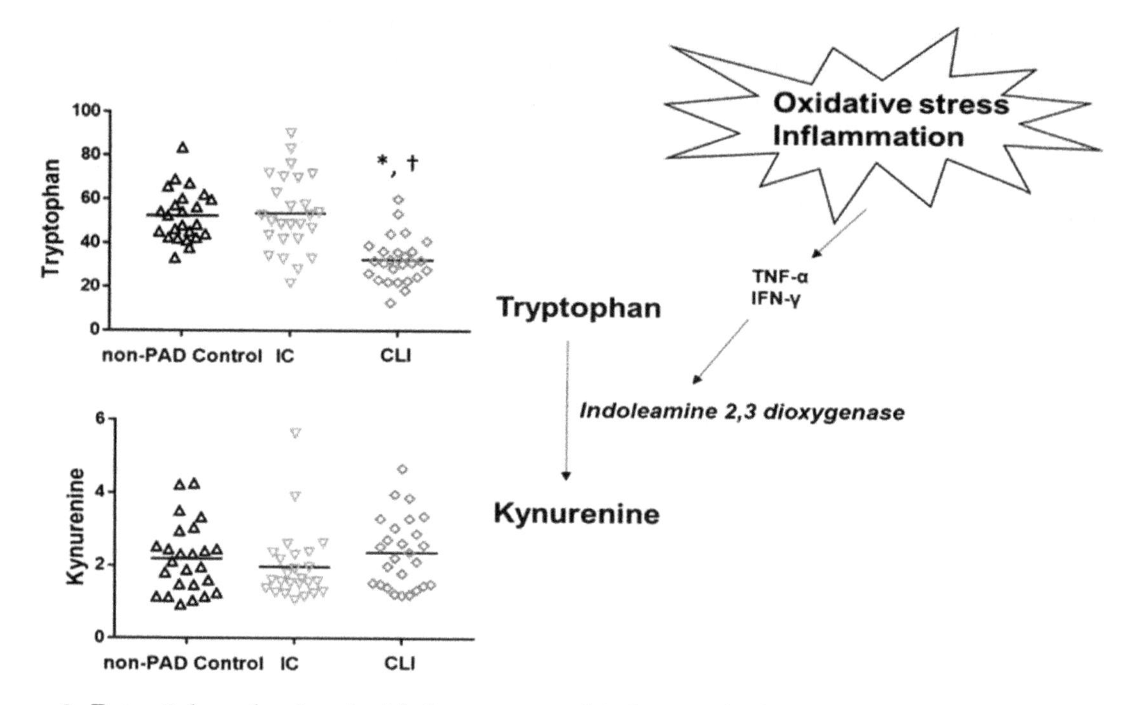

Figure 3. Potential mechanism (oxidative stress and inflammation) operating to produce decreased tryptophan levels in CLI. Note: Accelerated conversion of tryptophan to kynurenine is induced by inflammatory cytokines. Tryptophan is converted to kynurenine by the enzyme indoleamine 2,3 dioxygenase (IDO). IDO expression and activity are enhanced by tumor necrosis factor-alpha (TNF-α) and interferon-gamma (IFN-γ). Elevations in these cytokines may explain an increased conversion of tryptophan to kynurenine in CLI patients. * denotes a significant difference from non-PAD controls and † denotes a significant difference from IC.

Several carnitine esters and members of the acyl carnitines, including hydroxypropionylcarnitine, propionylcarnitine, and tiglylcarnitine, were significantly elevated in both IC and CLI patients compared to non-PAD controls. During the metabolism of amino acids, carbohydrates, and fatty acids, these substrates are converted to acyl-CoA intermediates for oxidation in the Krebs cycle. Under functional metabolism, carnitine buffers acyl-CoA by forming acylcarnitines. However, during metabolic stress, acyl-CoA is incompletely oxidized and accumulates, and transfer of the acyl group to carnitine thus leads to accumulation of acylcarnitine. Therefore, accumulation of acylcarnitines can be an indication of dysfunctional metabolism [54]. Early studies in IC patients showed that short-chain acylcarnitines accumulate in plasma, which is inversely correlated with exercise performance [55]. In skeletal muscle tissue from patients with unilateral claudication, acylcarnitine accumulation was specific only to the affected limb, and interestingly, accumulation of acylcarnitine was shown to be a better indicator of exercise performance than even the ABI [56].

In patients with more severe PAD, however, a reduction in total and acylcarnitine content has been shown [57]. This is consistent with our study, in which CLI patients also demonstrated reduced total acylcarnitine levels, which has been thought to suggest dysfunctional fatty acid β-oxidation [58,59]. Additionally, in our study there was a weak positive association between the ABI and total acylcarnitine ($r = 0.378$). The rate-limiting step in the β-oxidation of long-chain fatty acids is the conjugation of carnitine to fatty acyl coenzyme A (coA) by the enzyme carnitine palmitoyltransferase (CPT1) [60]. Since acylcarnitine levels remain constant and only levels of free carnitine are affected by factors, such as age and sex, low acylcarnitine levels may suggest metabolic alterations due to decreased levels of total carnitine, reduced CPT1 activity, or decreased availability of acyl-coA [59]. Consistent with a potentially dysfunctional fatty acid β-oxidation, muscle tissue from CLI patients demonstrates reduced expression of oxidative phosphorylation proteins, as well as lower mitochondrial respiratory capacity [15]. However, other carnitine esters, including hydroxypropionylcarnitine, propionylcarnitine, and tigylcarnitine, were significantly elevated in both IC and CLI patients compared to non-PAD controls. Therefore, the role of carnitines in PAD warrants further exploration.

Sphingolipids are major components of cellular membranes, critical for the fluidity and architecture of the membrane. Sphingomyelins are a type of sphingolipid usually consisting of phosphocholine and ceramide. The metabolites of sphingolipids, such as ceramides, are important for regulating cell proliferation and survival, as well as the inflammatory responses [61]. In this study, levels of certain ceramides were markedly reduced in both IC and CLI patients. Further, CLI patients demonstrated reduced levels of sphingomyelins. Similar findings were reported for patients with sickle-cell disease, which is associated with a progressive vasculopathy, vascular occlusion, and endothelial dysfunction, all of which are pathophysiological aspects of PAD as well [39,62]. In contrast, however, other studies have shown that sphingomyelin and ceramides are independent risk factors for coronary heart disease and that higher levels are associated with atherosclerosis and the development of metabolic disease [63–66]. Future research is needed to clarify the alternations in sphingolipid metabolism in CLI patients. Phosphatidylcholine levels were lower in CLI patients, which is consistent with a study in patients with atherosclerosis, where reduced phosphatidylcholine levels were correlated with increased arterial stiffness, increased resting heart rate, and/or worsened endothelial function [67]. Interestingly, the hydrolysis of phosphatidylcholine to phosphatidic acid and choline is catalyzed by phospholipase D (PLD), and high PLD activity is associated with oxidative stress, inflammation, hypoxia, and atherosclerosis [68]. Finally, several cholesteryl ester species were lower in CLI patients as well. Of note, the ratio of cholesteryl ester CE (18:1)/CE (18:2) was significantly increased in both IC and CLI patients, which is consistent with findings in high fat diet-induced obese mice [29]. Since CE (18:1) is considered the preferred fatty acid of ACAT, this suggests higher ACAT activity, which is consistent with obesity and hypercholesterolemia [30].

Currently available options (risk factor management, medications, exercise therapy, and revascularization operations) for the management of PAD are limited. There are two medications, with only modest efficacy, approved for claudication, and operations are associated with considerable morbidity and poor durability [69,70]. PAD patients suffer from high rates of cardiovascular events, including stroke and myocardial infarction [71], and PAD also significantly impairs quality of life and leads to functional impairment and decline [72]. This highlights the importance of identifying novel targets for intervention for this population. In this study, we identified several metabolites that are altered in symptomatic PAD patients compared to non-PAD controls while also identifying a distinct metabolomic signature associated with only CLI [15].

One important limitation of this study is the sample size was relatively small. Thus, external validation from a larger sample could help add to the translational impact of the study results. Furthermore, while there is an emerging use of metabolomics in clinical settings, complexities and challenges, for example, related to testing strategies and quality control, limit its immediate clinical impact. Thus far, the field of metabolomics has primarily been limited to biomedical research and biomarker discovery; however, greater considerations must be taken into account for use as a clinical test. Therefore, this may also affect the translational impact of this study.

Another important point to note is the use of only serum may limit the generalizability of these findings to other fluids and tissues. Specifically, during centrifugation to separate serum from coagulated blood, platelets release proteins that include cytokines and metabolites into the serum [73]. Since anticoagulants are added before the removal of blood cells to obtain plasma, there may be differences between human plasma and serum metabolites. However, in a large study that compared metabolite concentrations between plasma and serum, although there were differences in the exact concentrations between blood matrices, the changes between groups were proportional and the correlation was high between plasma and serum [73]. This study also concluded that reproducibility was high in both plasma and serum and that either will lead to similar results in clinical studies (as long as the same matrix is used throughout), with serum potentially providing greater sensitivity in biomarker studies, thus supporting our use of serum in this study [73].

5. Conclusions

In conclusion, we identified a number of metabolites that are altered in PAD. To our knowledge, this is the first time that a complete metabolomic profiling comparing patients with different severities of PAD and non-PAD controls is presented. These data provide unique metabolomic fingerprints that may be helpful in screening for the presence of PAD, and may also be useful in risk-stratifying PAD patients and predicting their clinical outcomes. Further, these alterations provide insight into the disrupted pathways that underlie the pathophysiology of PAD and may contribute to a better understanding of the disease and to the development of novel therapeutic interventions for PAD patients.

Author Contributions: A.I., M.E.F., R.L. and P.K. designed the study. M.F., R.S.S., W.T.B. and I.I.P. recruited the patients and collected the blood. I.I.P. was the Principal investigator of the clinical recruitment protocol. Metabolomics were performed and evaluated by R.L., P.K., G.P.C., E.P., I.S., C.J.M. Statistical analysis was performed and evaluated by G.R.H., A.I., and P.K., A.I., R.L., I.I.P. and P.K. wrote the manuscript and all authors contributed to the final version of the manuscript.

Acknowledgments: The authors would like to thank Alejandro Ramirez for technical support and to acknowledge the Baylor University Mass Spectrometry Center (Waco, Texas) for support during this work.

References

1. Criqui, M.H.; Aboyans, V. Epidemiology of peripheral artery disease. *Circ. Res.* **2015**, *116*, 1509–1526. [CrossRef] [PubMed]
2. Shu, J.; Santulli, G. Update on peripheral artery disease: Epidemiology and evidence-based facts. *Atherosclerosis* **2018**, *275*, 379–381. [CrossRef] [PubMed]
3. Gerhard-Herman, M.D.; Gornik, H.L.; Barrett, C.; Barshes, N.R.; Corriere, M.A.; Drachman, D.E.; Fleisher, L.A.; Fowkes, F.G.; Hamburg, N.M.; Kinlay, S.; et al. 2016 AHA/ACC Guideline on the Management of Patients With Lower Extremity Peripheral Artery Disease: Executive Summary: A Report of the American College of Cardiology/American Heart Association Task Force on Clinical Practice Guidelines. *Circulation* **2017**, *135*, e686–e725. [CrossRef] [PubMed]
4. Dua, A.; Lee, C.J. Epidemiology of Peripheral Arterial Disease and Critical Limb Ischemia. *Tech. Vasc. Interv. Radiol.* **2016**, *19*, 91–95. [CrossRef] [PubMed]
5. Pipinos, I.I.; Judge, A.R.; Selsby, J.T.; Zhu, Z.; Swanson, S.A.; Nella, A.A.; Dodd, S.L. The myopathy of peripheral arterial occlusive disease: Part 1. Functional and histomorphological changes and evidence for mitochondrial dysfunction. *Vasc. Endovascular Surg.* **2007**, *41*, 481–489. [CrossRef] [PubMed]
6. Pipinos, I.I.; Judge, A.R.; Selsby, J.T.; Zhu, Z.; Swanson, S.A.; Nella, A.A.; Dodd, S.L. The myopathy of peripheral arterial occlusive disease: Part 2. Oxidative stress, neuropathy, and shift in muscle fiber type. *Vasc. Endovascular Surg.* **2008**, *42*, 101–112. [CrossRef] [PubMed]
7. Brass, E.P.; Hiatt, W.R. Acquired skeletal muscle metabolic myopathy in atherosclerotic peripheral arterial disease. *Vasc. Med.* **2000**, *5*, 55–59. [CrossRef]
8. Rontoyanni, V.G.; Nunez Lopez, O.; Fankhauser, G.T.; Cheema, Z.F.; Rasmussen, B.B.; Porter, C. Mitochondrial Bioenergetics in the Metabolic Myopathy Accompanying Peripheral Artery Disease. *Front. Physiol.* **2017**, *8*, 141. [CrossRef]
9. Brass, E.P. Skeletal muscle metabolism as a target for drug therapy in peripheral arterial disease. *Vasc. Med.* **1996**, *1*, 55–59. [CrossRef]
10. Gardner, A.W.; Killewich, L.A.; Katzel, L.I.; Womack, C.J.; Montgomery, P.S.; Otis, R.B.; Fonong, T. Relationship between free-living daily physical activity and peripheral circulation in patients with intermittent claudication. *Angiology* **1999**, *50*, 289–297. [CrossRef]

11. Gardner, A.W.; Montgomery, P.S.; Scott, K.J.; Afaq, A.; Blevins, S.M. Patterns of ambulatory activity in subjects with and without intermittent claudication. *J. Vasc. Surg.* **2007**, *46*, 1208–1214. [CrossRef] [PubMed]
12. Myers, S.A.; Johanning, J.M.; Stergiou, N.; Lynch, T.G.; Longo, G.M.; Pipinos, I.I. Claudication distances and the Walking Impairment Questionnaire best describe the ambulatory limitations in patients with symptomatic peripheral arterial disease. *J. Vasc. Surg.* **2008**, *47*, 550–555. [CrossRef] [PubMed]
13. McDermott, M.M.; Ferrucci, L.; Guralnik, J.; Tian, L.; Liu, K.; Hoff, F.; Liao, Y.; Criqui, M.H. Pathophysiological changes in calf muscle predict mobility loss at 2-year follow-up in men and women with peripheral arterial disease. *Circulation* **2009**, *120*, 1048–1055. [CrossRef] [PubMed]
14. McDermott, M.M.; Guralnik, J.M.; Ferrucci, L.; Tian, L.; Pearce, W.H.; Hoff, F.; Liu, K.; Liao, Y.; Criqui, M.H. Physical activity, walking exercise, and calf skeletal muscle characteristics in patients with peripheral arterial disease. *J. Vasc. Surg.* **2007**, *46*, 87–93. [CrossRef] [PubMed]
15. Ryan, T.E.; Yamaguchi, D.J.; Schmidt, C.A.; Zeczycki, T.N.; Shaikh, S.R.; Brophy, P.; Green, T.D.; Tarpey, M.D.; Karnekar, R.; Goldberg, E.J.; et al. Extensive skeletal muscle cell mitochondriopathy distinguishes critical limb ischemia patients from claudicants. *JCI Insight* **2018**, *3*. [CrossRef] [PubMed]
16. Shammas, N.W. Epidemiology, classification, and modifiable risk factors of peripheral arterial disease. *Vasc. Health Risk Manag.* **2007**, *3*, 229–234. [CrossRef]
17. Selvin, E.; Erlinger, T.P. Prevalence of and risk factors for peripheral arterial disease in the United States: Results from the National Health and Nutrition Examination Survey, 1999–2000. *Circulation* **2004**, *110*, 738–743. [CrossRef]
18. Garcia-Fontana, B.; Morales-Santana, S.; Diaz Navarro, C.; Rozas-Moreno, P.; Genilloud, O.; Vicente Perez, F.; Perez del Palacio, J.; Munoz-Torres, M. Metabolomic profile related to cardiovascular disease in patients with type 2 diabetes mellitus: A pilot study. *Talanta* **2016**, *148*, 135–143. [CrossRef]
19. Trabado, S.; Al-Salameh, A.; Croixmarie, V.; Masson, P.; Corruble, E.; Feve, B.; Colle, R.; Ripoll, L.; Walther, B.; Boursier-Neyret, C.; et al. The human plasma-metabolome: Reference values in 800 French healthy volunteers; impact of cholesterol, gender and age. *PLoS ONE* **2017**, *12*, e0173615. [CrossRef]
20. Shah, S.H.; Kraus, W.E.; Newgard, C.B. Metabolomic profiling for the identification of novel biomarkers and mechanisms related to common cardiovascular diseases: Form and function. *Circulation* **2012**, *126*, 1110–1120. [CrossRef]
21. Fiehn, O.; Kopka, J.; Dormann, P.; Altmann, T.; Trethewey, R.N.; Willmitzer, L. Metabolite profiling for plant functional genomics. *Nat. Biotechnol.* **2000**, *18*, 1157–1161. [CrossRef] [PubMed]
22. Liu, X.; Xu, G. Recent advances in using mass spectrometry for mitochondrial metabolomics and lipidomics—A review. *Anal. Chim. Acta* **2018**, *1037*, 3–12. [CrossRef] [PubMed]
23. Dona, A.C.; Coffey, S.; Figtree, G. Translational and emerging clinical applications of metabolomics in cardiovascular disease diagnosis and treatment. *Eur. J. Prev. Cardiol.* **2016**, *23*, 1578–1589. [CrossRef] [PubMed]
24. Puchades-Carrasco, L.; Pineda-Lucena, A. Metabolomics Applications in Precision Medicine: An Oncological Perspective. *Curr. Top. Med. Chem.* **2017**, *17*, 2740–2751. [CrossRef] [PubMed]
25. Huang, C.C.; McDermott, M.M.; Liu, K.; Kuo, C.H.; Wang, S.Y.; Tao, H.; Tseng, Y.J. Plasma metabolomic profiles predict near-term death among individuals with lower extremity peripheral arterial disease. *J. Vasc. Surg.* **2013**, *58*, 989–996.e1. [CrossRef] [PubMed]
26. Zagura, M.; Kals, J.; Kilk, K.; Serg, M.; Kampus, P.; Eha, J.; Soomets, U.; Zilmer, M. Metabolomic signature of arterial stiffness in male patients with peripheral arterial disease. *Hypertens Res.* **2015**, *38*, 840–846. [CrossRef]
27. Saleem, F.; Bouatra, S.; Guo, A.C.; Psychogios, N.; Mandal, R.; Dunn, S.M.; Ametaj, B.N.; Wishart, D.S. The bovine ruminal fluid metabolome. *Metabolomics* **2013**, *9*, 360–378. [CrossRef]
28. Ormstad, H.; Verkerk, R.; Sandvik, L. Serum Phenylalanine, Tyrosine, and their Ratio in Acute Ischemic Stroke: On the Trail of a Biomarker? *J. Mol. Neurosci.* **2016**, *58*, 102–108. [CrossRef]
29. Eisinger, K.; Liebisch, G.; Schmitz, G.; Aslanidis, C.; Krautbauer, S.; Buechler, C. Lipidomic analysis of serum from high fat diet induced obese mice. *Int. J. Mol. Sci.* **2014**, *15*, 2991–3002. [CrossRef]
30. Roberts, C.K.; Liang, K.; Barnard, R.J.; Kim, C.H.; Vaziri, N.D. HMG-CoA reductase, cholesterol 7alpha-hydroxylase, LDL receptor, SR-B1, and ACAT in diet-induced syndrome X. *Kidney Int.* **2004**, *66*, 1503–1511. [CrossRef]

31. Lee, R.G.; Kelley, K.L.; Sawyer, J.K.; Farese, R.V., Jr.; Parks, J.S.; Rudel, L.L. Plasma cholesteryl esters provided by lecithin:cholesterol acyltransferase and acyl-coenzyme a:cholesterol acyltransferase 2 have opposite atherosclerotic potential. *Circ. Res.* **2004**, *95*, 998–1004. [CrossRef] [PubMed]
32. Xia, J.; Wishart, D.S. Web-based inference of biological patterns, functions and pathways from metabolomic data using MetaboAnalyst. *Nat. Protoc.* **2011**, *6*, 743. [CrossRef] [PubMed]
33. Hastie, T.; Tibshirani, R.; Friedman, J.H. *The Elements of Statistical Learning: Data Mining, Inference, and Prediction*, 2nd ed.; Springer: New York, NY, USA, 2009.
34. Krishna, S.M.; Moxon, J.V.; Golledge, J. A review of the pathophysiology and potential biomarkers for peripheral artery disease. *Int. J. Mol. Sci.* **2015**, *16*, 11294–11322. [CrossRef] [PubMed]
35. Joosten, M.M.; Pai, J.K.; Bertoia, M.L.; Gansevoort, R.T.; Bakker, S.J.; Cooke, J.P.; Rimm, E.B.; Mukamal, K.J. beta2-microglobulin, cystatin C, and creatinine and risk of symptomatic peripheral artery disease. *J. Am. Heart Assoc.* **2014**, *3*. [CrossRef] [PubMed]
36. Hess, S.; Baker, G.; Gyenes, G.; Tsuyuki, R.; Newman, S.; Le Melledo, J.M. Decreased serum L-arginine and L-citrulline levels in major depression. *Psychopharmacology (Berl.)* **2017**, *234*, 3241–3247. [CrossRef] [PubMed]
37. Morris, C.R.; Poljakovic, M.; Lavrisha, L.; Machado, L.; Kuypers, F.A.; Morris, S.M., Jr. Decreased arginine bioavailability and increased serum arginase activity in asthma. *Am. J. Respir. Crit. Care Med.* **2004**, *170*, 148–153. [CrossRef] [PubMed]
38. Kayanoki, Y.; Kawata, S.; Yamasaki, E.; Kiso, S.; Inoue, S.; Tamura, S.; Taniguchi, N.; Matsuzawa, Y. Reduced nitric oxide production by L-arginine deficiency in lysinuric protein intolerance exacerbates intravascular coagulation. *Metab. Clin. Exp.* **1999**, *48*, 1136–1140. [CrossRef]
39. Ismaeel, A.; Brumberg, R.S.; Kirk, J.S.; Papoutsi, E.; Farmer, P.J.; Bohannon, W.T.; Smith, R.S.; Eidson, J.L.; Sawicki, I.; Koutakis, P. Oxidative Stress and Arterial Dysfunction in Peripheral Artery Disease. *Antioxidants* **2018**, *7*, 145. [CrossRef]
40. Barbato, J.E.; Tzeng, E. Nitric oxide and arterial disease. *J. Vasc. Surg.* **2004**, *40*, 187–193. [CrossRef]
41. Koutakis, P.; Ismaeel, A.; Farmer, P.; Purcell, S.; Smith, R.S.; Eidson, J.L.; Bohannon, W.T. Oxidative stress and antioxidant treatment in patients with peripheral artery disease. *Physiol. Rep.* **2018**, *6*, e13650. [CrossRef]
42. Brevetti, G.; Giugliano, G.; Brevetti, L.; Hiatt, W.R. Inflammation in peripheral artery disease. *Circulation* **2010**, *122*, 1862–1875. [CrossRef] [PubMed]
43. Ozaki, Y.; Imanishi, T.; Akasaka, T. Inflammatory Biomarkers in Peripheral Artery Disease: Diagnosis, Prognosis, and Therapeutic Challenges. *Curr. Med. Chem.* **2015**, *22*, 2744–2753. [CrossRef]
44. Signorelli, S.S.; Anzaldi, M.; Fiore, V. Inflammation in peripheral arterial disease (PAD). *Curr. Pharm. Des.* **2012**, *18*, 4350–4357. [CrossRef] [PubMed]
45. Signorelli, S.S.; Scuto, S.; Marino, E.; Xourafa, A.; Gaudio, A. Oxidative Stress in Peripheral Arterial Disease (PAD) Mechanism and Biomarkers. *Antioxidants* **2019**, *8*, 367. [CrossRef] [PubMed]
46. Yu, B.; Li, A.H.; Muzny, D.; Veeraraghavan, N.; de Vries, P.S.; Bis, J.C.; Musani, S.K.; Alexander, D.; Morrison, A.C.; Franco, O.H.; et al. Association of Rare Loss-Of-Function Alleles in HAL, Serum Histidine: Levels and Incident Coronary Heart Disease. *Circ. Cardiovasc. Genet.* **2015**, *8*, 351–355. [CrossRef]
47. Feng, R.N.; Niu, Y.C.; Sun, X.W.; Li, Q.; Zhao, C.; Wang, C.; Guo, F.C.; Sun, C.H.; Li, Y. Histidine supplementation improves insulin resistance through suppressed inflammation in obese women with the metabolic syndrome: A randomised controlled trial. *Diabetologia* **2013**, *56*, 985–994. [CrossRef] [PubMed]
48. Watanabe, M.; Suliman, M.E.; Qureshi, A.R.; Garcia-Lopez, E.; Barany, P.; Heimburger, O.; Stenvinkel, P.; Lindholm, B. Consequences of low plasma histidine in chronic kidney disease patients: Associations with inflammation, oxidative stress, and mortality. *Am. J. Clin. Nutr.* **2008**, *87*, 1860–1866. [CrossRef] [PubMed]
49. Weiss, D.J.; Casale, G.P.; Koutakis, P.; Nella, A.A.; Swanson, S.A.; Zhu, Z.; Miserlis, D.; Johanning, J.M.; Pipinos, I.I. Oxidative damage and myofiber degeneration in the gastrocnemius of patients with peripheral arterial disease. *J. Transl. Med.* **2013**, *11*, 230. [CrossRef] [PubMed]
50. Koutakis, P.; Weiss, D.J.; Miserlis, D.; Shostrom, V.K.; Papoutsi, E.; Ha, D.M.; Carpenter, L.A.; McComb, R.D.; Casale, G.P.; Pipinos, I.I. Oxidative damage in the gastrocnemius of patients with peripheral artery disease is myofiber type selective. *Redox. Biol.* **2014**, *2*, 921–928. [CrossRef]
51. Murr, C.; Grammer, T.B.; Kleber, M.E.; Meinitzer, A.; Marz, W.; Fuchs, D. Low serum tryptophan predicts higher mortality in cardiovascular disease. *Eur. J. Clin. Investig.* **2015**, *45*, 247–254. [CrossRef]

52. Schrocksnadel, K.; Wirleitner, B.; Winkler, C.; Fuchs, D. Monitoring tryptophan metabolism in chronic immune activation. *Clin. Chim. Acta* **2006**, *364*, 82–90. [CrossRef] [PubMed]
53. Kinscherf, R.; Hack, V.; Fischbach, T.; Friedmann, B.; Weiss, C.; Edler, L.; Bartsch, P.; Droge, W. Low plasma glutamine in combination with high glutamate levels indicate risk for loss of body cell mass in healthy individuals: The effect of N-acetyl-cysteine. *J. Mol. Med.* **1996**, *74*, 393–400. [CrossRef] [PubMed]
54. Bieber, L.L. Carnitine. *Annu. Rev. Biochem.* **1988**, *57*, 261–283. [CrossRef] [PubMed]
55. Hiatt, W.R.; Nawaz, D.; Brass, E.P. Carnitine metabolism during exercise in patients with peripheral vascular disease. *J. Appl. Physiol.* **1987**, *62*, 2383–2387. [CrossRef] [PubMed]
56. Hiatt, W.R.; Wolfel, E.E.; Regensteiner, J.G.; Brass, E.P. Skeletal muscle carnitine metabolism in patients with unilateral peripheral arterial disease. *J. Appl. Physiol.* **1992**, *73*, 346–353. [CrossRef] [PubMed]
57. Brevetti, G.; Angelini, C.; Rosa, M.; Carrozzo, R.; Perna, S.; Corsi, M.; Matarazzo, A.; Marcialis, A. Muscle carnitine deficiency in patients with severe peripheral vascular disease. *Circulation* **1991**, *84*, 1490–1495. [CrossRef] [PubMed]
58. Saiki, S.; Hatano, T.; Fujimaki, M.; Ishikawa, K.I.; Mori, A.; Oji, Y.; Okuzumi, A.; Fukuhara, T.; Koinuma, T.; Imamichi, Y.; et al. Decreased long-chain acylcarnitines from insufficient beta-oxidation as potential early diagnostic markers for Parkinson's disease. *Sci. Rep.* **2017**, *7*, 7328. [CrossRef]
59. Miyagawa, T.; Miyadera, H.; Tanaka, S.; Kawashima, M.; Shimada, M.; Honda, Y.; Tokunaga, K.; Honda, M. Abnormally low serum acylcarnitine levels in narcolepsy patients. *Sleep* **2011**, *34*, 349–353A. [CrossRef]
60. McGarry, J.D.; Brown, N.F. The mitochondrial carnitine palmitoyltransferase system. From concept to molecular analysis. *Eur. J. Biochem.* **1997**, *244*, 1–14. [CrossRef]
61. Presa, N.; Gomez-Larrauri, A.; Rivera, I.G.; Ordonez, M.; Trueba, M.; Gomez-Munoz, A. Regulation of cell migration and inflammation by ceramide 1-phosphate. *Biochim. Biophys. Acta* **2016**, *1861*, 402–409. [CrossRef]
62. Aslan, M.; Kirac, E.; Kaya, S.; Ozcan, F.; Salim, O.; Kupesiz, O.A. Decreased Serum Levels of Sphingomyelins and Ceramides in Sickle Cell Disease Patients. *Lipids* **2018**, *53*, 313–322. [CrossRef] [PubMed]
63. Jiang, X.C.; Paultre, F.; Pearson, T.A.; Reed, R.G.; Francis, C.K.; Lin, M.; Berglund, L.; Tall, A.R. Plasma sphingomyelin level as a risk factor for coronary artery disease. *Arterioscl. Throm. Vas.* **2000**, *20*, 2614–2618. [CrossRef] [PubMed]
64. Nelson, J.; Jiang, X.C.; Tabas, I.; Tall, A.; Shea, S. Plasma sphingomyelin and subclinical atherosclerosis: Findings from the multi-ethnic study of atherosclerosis. *Am. J. Epidemiol.* **2006**, *163*, 903–912. [CrossRef] [PubMed]
65. Hanamatsu, H.; Ohnishi, S.; Sakai, S.; Yuyama, K.; Mitsutake, S.; Takeda, H.; Hashino, S.; Igarashi, Y. Altered levels of serum sphingomyelin and ceramide containing distinct acyl chains in young obese adults. *Nutr. Diabetes* **2014**, *4*, e141. [CrossRef] [PubMed]
66. Holland, W.L.; Summers, S.A. Sphingolipids, insulin resistance, and metabolic disease: New insights from in vivo manipulation of sphingolipid metabolism. *Endocr. Rev.* **2008**, *29*, 381–402. [CrossRef] [PubMed]
67. Paapstel, K.; Kals, J.; Eha, J.; Tootsi, K.; Ottas, A.; Piir, A.; Jakobson, M.; Lieberg, J.; Zilmer, M. Inverse relations of serum phosphatidylcholines and lysophosphatidylcholines with vascular damage and heart rate in patients with atherosclerosis. *Nutr. Metab. Cardiovasc. Dis.* **2018**, *28*, 44–52. [CrossRef] [PubMed]
68. Tappia, P.S.; Dent, M.R.; Dhalla, N.S. Oxidative stress and redox regulation of phospholipase D in myocardial disease. *Free Radic. Biol. Med.* **2006**, *41*, 349–361. [CrossRef]
69. Roset, P.N. Systematic review of the efficacy of cilostazol, naftidrofuryl oxalate and pentoxifylline for the treatment of intermittent claudication (*Br J Surg* 2012; 99: 1630–1638). *Br. J. Surg.* **2013**, *100*, 1838. [CrossRef]
70. Nowygrod, R.; Egorova, N.; Greco, G.; Anderson, P.; Gelijns, A.; Moskowitz, A.; McKinsey, J.; Morrissey, N.; Kent, K.C. Trends, complications, and mortality in peripheral vascular surgery. *J. Vasc. Surg.* **2006**, *43*, 205–216. [CrossRef]
71. Steg, P.G.; Bhatt, D.L.; Wilson, P.W.; D'Agostino, R., Sr.; Ohman, E.M.; Rother, J.; Liau, C.S.; Hirsch, A.T.; Mas, J.L.; Ikeda, Y.; et al. One-year cardiovascular event rates in outpatients with atherothrombosis. *JAMA* **2007**, *297*, 1197–1206. [CrossRef]
72. McDermott, M.M. Functional impairment in peripheral artery disease and how to improve it in 2013. *Curr. Cardiol. Rep.* **2013**, *15*, 347. [CrossRef] [PubMed]
73. Yu, Z.H.; Kastenmuller, G.; He, Y.; Belcredi, P.; Moller, G.; Prehn, C.; Mendes, J.; Wahl, S.; Roemisch-Margl, W.; Ceglarek, U.; et al. Differences between Human Plasma and Serum Metabolite Profiles. *PLoS ONE* **2011**, *6*. [CrossRef] [PubMed]

4

Functional Role of Natriuretic Peptides in Risk Assessment and Prognosis of Patients with Mitral Regurgitation

Giovanna Gallo [1], Maurizio Forte [2], Rosita Stanzione [2], Maria Cotugno [2], Franca Bianchi [2], Simona Marchitti [2], Andrea Berni [1], Massimo Volpe [1,2] and Speranza Rubattu [1,2,*]

1 Department of Clinical and Molecular Medicine, School of Medicine and Psychology, Sapienza University of Rome, 00189 Rome, Italy; giovanna.gallo@uniroma1.it (G.G.); andrea.berni@uniroma1.it (A.B.); massimo.volpe@uniroma1.it (M.V.)
2 IRCCS Neuromed, 86077 Pozzilli (Isernia), Italy; maurizio.forte@neuromed.it (M.F.); stanzione@neuromed.it (R.S.); maria.cotugno@neuromed.it (M.C.); franca.bianchi@neuromed.it (F.B.); simona.marchitti@neuromed.it (S.M.)
* Correspondence: rubattu.speranza@neuromed.it

Abstract: The management of mitral valve regurgitation (MR), a common valve disease, represents a challenge in clinical practice, since the indication for either surgical or percutaneous valve replacement or repair are guided by symptoms and by echocardiographic parameters which are not always feasible. In this complex scenario, the use of natriuretic peptide (NP) levels would serve as an additive diagnostic and prognostic tool. These biomarkers contribute to monitoring the progression of the valve disease, even before the development of hemodynamic consequences in a preclinical stage of myocardial damage. They may contribute to more accurate risk stratification by identifying patients who are more likely to experience death from cardiovascular causes, heart failure, and cardiac hospitalizations, thus requiring surgical management rather than a conservative approach. This article provides a comprehensive overview of the available evidence on the role of NPs in the management, risk evaluation, and prognostic assessment of patients with MR both before and after surgical or percutaneous valve repair. Despite largely positive evidence, a series of controversial findings exist on this relevant topic. Recent clinical trials failed to assess the role of NPs following the interventional procedure. Future larger studies are required to enable the introduction of NP levels into the guidelines for the management of MR.

Keywords: natriuretic peptides; mitral valve regurgitation; valve repair; valve replacement; risk prediction

---

1. Introduction

Mitral regurgitation (MR) represents one of the most frequent valve diseases with an indication for valve replacement or repair, both as surgical or transcatheter interventional management [1].

The etiology of mitral dysfunction, namely primary or secondary regurgitation, should be clearly identified. In primary or organic MR, the valve apparatus is directly affected as a consequence of a degenerative (i.e., fail leaflet or prolapse) or infective (i.e., endocarditis) process. In secondary or functional MR, the structure of the components of the valve apparatus, such as leaflets and chordae, is preserved, but an impaired left ventricular (LV) geometry is responsible of an altered balance between closing and tethering forces on the valve. In both abovementioned conditions, MR is responsible for or contributes to the development of LV and left atrial (LA) overload, leading to hemodynamic alterations.

According to the most recent European Guidelines [2], urgent surgery is recommended in cases of acute severe MR. In chronic primary MR, valve replacement or repair is indicated in symptomatic patients and, in the absence of symptoms, in the presence of LV ejection fraction (LVEF) <60%, LV end-systolic diameter (LVESD) ≥45 mm, atrial fibrillation (AF), and systolic pulmonary pressure ≥50 mmHg. Valve repair should be preferred if feasible and able to achieve a durable result with a low risk of re-intervention, such as in segmental valve prolapse. Rheumatic lesions, leaflets, or extensive annular calcifications more often require valvular replacement, preferably preserving sub-valvular apparatuses. In patients with high surgical risk, percutaneous edge-to-edge mitral repair is currently widely adopted and recommended by international Guidelines [2,3].

In secondary MR, due to significant operative mortality, high rates of recurrent MR, and the absence of a definite survival benefit, surgery is indicated when concomitant coronary revascularization is required. Even in this circumstance, percutaneous edge-to-edge repair may represent an efficacious option [4,5].

Although a "watchful waiting" strategy is considered safe and is accepted in asymptomatic patients, the assessment of correct and univocal timing of surgeries still remains a challenge. The identification of symptoms may be difficult due to its subjective nature and to the risk that patients could minimize their clinical manifestations in order to delay surgery, or could progressively reduce their activities as a consequence of an impaired functional capacity. In addition, symptoms may become clear when LV dysfunction is irreversible [6].

In this complex scenario, one of the unmet needs is a more accurate risk stratification, in which biomarkers may represent a useful tool to identify patients with a possibly unfavorable prognosis under conservative management or after mitral valve (MV) surgery.

Among several biomarkers available in clinical practice, natriuretic peptides (NPs) have a well-established role in cardiovascular diseases and, particularly, in heart failure (HF) where they reflect cardiac overload, LV systolic and diastolic dysfunctions, and are associated to cardiovascular outcomes [7].

Atrial natriuretic peptide (ANP), brain natriuretic peptide (BNP), and their inactive *N*-terminal portions (NT-proANP and NT-proBNP) are released in response to increased myocardial stretch, as a consequence of volume or pressure overload. NPs exert several cardiovascular and renal actions mediated by the type A natriuretic peptide receptor through the second messenger cGMP. The effects of NPs are able to counterbalance hemodynamic congestion through the regulation of electrolytes, water balance, and permeability of systemic vasculature. Moreover, they inhibit the renin–angiotensin–aldosterone system and the sympathetic nervous system. At the cellular level, a modulatory role on cellular growth and proliferation is recognized [8–10]. Some differences exist among NPs. ANP is stored in granules as a previously synthesized pool within the atrial cardiomyocytes and is quickly released upon request. BNP production is regulated by gene expression in ventricular cardiomyocytes, secreted as a prohormone, then cleaved into the active peptide and the NT-proBNP. As compared to ANP, BNP has a longer half-life (1–2 hours compared to approximately 22 minutes) and greater plasma concentrations (about 10-fold higher) [11,12]. Moreover, it has been proposed that NPs' responses may depend on the specific pathophysiology of the underlying cardiac stress, suggesting that ANP may be more sensitive in the case of subclinical damage, whereas the BNP level shows a greater increase in acute conditions [13,14].

The aim of our review is to analyze the current available evidence on the role of NPs in the management, risk evaluation, and prognostic assessment of patients with MR before and after surgical or percutaneous valve repair.

2. NPs and Risk Assessment in MR

Several studies have investigated the association between increased levels of NPs in patients with MR, parameters of LV dysfunction, and cardiovascular outcomes.

An analysis of data obtained in 1399 patients from 15 studies found a positive relationship between levels of NPs and LV end-systolic parameters, such as the LV end-systolic index (LVESI) and LVESD [15]. BNP level was also associated with the myocardial performance index (MPI), an echocardiographic index of systolic and diastolic function [16]. Mayer and colleagues documented that patients with severe MR and BNP values >409 pg/mL had a mean LVESD of 40 mm [17], which represents a criterion for surgery according to U.S. Guidelines [3]. A linear relationship between the LVESD value of 40 mm and NT-proBNP level >292 pg/mL was identified by Potocki et al. [18]. An elevated BNP level has been documented in patients with pulmonary artery pressure >50 mmHg [18], this parameter being another indication for valve replacement or repair [2,3]. NT-proBNP values were directly related to HF functional classes in MR, with mean levels of 97 pg/mL for New York Heart Association (NYHA) class I, 170 pg/mL for class II, and 458 pg/mL for class III [19]. The addition of BNP to the Society of Thoracic Surgeons (STS) score improved the risk stratification in patients with primary MR and preserved LVEF [20].

In a prospective study conducted in 124 patients with chronic primary MR, Detaint and colleagues analyzed the relationship between BNP level, MR degree, LV and LA remodeling, and prognosis [21]. BNP level was associated to the LV end-systolic volume index, LA volume, and symptoms, and it was able to predict prognosis independently from age, sex, functional class, MR severity, and LVEF. At the 5-year follow-up, survival was significantly worse in patients with BNP level >31 pg/mL, showing a higher incidence of the combined end-point of death and HF [21].

In another study, BNP level >105 pg/mL had stronger predictive power compared to the most common parameters of MR severity, such as an effective orifice regurgitant area (EROA) and LVESD [22]. In 49 patients with MR and preserved ejection fraction (>55%), BNP > 41 pg/mL and NT-proBNP > 173 pg/mL showed the best accuracy in predicting the development of symptoms [23]. In 87 patients with severe MR, BNP below 80 pg/mL and NT-proBNP lower than 200 pg/mL showed the greatest negative predictive value of 98% for the development of symptoms or LV dysfunction during follow-up [24].

The prognostic role of BNP level in the management of MR has also been examined during exercise.

Exercise BNP level was strongly correlated with those measured at rest [25]. Patients with higher BNP values showed more severe MR, greater LA volume, more elevated systolic pulmonary pressure, and LV filling pressure estimated as an E/e′ ratio. Moreover, detected exercise BNP levels were higher in patients who developed symptoms and had an increased incidence of cardiac events, independently from age, gender, and body mass index. In patients with moderate MR, only the exercise LV global longitudinal strain, but neither resting nor exercise LVEF, was an independent determinant of exercise BNP level. A plausible explanation of these findings is that the BNP level has been assessed in patients with degenerative MR and not in MR secondary to LV dilatation, in which levels of NPs were measured before the development of LV systolic dysfunction [25]. A cut-off of 64 pg/mL was identified as the best cut-off value for exercise BNP level to behave as an independent predictor of worse cardiovascular outcomes [25]. Other studies have consistently demonstrated that an increase in BNP level during exercise is related to the development of HF, to subclinical LV dysfunction, and to reduced performance capacity [26,27].

According to the abovementioned results, BNP level may be used in clinical practice as a complementary tool for echocardiographic exams and exercise tests in order to identify those patients who are more likely to experience death from cardiovascular causes, and HF and cardiac hospitalizations, thus requiring surgical management, rather than a conservative approach. In addition, NPs may represent an essential tool to monitor the progression of the valve disease before the development of hemodynamic consequences in a preclinical stage of myocardial damage.

However, some controversial aspects deserve to be better-clarified. First of all, as documented by the abovementioned studies, it is still difficult to establish a univocal cut-off level able to identify MR patients at elevated cardiovascular risk, since different levels of NPs have been identified in the different studies. To overcome this problem, Clavel et al. introduced the BNP ratio, which is derived from a measured BNP value divided by the expected value related to the age and sex of each patient [26].

This parameter behaves as a significant independent prognostic marker of outcomes in valve heart disease patients, including MR patients under medical treatment [28,29]. However, it failed to maintain its role after surgery [28]. Interestingly, the BNP/ANP ratio revealed a prognostic role in one study, being significantly higher in the presence of clinical and echocardiographic criteria used for surgery recommendation, such as LVESD ≥ 45 mm, LVEF ≤ 60%, NYHA class II or greater, and AF [30].

Other critical issues relate to the appropriate time interval that should be considered for the subsequent measurements of the NP level, and the magnitude of changes of NP values between baseline and subsequent assessments, which may be related to a poor clinical outcome. In addition, age, AF, renal function, and body weight are known modulators of NP levels, thus representing potential confounders [31]. Finally, since a high BNP level may also be detected in patients with moderate MR, it cannot be used as a surrogate for MR quantification. On the other hand, it should be pointed out that, in the presence of good hemodynamic compensation with a normal NP level, regardless of LV dimension, the need for an interventional strategy may be missed.

3. The Role of NPs to Predict Outcome after MV Surgery or Percutaneous Repair

During the last few years, percutaneous edge-to-edge MV repair with the MitraClip (Abbott Vascular, CA USA) device has acquired increasing importance as a treatment option, especially in patients with HF with an elevated surgical risk. However, many patients are still being treated with the surgical MV repair or replacement, which represents the gold-standard procedure. Apart from the reduction of MR, both percutaneous and surgical interventions may produce several hemodynamic benefits, reducing LV and LA pressure and volume overload and, as a consequence, the myocardial wall stretch [2,3].

In this context, several studies have assessed the role of NPs in the management of patients treated with MV repair or replacement, investigating the sensibility of these biomarkers in identifying subjects with a worse response to the performed interventional procedure and with a lower chance of survival.

In a study involving 65 patients treated with edge-to-edge valve repair, a low NT-proBNP level, measured 6 months after the procedure, was associated with a significant reduction in LV end-diastolic volume (LVEDV) and end-systolic volume (LVESV) and to an improvement in LV and LA longitudinal strain [32]. Worse renal function, larger LVEDV, and a higher transmitral gradient after MitraClip (Abbott Vascular, CA USA) implantation were independently associated with a higher level of NT-proBNP at follow-up. Patients with low and medium NT-proBNP tertiles experienced a significantly greater reduction in NYHA functional class symptoms and quality of life score compared to those with a higher NT-proBNP level. At the 6-month follow-up, successful MR reduction was observed in a higher number of patients with low and medium NT-proBNP tertiles, whereas severe MR more often persisted in the high NT-proBNP tertile group (43%) [32].

After percutaneous valve repair, improvements in 6-minute walking distances and a decrease in LV volumes were paralleled by a significant reduction of NT-proBNP level [33].

Hwang and colleagues identified a BNP cut-off level of 125 pg/mL associated with a higher risk of cardiac death and re-hospitalization for cardiac causes in 117 patients who underwent surgical MV replacement [34]. Interestingly, a study conducted with 44 patients treated with transcatheter valve repair, as well as baseline levels of mid-regional proANP and NT-proBNP were significantly higher in those who experienced death or re-hospitalization for HF during a median follow-up of 211 days [35]. In a cohort of 174 retrospectively examined patients, the NT-proBNP level was significantly associated to survival at univariate analysis, but the independent predictive power of NT-proBNP was not confirmed at multivariate analysis [36]. However, the post-operative NT-proBNP level maintained its predictive role for a clinical outcome at multivariate analysis in other studies [37–39].

As for the pre-operative level, controversial findings were frequently reported with regard to the post-operative level. In 59 patients who underwent percutaneous MV repair, achieving a reduction of MR, an improvement of functional class, and structural reverse cardiac remodeling (reduced LA volume and LVESD and increased LVEF), the NT-proBNP level did not decrease significantly [40].

Similar findings were provided by Yoon et al. in a cohort of 144 patients successfully treated with edge-to-edge repair, in which the NT-proBNP level did not significantly decrease after MV clipping. In addition, NT-proBNP changes were not related to baseline LVEF and LV diameter and were not able to predict cardiovascular outcomes during a 6-month follow-up [41]. Furthermore, in a study which enrolled 194 patients treated with percutaneous valve repair, the NT-proBNP level remained elevated (≥10,000 pg/mL) in those patients who achieved a reduction of MR to grade ≤2 (21%) [42]. These controversial results may be explained by differences in the sample size of the enrolled populations, in the characteristics of the included patients (baseline LVEF, pulmonary artery pressure, LV diameter and diastolic function), in the duration of the follow-up, and also the rhythm status (i.e., sinus rhythm or AF) [43].

Finally, as for the pre-surgical management, it has not been clearly established which biomarker should be chosen, which cut-off value should be considered for the risk assessment of the patients, and which interval for serial monitoring of NPs has the best accuracy.

4. NPs Levels in MITRA-FR and COAPT Trials

Two recent trials have become available in patients subjected to MV repair. The MITRA-FR (Percutaneous Repair with the MitraClip Device (Abbott Vascular, CA USA) for Severe Functional/Secondary Mitral Regurgitation) trial, conducted in patients with severe secondary MR, showed that percutaneous MV repair added to standard pharmacological therapy was unable to reduce the rate of death or unplanned hospitalizations for HF at 1 year compared to those who received medical therapy alone [44].

The Cardiovascular Outcomes Assessment of the MitraClip Percutaneous Therapy for Heart Failure Patients with Functional Mitral Regurgitation (COAPT) study demonstrated that the transcatheter MV repair reduced the rate of hospitalizations for HF and all-cause mortality within 12 and 24 months of follow-up [45]. Although the MITRA-FR and COAPT trials enrolled comparable populations of patients with secondary MR, they obtained diametrically opposed results [44,45].

Several possible mechanisms have been proposed to explain the discrepant findings, mostly focusing on the different echocardiographic characteristics of the subjects included in the two trials [46,47]. The COAPT excluded patients with very severe LV dilation (LVESD < 70 mm), whereas LV diameter did not represent an exclusion criterion in MITRA-FR. This resulted in a significant difference in the documented mean LV volume (LVEDV 135 ± 35 mL/m^2 in MITRA-FR vs. 101 ± 34 mL/m^2 in COAPT) [44–47]. More interestingly, the two populations had a different degree of MR, the EROA being significantly greater in COAPT as compared with MITRA-FR (41 ± 15 mm^2 vs. 31 ± 10 mm^2, respectively) [44–47]. According to these considerations, it has been supposed that the underlying cardiac disease was probably the main cause of HF and the determinant of prognosis in MITRA-FR, with MR being a marker of adverse LV remodeling. In contrast, the LV dysfunction was more related to MR severity in COAPT, which also represented the main contributor to outcomes [48]. In such a context, it has been proposed that the degree of MR was "proportionate" to the degree of LV dilatation in MITRA-FR, whereas it was "disproportionate" in COAPT, and this parameter may have influenced the different clinical response to the percutaneous repair procedure [46,47].

In this complex scenario, the differences in the baseline NP levels between the two studies may mirror the different pathophysiological mechanisms. In the COAPT trial, both NT-proBNP and BNP levels were significantly higher than in MITRA-FR (median NT-proBNP > 5100 vs. 3200 pg/mL and median BNP >1000 vs. >760 pg/mL, respectively), and it may be argued that they were more related to MR severity than to either LVEF or LV diameter [44,45]. In fact, a higher degree of MR may have produced an increase in atrial and ventricular loading conditions, leading to a higher NP level. Unfortunately, precise data about the LA dimension, diastolic function (i.e., assessed with E/e' ratio), and systolic pulmonary pressure were not provided in the two trial populations. Furthermore, the two studies did not obtain any information about overtime changes in NPs levels after the transcatheter

MV repair procedure. Therefore, their potential relationship to echocardiographic parameters and to clinical outcomes could not be assessed in these trials.

5. NPs and Other Biomarkers

The most plausible pathophysiological explanation for the better association of NPs with pre- and post-procedural outcomes may be their optimal capacity to reflect cardiac performance in different hemodynamic conditions. Of note, lack of a sufficient number of studies using ANP as a marker in the management of MR does not currently allow to make a robust comparison with BNP.

Several efforts have been made over the last few years to investigate the role of other biomarkers in the MR condition, and have been previously reviewed [49]. More recently, other biomarkers have been investigated with some interesting insights.

The neutrophil gelatinase-associated lipocalin (NGAL) and cystatin C, both markers of functional and structural kidney damage, were shown to predict mortality in high-risk patients undergoing percutaneous MV repair [50]. However, they had low accuracy, probably due to a lack of relationship with the hemodynamic balance [35]. Similarly, the highly sensitive C-reactive protein (hsCRP), a biomarker able to improve risk prediction for cardiovascular diseases, showed low performance in the prognostic assessment of the MR patients [35]. On the other hand, the pre-operative level of soluble ST-2, a member of the interleukin-1 receptor family previously described as a stronger biomarker of myocardial stretch in HF, was correlated with LV function and structure after MV repair, thus providing complementary prognostic information to NT-proBNP level [35]. The level of galectin-3, a well-established marker of LV fibrosis, has been associated with worse cardiovascular outcomes after MV repair [35]. Interestingly, low galectin-3 and ST2 plasma levels were predictors of therapeutic success in 210 patients treated with percutaneous MV repair (PMVR) [51]. Of note, a lower galectin-3 level was a predictor of MR improvement after cardiac resynchronization therapy (CRT) [52]. In addition, biomarkers reflecting inflammation (hsCRP, interleukin-6) and cardiac remodeling processes (matrix metalloproteinases (MMP-2 and MMP-9)) were associated with a higher risk of mortality following the procedure [53]. The highly sensitive troponin T showed strong prognostic power in predicting survival after transcatheter MV repair, with an accuracy comparable to that of a mid-regional proANP level [35].

Of note, some evidence of the role of other parameters in the outcome prediction of MR patients has been collected. For instance, it was found that abnormalities of the calcium-phosphate metabolism may influence the health-related quality of life in patients with severe MR [54]. Amelioration of oxidative stress and endothelial dysfunction may be indicators of successful MV repair in patients with MV prolapse [55].

Finally, one study reported the negative prognostic impact of pre-procedural anemia in patients who underwent PMVR with a higher baseline NT-proBNP level [56].

Based on the evidence collected so far, markers of mechanisms involved in the cardiac remodeling process may be considered as complementary prognostic tools to the NP level.

6. Conclusions

The management of MR still represents a real challenge for physicians, since the assessment of symptoms is difficult and the recommended diagnostic exams, such as the echocardiogram, are often not accurately performed. It is well-known that NP secretion occurs in the presence of atrial and ventricular stretch, as a consequence of pressure and volume overload, and that NPs are independent predictors of mortality and morbidity in patients with severe MR. Due to their feasible measurement and to their significant association with echocardiographic parameters of LV dysfunction and of impaired filling, these biomarkers may represent an important tool to identify patients at elevated risk of adverse clinical outcomes, in which early surgical or percutaneous intervention should be considered (Figures 1 and 2).

Moreover, the NP level has also been documented to be a powerful independent predictor of reduced cardiac event-free survival in patients treated with surgical or transcatheter valve repair or replacement, thus representing potential instruments to significantly improve the evaluation of a short- and long-term prognosis after these procedures.

Although some controversies still exist, the majority of findings discussed in our review article are encouraging, and indicate NPs as potentially useful biomarkers for the clinical management of MR. Further larger studies are needed to solve key issues, that is, to better define which biomarker should preferably be used among NPs, which rest and eventually stress cut-off levels could clearly identify high-risk patients, and which degree of variation between serial measurements may have the best clinical accuracy. It is hoped that these future studies will allow the introduction of NP levels into the guidelines for the management of MR.

Figure 1

- ❖ NPs level is related to cardiac remodeling in MR.
- ❖ NPs level may be used to monitor the progression of MR, before the development of hemodynamic consequences.
- ❖ NPs may represent an important tool in the risk stratification of patients with severe MR.
- ❖ NPs level may contribute to identify patients who are more likely to have a poor clinical outcome and who should benefit from an invasive management rather than a conservative approach.
- ❖ NPs levels may predict adverse LV remodeling and higher CV risk after MV surgery or percutaneous repair.
- ❖ Most accurate cut-off values and intervals for serial monitoring of NPs should be better defined by further studies.

Figure 1. Summary of the main topics discussed in this review. Abbreviation legends: CV = cardiovascular; MR = mitral regurgitation; MV = mitral valve; NPs = natriuretic peptides.

Figure 2

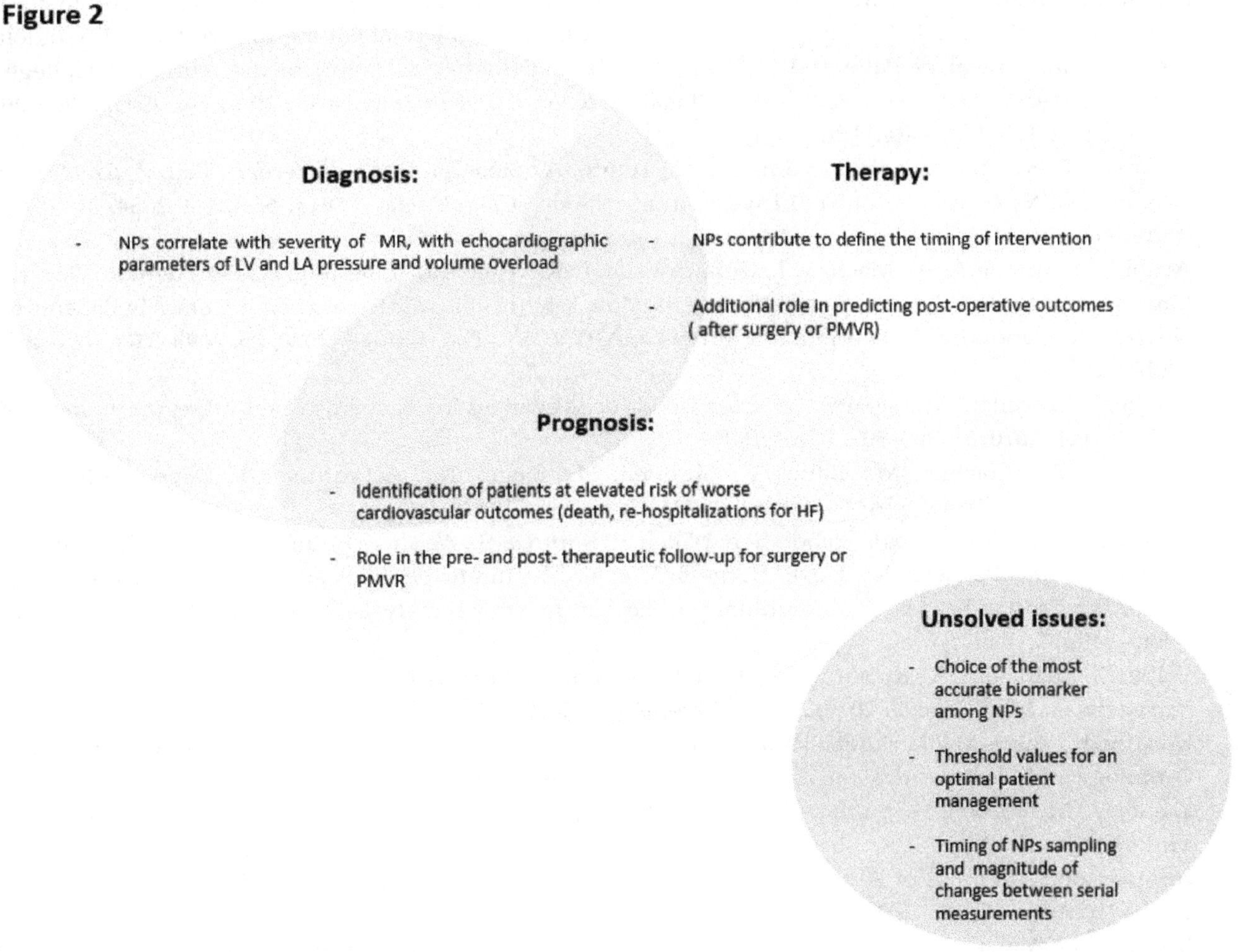

Diagnosis:

- NPs correlate with severity of MR, with echocardiographic parameters of LV and LA pressure and volume overload

Therapy:

- NPs contribute to define the timing of intervention
- Additional role in predicting post-operative outcomes (after surgery or PMVR)

Prognosis:

- Identification of patients at elevated risk of worse cardiovascular outcomes (death, re-hospitalizations for HF)
- Role in the pre- and post- therapeutic follow-up for surgery or PMVR

Unsolved issues:

- Choice of the most accurate biomarker among NPs
- Threshold values for an optimal patient management
- Timing of NPs sampling and magnitude of changes between serial measurements

Figure 2. Main clinical implications of NPs in MR. Abbreviation legends: HF = Heart failure; LA = left atrium; LV = left ventricle; NPs = natriuretic peptides; PMVR = percutaneous mitral valve repair.

Author Contributions: Conceptualization, G.G. and S.R.; methodology, G.G., M.F., R.S., M.C., F.B., S.M. and S.R.; formal analysis, G.G., M.F., R.S., M.C., F.B., S.M. and S.R.; investigation, G.G., M.F., R.S., M.C., F.B., S.M. and S.R.; resources, S.R. and M.V.; data curation, G.G., M.F., R.S., M.C., F.B., S.M. and S.R.; writing—original draft preparation, G.G. and S.R.; writing—review and editing, S.R., A.B. and M.V.; visualization, G.G. and S.R.; supervision, S.R.; project administration, S.R.; funding acquisition, S.R. and M.V. All authors have read and agreed to the published version of the manuscript.

References

1. Iung, B.; Baron, G.; Butchart, E.G.; Delahaye, F.; Gohlke-Bärwolf, C.; Levang, O.W.; Tornos, P.; Vanoverschelde, J.L.; Vermeer, F.; Boersma, E.; et al. A prospective survey of patients with valvular heart disease in Europe: The Euro Heart Survey on Valvular Heart Disease. *Eur. Heart J.* **2003**, *24*, 1231–1243. [CrossRef]
2. Baumgartner, H.; Falk, V.; Bax, J.J.; De Bonis, M.; Hamm, C.; Holm, P.J.; Iung, B.; Lancellotti, P.; Lansac, E.; Muñoz, D.R.; et al. ESC/EACTS Guidelines for the management of valvular heart disease. *Eur. Heart J.* **2017**, *38*, 2739–2791. [CrossRef] [PubMed]

3. Nishimura, R.A.; Otto, C.M.; Bonow, R.O.; Carabello, B.A.; Erwin, J.P. III; Fleisher, L.A.; Jneid, H.; Mack, M.J.; McLeod, C.J.; O'Gara, P.T.; et al. AHA/ACC Focused Update of the 2014 AHA/ACC Guideline for the Management of Patients With Valvular Heart Disease: A Report of the American College of Cardiology/American Heart Association Task Force on Clinical Practice Guidelines. *Circulation* **2017**, *135*, e1159–e1195. [CrossRef] [PubMed]
4. Feldman, T.; Kar, S.; Elmariah, S.; Smart, S.C.; Trento, A.; Siegel, R.J.; Apruzzese, P.; Fail, P.; Rinaldi, M.J.; Smalling, R.W.; et al. EVEREST II Investigators. *J. Am. Coll. Cardiol.* **2015**, *66*, 2844–2854. [CrossRef] [PubMed]
5. Arnold, S.V.; Stone, G.W.; Mack, M.J.; Chhatriwalla, D.K.; Austin, B.A.; Zhang, Z.; Ben-Yehuda, O.; Kar, S.; Lim, D.S.; Lindenfeld, J.A.; et al. COAPT Investigators Health Status Changes and Outcomes in Patients with Heart Failure and Mitral Regurgitation: From COAPT. *J. Am. Coll. Cardiol.* **2020**, *75*, 2099–2106. [CrossRef] [PubMed]
6. Magne, J.; Lancellotti, P.; Piérard, L.A. Exercise-induced changes in degenerative mitral regurgitation. *J. Am. Coll. Cardiol.* **2010**, *56*, 300–309. [CrossRef]
7. Flint, N.; Raschpichler, M.; Rader, F.; Shmueli, H.; Siegel, R.J. Asymptomatic Degenerative Mitral Regurgitation: A Review. *JAMA Cardiol.* **2020**. [CrossRef]
8. Natriuretic Peptides Studies Collaboration; Willeit, P.; Kaptoge, S.; Welsh, P.; Butterworth, A.S.; Chowdhury, R.; Spackman, S.A.; Pennells, L.; Gao, P.; Burgess, S.; et al. Natriuretic peptides and integrated risk assessment for cardiovascular disease: An individual-participant-data meta-analysis. *Lancet Diabetes Endocrinol.* **2016**, *4*, 840–849. [CrossRef]
9. Volpe, M.; Battistoni, A.; Rubattu, S. Natriuretic peptides in heart failure: Current achievements and future perspectives. *Int. J. Cardiol.* **2019**, *281*, 186–189. [CrossRef]
10. Rubattu, S.; Volpe, M. Natriuretic Peptides in the Cardiovascular System: Multifaceted Roles in Physiology, Pathology and Therapeutics. *Int. J. Mol. Sci.* **2019**, *20*, 3991. [CrossRef]
11. Yasue, H.; Yoshimura, H.; Sumida, H.; Kikuta, K.; Kugiyama, K.; Jougasaki, M.; Ogawa, H.; Okumura, K.; Mukoyama, M.; Nakao, K. Localization and mechanism of secretion of B-type natriuretic peptide in comparison with those of A-type natriuretic peptide in normal subjects and patients with heart failure. *Circulation* **1994**, *90*, 195–203. [CrossRef] [PubMed]
12. Xu-Cai, Y.O.; Wu, Q. Molecular forms of natriuretic peptides in heart failure and their implications. *Heart* **2010**, *96*, 419–424. [CrossRef] [PubMed]
13. Karakas, M.; Jaensch, A.; Breitling, L.P.; Brenner, H.; Koenig, W.; Rothenbacher, D. Prognostic value of midregional pro-A-type natriuretic peptide and N-terminal pro-B-type natriuretic peptide in patients with stable coronary heart disease followed over 8 years. *Clin. Chem.* **2014**, *60*, 1441–1449. [CrossRef] [PubMed]
14. Lugnier, C.; Meyer, A.; Charloux, A.; Andrès, E.; Gény, B.; Talha, S. The Endocrine Function of the Heart: Physiology and Involvements of Natriuretic Peptides and Cyclic Nucleotide Phosphodiesterases in Heart Failure. *J. Clin. Med.* **2019**, *8*, 1746. [CrossRef] [PubMed]
15. Johl, M.M.; Malhotra, P.; Kehl, D.W.; Rader, F.; Siegel, R.J. Natriuretic peptides in the evaluation and management of degenerative mitral regurgitation: A systematic review. *Heart* **2017**, *103*, 738–744. [CrossRef] [PubMed]
16. Sayar, N.; Lütfullah Orhan, A.; Cakmak, N.; Yılmaz, H.; Atmaca, H.; Tangürek, B.; Hasdemir, H.; Nurkalem, Z.; Ergelen, M.; Aksu, H.; et al. Correlation of the myocardial performance index with plasma B-type natriuretic peptide levels in patients with mitral regurgitation. *Int. J. Cardiovasc. Imag.* **2008**, *24*, 151–157. [CrossRef]
17. Mayer, S.A.; De Lemos, J.A.; Murphy, S.A.; Brooks, S.; Roberts, B.J.; Paul, A.; Grayburn, P.A. Comparison of B-type natriuretic peptide levels in patients with heart failure with versus without mitral regurgitation. *Am. J. Cardiol.* **2004**, *93*, 1002–1006. [CrossRef]
18. Potocki, M.; Mair, J.; Weber, M.; Hamm, C.; Burkard, T.; Hiemetzberger, R.; Peters, K.; Jander, N.; Cron, T.A.; Hess, N.; et al. Relation of N-terminal pro-B-type natriuretic peptide to symptoms, severity, and left ventricular remodeling in patients with organic mitral regurgitation. *Am. J. Cardiol.* **2009**, *104*, 559–564. [CrossRef]
19. Yusoff, R.; Clayton, N.; Keevil, B.; Morris, J.; Ray, S. Utility of plasma N-terminal brain natriuretic peptide as a marker of functional capacity in patients with chronic severe mitral regurgitation. *Am. J. Cardiol.* **2006**, *97*, 1498–1501. [CrossRef]

20. Mentias, A.; Patel, K.; Patel, H.; Gillinov, A.M.; Rodriguez, L.L.; Svensson, L.G.; Mihaljevic, T.; Sabik, J.F.; Griffin, B.P.; Desai, M.Y. Prognostic Utility of Brain Natriuretic Peptide in Asymptomatic Patients With Significant Mitral Regurgitation and Preserved Left Ventricular Ejection Fraction. *Am. J. Cardiol.* **2016**, *117*, 258–263. [CrossRef]
21. Detaint, D.; Messika-Zeitoun, D.; Avierinos, J.F.; Scott, C.; Chen, H.; Burnett, C.J., Jr.; Enriquez-Sarano, M. B-type natriuretic peptide in organic mitral regurgitation: Determinants and impact on outcome. *Circulation* **2005**, *111*, 2391–2397. [CrossRef]
22. Magne, J.; Mahjoub, H.; Pierard, L.A.; O'Connor, K.; Pirlet, C.; Pibarot, P.; Lancellotti, P. Prognostic importance of brain natriuretic peptide and left ventricular longitudinal function in asymptomatic degenerative mitral regurgitation. *Heart* **2012**, *98*, 584–591. [CrossRef] [PubMed]
23. Sutton, T.M.; Stewart, R.A.; Gerber, I.L.; West, T.M.; Richards, A.M.; Yandle, T.G.; Kerr, A.J. Plasma natriuretic peptide levels increase with symptoms and severity of mitral regurgitation. *J. Am. Coll. Cardiol.* **2003**, *41*, 2280–2287. [CrossRef]
24. Klaar, U.; Gabriel, H.; Bergler-Klein, J.; Pernicka, E.; Heger, M.; Mascherbauer, J.; Rosenhek, R.; Binder, T.; Maurer, G.; Baumgartner, H. Prognostic value of serial B-type natriuretic peptide measurement in asymptomatic organic mitral regurgitation. *Eur. J. Heart Fail.* **2011**, *13*, 163–169. [CrossRef]
25. Magne, J.; Mahjoub, H.; Pibarot, P.; Pirlet, C.; Pierard, L.A.; Lancellotti, P. Prognostic importance of exercise brain natriuretic peptide in asymptomatic degenerative mitral regurgitation. *Eur. J. Heart Fail.* **2012**, *14*, 1293–1302. [CrossRef] [PubMed]
26. Pascual-Figal, D.A.; Peñafiel, P.; de la Morena, G.; Redondo, B.; Nicolás, F.; Casas, T.; Valdés, M. Relation of B-type natriuretic peptide levels before and after exercise and functional capacity in patients with idiopathic dilated cardiomyopathy. *Am. J. Cardiol.* **2007**, *99*, 1279–1283. [CrossRef]
27. Kato, M.; Kinugawa, T.; Ogino, K.; Redondo, B.; Nicolás, F.; Casas, T.; Valdés, M. Augmented response in plasma brain natriuretic peptide to dynamic exercise in patients with left ventricular dysfunction and congestive heart failure. *J. Intern. Med.* **2000**, *248*, 309–315. [CrossRef]
28. Clavel, M.A.; Tribouilloy, C.; Vanoverschelde, J.L.; Pizarro, R.; Suri, R.M.; Szymanski, C.; Lazam, S.; Oberti, P.; Michelena, H.I.; Jaffe, A.; et al. Association of B-Type Natriuretic Peptide With Survival in Patients With Degenerative Mitral Regurgitation. *J. Am. Coll. Cardiol.* **2016**, *68*, 1297–1307. [CrossRef]
29. Zhang, B.; Xu, H.; Zhang, H.; Liu, Q.; Ye, Y.; Hao, J.; Zhao, Q.; Qi, X.; Liu, S.; Zhang, E.; et al. CHINA-DVD CollaboratorsPrognostic Value of N-Terminal Pro-B-Type Natriuretic Peptide in Elderly Patients With Valvular Heart Disease. *J. Am. Coll. Cardiol.* **2020**, *75*, 1659–1672. [CrossRef]
30. Shimamoto, K.; Kusumoto, M.; Sakai, R.; Watanabe, H.; Ihara, S.; Koike, N.; Kawana, M. Usefulness of the brain natriuretic peptide to atrial natriuretic peptide ratio in determining the severity of mitral regurgitation. *Can. J. Cardiol.* **2007**, *23*, 295–300. [CrossRef]
31. Kaneko, H.; Neuss, M.; Schau, T.; Weissenborn, J.; Butter, C. Interaction between renal function and percutaneous edge-to-edge mitral valve repair using MitraClip. *J. Cardiol.* **2017**, *69*, 476–482. [CrossRef]
32. Van Wijngaarden, S.E.; Kamperidis, V.; Al-Amri, I.; van der Kley, F.; Schalij, M.J.; Ajmone Marsan, N.; Bax, J.J.; Delgado, V. Effects of Transcatheter Mitral Valve Repair With MitraClip on Left Ventricular and Atrial Hemodynamic Load and Myocardial Wall Stress. *J. Card. Fail.* **2018**, *24*, 137–145. [CrossRef]
33. Franzen, O.; van der Heyden, J.; Baldus, S.; Schlüter, M.; Schillinger, W.; Butter, C.; Hoffmann, R.; Corti, R.; Pedrazzini, G.; Swaans, M.J.; et al. MitraClip®therapy in patients with end-stage systolic heart failure. *Eur. J. Heart Fail.* **2011**, *13*, 569–576. [CrossRef] [PubMed]
34. Hwang, I.C.; Kim, Y.J.; Kim, K.H.; Lee, S.P.; Kim, Y.K.; Sohn, D.W.; Oh, B.H.; Parket, Y.B. Prognostic value of B-type natriuretic peptide in patients with chronic mitral regurgitation undergoing surgery: Mid-term follow-up results. *Eur. J. Cardiothorac. Surg.* **2013**, *43*, e1–e6. [CrossRef] [PubMed]
35. Wöhrle, J.; Karakas, M.; Trepte, U.; Seeger, J.; Gonska, B.; Koenig, W.; Rottbauer, W. Midregional-proAtrial Natriuretic Peptide and High Sensitive Troponin T Strongly Predict Adverse Outcome in Patients Undergoing Percutaneous Repair of Mitral Valve Regurgitation. *PLoS ONE* **2015**, *10*, e0137464. [CrossRef] [PubMed]
36. Kreusser, M.M.; Geis, N.A.; Berlin, N.; Greiner, S.; Pleger, S.T.; Bekeredjian, R.; Katus, K.A.; Raake, P.W. Invasive hemodynamics and cardiac biomarkers to predict outcomes after percutaneous edge-to-edge mitral valve repair in patients with severe heart failure. *Clin. Res. Cardiol.* **2019**, *108*, 375–387. [CrossRef]

37. Triantafyllis, A.S.; Kortlandt, F.; Bakker, A.L.; Swaans, M.J.; Eefting, F.D.; van der Heyden, J.A.S.; Post, M.C.; Rensing, B.W.J.M. Long-term survival and preprocedural predictors of mortality in high surgical risk patients undergoing percutaneous mitral valve repair. *Catheter Cardiovasc. Interv.* **2016**, *87*, 467–475. [CrossRef]
38. Toggweiler, S.; Zuber, M.; Sürder, D.; Biaggi, P.; Gstrein, C.; Moccetti, T.; Pasotti, E.; Gaemperli, O.; Faletra, F.; Petrova-Slater, I.; et al. Two-year outcomes after percutaneous mitral valve repair with the MitraClip system: Durability of the procedure and predictors of outcome. *Open Heart* **2014**, *1*, e000056. [CrossRef]
39. Perreas, K.; Samanidis, G.; Dimitriou, S.; Athanasiou, A.; Balanika, M.; Smirli, A.; Antzaka, C.; Politis, K.; Khoury, M.; Michalis, A. NT-proBNP in the mitral valve surgery. *Critl. Pathw. Cardiol.* **2014**, *13*, 55–61. [CrossRef]
40. Pleger, S.T.; Schulz-Schönhagen, M.; Geis, N.; Chorianopoulos, E.; Antaredja, M.; Lewening, M.; Katus, H.A.; Bekeredjian, R. One year clinical efficacy and reverse cardiac remodelling in patients with severe mitral regurgitation and reduced ejection fraction after MitraClip implantation. *Eur. J. Heart Fail.* **2013**, *15*, 919–927. [CrossRef]
41. Yoon, J.N.; Frangieh, A.H.; Attinger-Toller, A.; Gruner, C.; Tanner, F.C.; Taramasso, M.; Corti, R.; Lüscher, T.F.; Ruschitzka, F.; Bettex, D.; et al. Changes in serum biomarker profiles after percutaneous mitral valve repair with the MitraClip system. *Cardiol. J.* **2016**, *23*, 384–392. [CrossRef] [PubMed]
42. Schau, T.; Isotani, A.; Neuss, M.; Schöpp, M.; Seifert, M.; Höpfner, C.; Burkhoff, D.; Butter, C. Long-term survival after Mitraclip therapy in patients with severe mitral regurgitation and severe congestive heart failure: A comparison among survivals predicted by heart failure models. *J. Cardiol.* **2016**, *67*, 287–294. [CrossRef] [PubMed]
43. Hwang, I.C.; Kim, D.H.; Kim, Y.J.; Kim, K.H.; Lee, S.P.; Kim, Y.K.; Sohn, D.W.; Oh, B.H.; Park, Y.B. Change of B-type natriuretic peptide after surgery and its association with rhythm status in patients with chronic severe mitral regurgitation. *Can. J. Cardiol.* **2013**, *29*, 704–711. [CrossRef] [PubMed]
44. Obadia, J.F.; Messika-Zeitoun, D.; Leurent, G.; Iung, B.; Bonnet, G.; Piriou, N.; Lefèvre, T.; Piot, C.; Rouleau, F.; Carrié, D.; et al. MITRA-FR Investigators.Percutaneous Repair or Medical Treatment for Secondary Mitral Regurgitation. *N. Engl. J. Med.* **2018**, *379*, 2297–2306. [CrossRef]
45. Stone, G.W.; Lindenfeld, J.; Abraham, W.T.; Kar, S.; Lim, D.S.; Mishell, J.M.; Whisenant, B.; Grayburn, P.A.; Rinaldi, M.; Kapadia, S.R.; et al. COAPT Investigators.Transcatheter Mitral-Valve Repair in Patients with Heart Failure. *N. Engl. J. Med.* **2018**, *379*, 2307–2318. [CrossRef]
46. Pibarot, P.; Delgado, V.; Bax, J.J. MITRA-FR vs. COAPT: Lessons from two trials with diametrically opposed results. *Eur. Heart J. Cardiovasc. Imag.* **2019**, *20*, 620–624. [CrossRef]
47. Hagendorff, A.; Doenst, T.; Falk, V. Echocardiographic assessment of functional mitral regurgitation: Opening Pandora's box? *ESC Heart Fail.* **2019**, *6*, 678–685. [CrossRef]
48. Grayburn, P.A.; Sannino, A.; Packer, M. Proportionate and Disproportionate Functional Mitral Regurgitation: A New Conceptual Framework That Reconciles the Results of the MITRA-FR and COAPT Trials. *JACC Cardiovasc. Imag.* **2019**, *12*, 353–362. [CrossRef]
49. Bäck, M.; Pizarro, R.; Clavel, M.A. Biomarkers in Mitral Regurgitation. *Prog. Cardiovasc. Dis.* **2017**, *60*, 334–341. [CrossRef]
50. Dörr, O.; Walther, C.; Liebetrau, C.; Keller, T.; Ortlieb, R.M.; Boeder, N.; Bauer, P.; Möllmann, H.; Gaede, L.; Troidl, C.; et al. Evaluation of cystatin C and neutrophil gelatinase-associated lipocalin as predictors of mortality in patients undergoing percutaneous mitral valve repair (MitraClip). *Clin. Cardiol.* **2018**, *41*, 1474–1479. [CrossRef]
51. Dörr, O.; Walther, C.; Liebetrau, C.; Keller, T.; Ortlieb, R.M.; Boeder, N.; Bauer, P.; Möllmann, H.; Gaede, L.; Troidl, C.; et al. Galectin-3 and ST2 as predictors of therapeutic success in high-risk patients undergoing percutaneous mitral valve repair (MitraClip). *Clin. Cardiol.* **2018**, *41*, 1164–1169. [CrossRef] [PubMed]
52. Beaudoin, J.; Singh, J.P.; Szymonifka, J.; Zhou, Q.; Levine, R.A.; Januzzi, J.L.; Truong, Q.A. Novel Heart Failure Biomarkers Predict Improvement of Mitral Regurgitation in Patients Receiving Cardiac Resynchronization Therapy-The BIOCRT Study. *Can. J. Cardiol.* **2016**, *32*, 1478–1484. [CrossRef] [PubMed]
53. Dörr, O.; Walther, C.; Liebetrau, C.; Keller, T.; Ortlieb, R.M.; Boeder, N.; Bauer, P.; Möllmann, H.; Gaede, L.; Troidl, C.; et al. Specific biomarkers of myocardial inflammation and remodeling processes as predictors of mortality in high-risk patients undergoing percutaneous mitral valve repair (MitraClip). *Clin. Cardiol.* **2018**, *41*, 481–487. [CrossRef] [PubMed]

54. Mozenska, O.; Bil, J.; Segiet, A.; Kosior, D.A. The influence of calcium-phosphate metabolism abnormalities on the quality of life in patients with hemodynamically significant mitral regurgitation. *BMC Cardiovasc. Disord.* **2019**, *19*, 116. [CrossRef] [PubMed]
55. Porro, B.; Songia, P.; Myasoedova, V.A.; Valerio, V.; Moschetta, D.; Gripari, P.; Fusini, L.; Cavallotti, L.; Canzano, P.; Turnu, L.; et al. Endothelial Dysfunction in Patients with Severe Mitral Regurgitation. *J. Clin. Med.* **2019**, *8*, 835. [CrossRef] [PubMed]
56. Kaneko, H.; Neuss, M.; Okamoto, M.; Weissenborn, J.; Butter, C. Impact of Preprocedural Anemia on Outcomes of Patients with Mitral Regurgitation Who Underwent MitraClip Implantation. *Am. J. Cardiol.* **2018**, *122*, 859–865. [CrossRef]

5

Transient Laterality of Cerebral Oxygenation Changes in Response to Head-of-Bed Manipulation in Acute Ischemic Stroke

Naoki Katayama [1,2], Keiichi Odagiri [1,*], Akio Hakamata [1], Naoki Inui [1], Katsuya Yamauchi [3] and Hiroshi Watanabe [1]

[1] Department of Clinical Pharmacology and Therapeutics, Hamamatsu University School of Medicine, 1-20-1 Handayama, Higashi-ku, Hamamatsu 431-3192, Japan; katayama_20@yahoo.co.jp (N.K.); hakamata@hama-med.ac.jp (A.H.); inui@hama-med.ac.jp (N.I.); hwat@hama-med.ac.jp (H.W.)
[2] Department of Rehabilitation Medicine, Seirei Mikatahara General Hospital, 3453 Mikatahara-cho, Kita-ku, Hamamatsu 433-8558, Japan
[3] Department of Rehabilitation Medicine, Hamamatsu University Hospital, 1-20-1 Handayama, Higashi-ku, Hamamatsu 431-3192, Japan; yamakatu@hama-med.ac.jp
* Correspondence: kodagiri@hama-med.ac.jp

Abstract: Background: Cerebral oxygenation monitoring provides important information for optimizing individualized management in patients with acute ischemic stroke (AIS). Although changes in cerebral oxygenation are known to occur in response to head-of-bed (HOB) elevation within 72 h after onset, changes in cerebral oxygenation during stroke recovery are unclear. We compared changes in total- (tHb), oxygenated- (HbO_2), and deoxygenated-hemoglobin (deoxyHb) concentrations in response to HOB manipulation between the timeframes within 72 h and 7–10 days after AIS onset. Methods: We measured forehead ΔtHb, ΔHbO_2, and ΔdeoxyHb in response to HOB elevation (30°) within 72 h (first measurement) and 7–10 days (second measurement) after AIS onset using time-resolved near-infrared spectroscopy. Results: We enrolled 30 participants (mean age 72.8 ± 11.3 years; 13 women) with a first AIS. There were no significant differences in ΔtHb, ΔHbO_2, or ΔdeoxyHb measurements on the infarct or contra-infarct side. At the first measurement, ΔtHb, ΔHbO_2, and ΔdeoxyHb measured on the contra-infarct side did not correlate with those measured on the infarct side: ΔtHb ($r = 0.114$, $p = 0.539$); ΔHbO_2 ($r = 0.143$, $p = 0.440$); ΔdeoxyHb ($r = 0.227$, $p = 0.221$). Notably, at the second measurement, correlation coefficients of ΔtHb and ΔHbO_2 between the contra-infarct and infarct sides were statistically significant: ΔtHb ($r = 0.491$, $p = 0.008$); ΔHbO_2 ($r = 0.479$, $p = 0.010$); ΔdeoxyHb ($r = 0.358$, $p = 0.054$). Conclusion: Although changes in cerebral oxygenation in response to HOB elevation had a laterality difference between hemispheres within 72 h of AIS onset, the difference had decreased, at least partially, 7–10 days after AIS onset.

Keywords: cerebral blood volume; hemodynamics; near-infrared spectroscopy; optical imaging; rehabilitation; stroke

---

1. Introduction

Acute ischemic stroke (AIS) is a significant cause of permanent disability [1]. Early rehabilitation for AIS patients—considered an important issue in poststroke functional outcomes—has been recommended in recent guidelines [2,3]. A large-scale clinical trial; however, provided evidence that early intervention was not associated with disability outcomes [4]. It is also recognized that supine AIS patients have improved cerebral blood flow (CBF) and oxygenation, although with an increased risk of aspiration pneumonia [5–8]. Another clinical trial revealed that a head-up position initiated within

24 h of AIS onset was not associated with a disability outcome or severe adverse effects, including pneumonia [9]. Thus, the optimal head position in patients with AIS is still unknown.

Near-infrared spectroscopy (NIRS) noninvasively measures hemoglobin (Hb) levels in the brain [10]. Compared with other technologies, such as transcranial Doppler (TCD) and positron emission tomography (PET), NIRS has several advantages: (1) it allows flexible measurements in sitting, standing, and moving subjects; (2) it is an irradiation-based, completely noninvasive technique that does not cause adverse effects on the body during repeated measurements, even in children; (3) it has high time resolution; and (4) it is compact and portable. Because of these advantages, the use of NIRS, such as cerebral oxygen monitors, is increasing in the medical field despite its drawbacks (e.g., possible interferences caused by attachment of optodes, shallow measurement depth, effects of drugs influencing cerebral blood flow or cutaneous blood flow, artifacts of cutaneous blood flow, and narrow measurement territory depending on the attachment site of optode). This increase is because these systems are simple but enable the observation of changes in brain activity over time via monitoring of Hb levels, which reflect fluctuations in regional cerebral blood flow. Indeed, NIRS can be useful to detect the intraindividual fluctuation and the interindividual difference of cerebral hemodynamic response in response to posture change [11]. Thus, well-known applications of NIRS include the monitoring of cerebral blood flow and hypoxic conditions in a variety of clinical settings [12–14]. During the last two decades, several studies have used the NIRS system to evaluate changes in cerebral oxygenation in upright AIS patients [7,15–17]. Their findings provided important information for optimal individualized management, based on cerebral oxygenation monitoring in AIS patients. Nevertheless, correlation of the total- (tHb), oxygenated- (HbO_2), and deoxygenated-hemoglobin (deoxyHb) concentrations in response to head-of-bed (HOB) elevation between the infarct and contra-infarct sides have never been assessed, leaving the changes in cerebral oxygenation during stroke recovery not well understood. In the current exploratory study, we therefore aim to compare the changes in tHb (ΔtHb), HbO_2 (ΔHbO_2), and deoxyHb (ΔdeoxyHb) in response to HOB manipulation between the timeframes within 72 h and 7–10 days after AIS onset.

2. Methods

2.1. Study Design and Participants

This study was designed as a single-center exploratory study to compare the changes in cerebral oxygenation in response to HOB manipulation between different time points in AIS patients, and it was conducted at Seirei Mikatahara General Hospital, Hamamatsu, Japan. Study participants were consecutively recruited from among acute cerebral infarction patients hospitalized at our hospital from September 2016 to March 2017. Eligible patients were those having a first-ever ischemic stroke and who had been hospitalized within 24 h of symptoms onset. Main exclusion criteria were a patient with infratentorial stroke; a history of cerebral disease (prior stroke, brain contusion, brain tumor, brain infections, intracerebral hemorrhage and trauma); orthostatic hypotension; taking antihypertensive agents after hospitalization; or unable to participate in this study (could not maintain a 30° passive sitting position; presence of a skin disease (not suitable for applying a probe to the forehead); unable to follow verbal instructions).

2.2. Ethics and Study Registration

This study protocol complied with the Helsinki Declaration. The institutional research review board of Seirei Mikatahara General Hospital and Hamamatsu University School of Medicine approved the study (Approved number 16-15 and 16-001). Written informed consent was provided by all participants. The study was registered at the UMIN Clinical Trials Registry (URL: http://www.umin.ac.jp/ctr/index.htm. Unique identifier: UMIN 000022904).

2.3. Cerebral Hemoglobin Concentration Measurement by Time-Resolved NIRS

We used a single-channel, time-resolved NIRS system (TRS-10; Hamamatsu Photonics K.K., Hamamatsu, Japan) to measure bilateral forehead cerebral (prefrontal cortex) hemoglobin concentration. The temporal profile obtained from TRS-10 measurement was fitted with that obtained from the theoretical solution of the photon diffusion equation (DE) [18], because the DE-fit method could provide information about the hemodynamic changes in the depth direction [19]. The TRS-10 system consists of three pulsed laser diodes with wavelengths of 759, 797, and 833 nm, having a duration of 100 ps and repetition frequency of 5 MHz. An optode, which includes infrared light irradiation and reception probes in a single device, was fixed on the participant's head with Velcro and a headband so the irradiated infrared light was positioned at Fp1 and Fp2 according to the International 10-20 system. This NIRS device can measure the tHb, HbO_2, and deoxyHb of tissues within a semicircular area between the irradiation and reception probes. The measurement depth increases with increased distance between the irradiation and reception probes (limit of 5 cm), because the farther the distance, the weaker the light reaching the reception probe. One study reporting simultaneous measurements with TRS-10 and PET found that TRS-10 measurements with irradiation and reception probes 3 cm apart significantly correlated with PET measurements around gray matter [20]. We therefore set the distance between the irradiation and reception probes at 3 cm outside the infrared reception port on the optode.

2.4. Cerebral Blood Hemoglobin Concentration Measurements Protocol

Based on previous studies [21–24], we measured forehead tHb, HbO_2, and deoxyHb within 72 h (first measurement) and 7–10 days (second measurement) after AIS onset. After placing probes on the forehead, the participant laid on his/her back. Data were collected every 10 s for 5 min at each HOB angle (0°, 30°, 0°) sequentially. At each HOB angle, the mean tHb, HbO_2, and deoxyHb values were calculated after discarding data obtained during the first minute, because it took 15 s to change the HOB position of the bed. Because the TRS-10 system has a single channel, two consecutive measurements were conducted in each participant. We first measured forehead tHb, HbO_2, and deoxyHb on the contra-infarct side and then on the infarct side. Systemic blood pressure and heart rate were also measured for 1 min in each position using an automatic hemodynamometer (HBP1300; Omron Corp., Tokyo, Japan).

2.5. Statistical Analysis

Values are expressed as means ± standard deviations (SD) or medians (interquartile range) (nonparametrically distributed values) of the indicated numbers or proportions (%). Changes in systemic blood pressure, heart rate, tHb, HbO_2, and deoxyHb were compared with the baseline (HOB 0°). These measurement values at HOB 30° were compared with those at HOB 0° using the Wilcoxon signed-rank test. Correlations between the infarct and contra-infarct sides for each measurement were assessed using Spearman's rank correlation coefficient. The significance of the difference between the two correlation coefficients was evaluated using the Fisher r-to-z transformation. $p < 0.05$ was regarded as indicating statistical significance. All statistical analyses were performed using PASW Statistics version 18.0.0 (IBM Co., Armonk, NY, USA) and Microsoft Excel 2016 (Microsoft Co., Redmond, WA, USA).

3. Results

3.1. *Study Participants' Characteristics*

Altogether, 32 AIS patients met the inclusion criteria and were enrolled. Two participants died before the second measurements and were excluded from the analyses. The participants' characteristics are shown in Table 1.

Table 1. Patients' characteristics.

Characteristic	Value
Age, year	72.8 ± 11.3
Female sex, *n* (%)	13 (43.3)
Height (cm)	158.0 ± 11.6
Body weight (kg)	56.0 ± 14.4
Body mass index (kg/m^2)	22.1 ± 3.1
Stroke side (right/left)	11/19
NIHSS score	7.6 ± 4.9
TOAST classification, *n* (%)	
Large-artery atherosclerosis	10 (33.3)
Small-vessel occlusion	10 (33.3)
Cardioembolism	6 (20.0)
Stroke of other determined etiology	4 (13.3)
Stroke of undetermined etiology	0 (0)
Vascular territorial segmentation, *n* (%)	
Anterior cerebral artery	6 (20.0)
Middle cerebral artery	17 (56.7)
Posterior cerebral artery	7 (20.3)
Medical history *n* (%)	
Hypertension	18 (60.0)
Diabetes mellitus	8 (26.7)
Dyslipidemia	22 (73.3)
Chronic atrial fibrillation	4 (13.3)
Tobacco use	12 (40.0)

Data are expressed as means ± Standard deviation unless otherwise stated; TOAST—Trial of Org 10172 in Acute Stroke Treatment; NIHSS—National Institutes of Health Stroke Scale.

3.2. *Changes in Blood Pressure, Heart Rate, tHb, HbO$_2$, and deoxyHb with HOB Elevation*

Table 2 shows the changes in systolic (SBP) and diastolic (DBP) blood pressures and the heart rate in response to HOB elevations from 0° to 30°. These HOB elevations did not affect any hemodynamic parameters. There were also no intraindividual differences in the SBP or heart rate at baseline measurements (HOB 0°) at each measurement session (first measurement: SBP ($p = 0.74$), DBP ($p = 0.87$), heart rate ($p = 0.94$); second measurement: SBP ($p = 0.83$), DBP ($p = 0.94$), heart rate ($p = 0.30$).

Table 2. Comparisons of the systemic blood pressure and heart rate in response to HOB manipulation.

Parameters	Item Measured	HOB 0°	HOB 30°	Difference	*p*
First Measurement					
Contra-infarct Side	sBP (mmHg)	137.6 ± 20.9	137.7 ± 19.8	0.1 ± 4.1	0.90
	dBP(mmHg)	75.9 ± 11.7	76.9 ± 10.6	1.0 ± 5.4	0.91
	HR (bpm)	73.5 ± 10.4	73.5 ± 9.7	0.0 ± 3.5	0.95
Infarct Side	sBP (mmHg)	137.9 ± 20.6	137.3 ± 19.8	−0.6 ± 3.7	0.39
	dBP (mmHg)	75.9 ± 11.2	76.4 ± 10.9	0.5 ± 4.6	0.63
	HR (bpm)	73.6 ± 11.0	73.4 ± 11.4	−0.2 ± 3.6	0.86
Second Measurement					
Contra-Infarct Side	sBP (mmHg)	128.9 ± 16.5	129.8 ±15.0	0.9 ± 5.1	0.53
	dBP (mmHg)	71.0 ± 9.0	71.1 ± 8.6	0.0 ± 3.9	0.51
	HR (bpm)	75.6 ± 8.1	76.5 ± 7.8	0.9 ± 3.9	0.36
Infarct Side	sBP (mmHg)	129.5 ± 15.1	128.7 ± 15.6	−0.8 ±5.3	0.10
	dBP (mmHg)	71.0 ± 8.4	70.3 ± 8.3	−0.7 ± 4.6	0.24
	HR (bpm)	74.8 ± 8.4	75.1 ± 7.7	0.3 ± 3.1	0.21

Data are expressed as means ± Standard deviation; HOB—head-of-bed, sBP—systolic blood pressure; dBP—diastolic blood pressure; HR—heart rate; bpm—beats per minute; mmHg—millimeters of mercury.

3.3. Changes in Cerebral Hemoglobin Concentrations with HOB Elevation

Figure 1 shows the time-series changes in the tHb in response to HOB manipulation. Changes in the tHb showed large interindividual differences, which were also observed in the changes in the HbO_2 and deoxyHb (Figure 2; Figure 3). There were no significant differences in the ΔtHb, ΔHbO_2, or ΔdeoxyHb on either the infarct or the contra-infarct side between the two measurements.

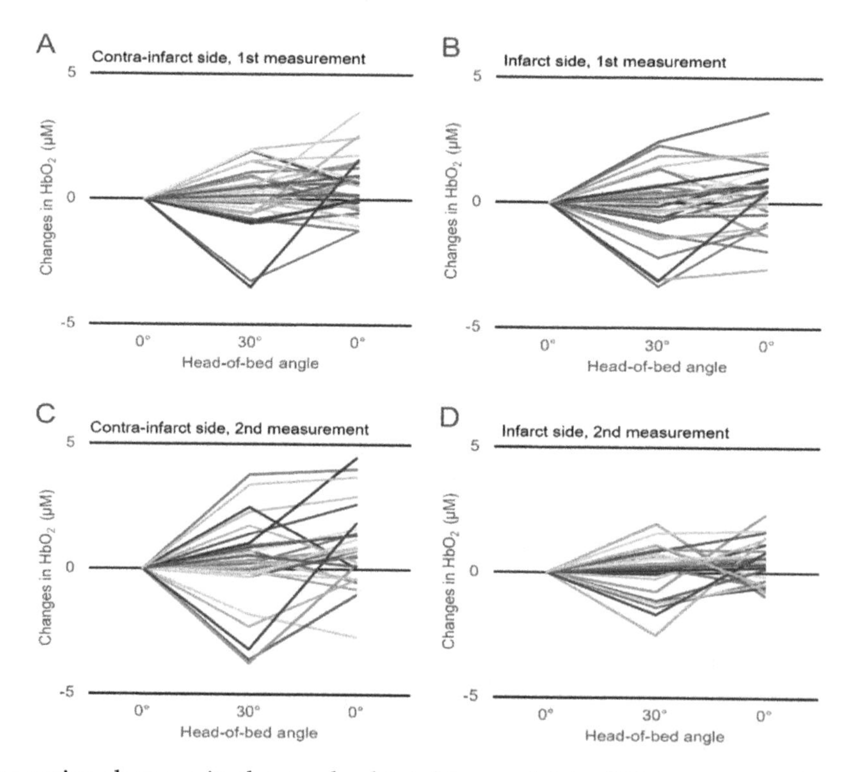

Figure 1. Time-series changes in the cerebral total hemoglobin (tHb) concentration in response to head-of-bed manipulation (from 0° to 30°) for 30 participants within 72 h of onset of acute ischemic stroke (AIS) (first measurement) on the contra-infarct (contralateral) side (**A**) and infarct side (**B**) and those measured 7–10 days after onset of AIS (second measurement) on the contra-infarct side (**C**) and infarct side (**D**).

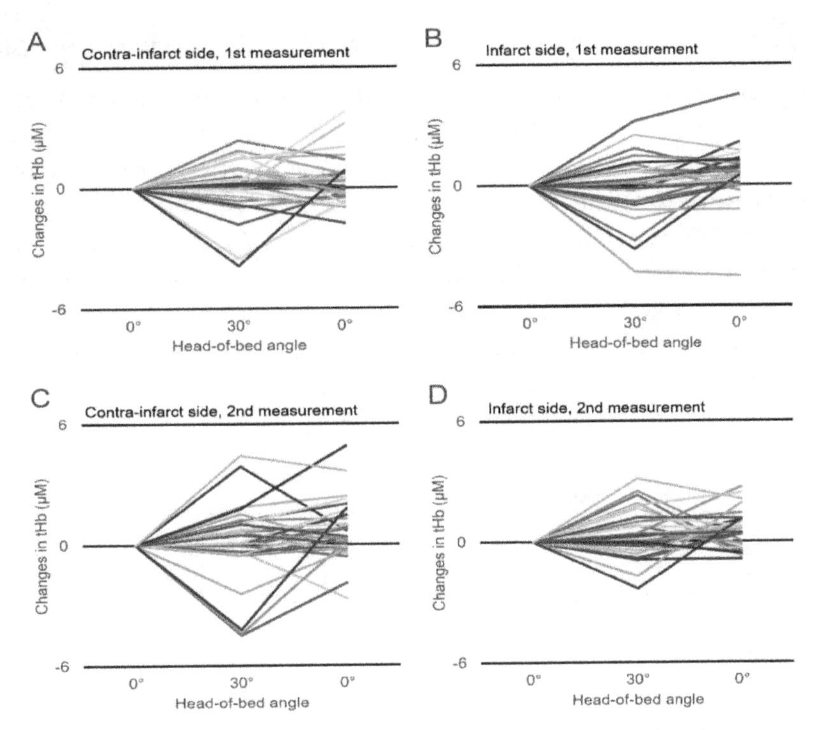

Figure 2. Time-series changes in the cerebral oxygenated-hemoglobin (HbO_2) concentration in response to head-of-bed manipulation for 30 participants within 72 h of AIS onset (first measurement) on the contra-infarct side (**A**) and infarct side (**B**) and those measured 7–10 days after AIS onset (second measurement) on the contra-infarct side (**C**) and infarct side (**D**).

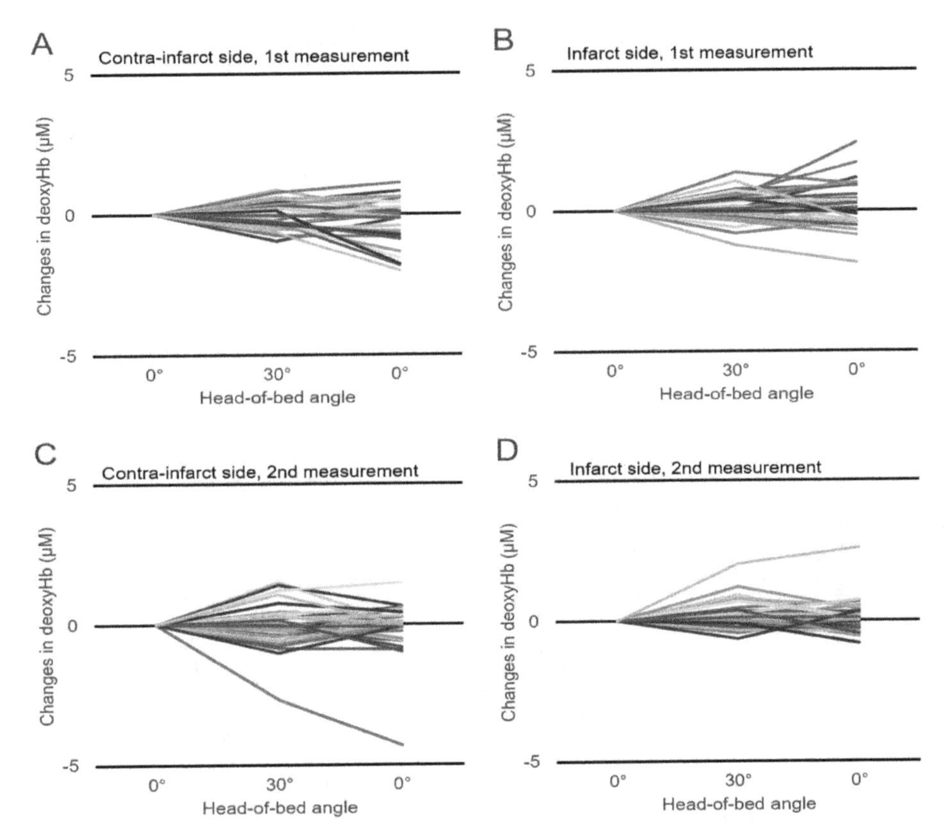

Figure 3. Time-series changes in the cerebral deoxygenated-hemoglobin (deoxyHb) concentration in response to head-of-bed manipulation for 30 participants within 72 h of AIS onset (first measurement) on the contra-infarct side (**A**) and infarct side (**B**) and those measured 7–10 days after onset of AIS (second measurement) on the contra-infarct side (**C**) and infarct side (**D**).

3.4. *Correlations of Hemoglobin Concentration Changes with HOB Elevation between Measurements*

Figure 4 shows the correlations of the ΔtHb, ΔHbO_2, and ΔdeoxyHb in response to HOB elevation between the first and second measurements for each hemisphere. The first measurements of the ΔtHb and ΔHbO_2 were significantly correlated with those at the second measurements for either hemisphere (ΔtHb: contra-infarct side ($r = 0.569, p = 0.020$), infarct side ($r = 0.408, p = 0.028$); ΔHbO_2: contra-infarct side ($r = 0.576, p = 0.020$), infarct side ($r = 0.378, p = 0.042$)). Although correlation coefficients in the contra-infarct side seemed to indicate a stronger relation than those in the infarct side, there were no statistically significant differences for ΔtHb or ΔHbO_2 (ΔtHb ($z = 0.772, p = 0.441$); ΔHbO_2 ($z = 0.955, p = 0.342$)), ΔdeoxyHb did not show a significant correlation between the first and second measurements (contra-infarct side ($z = 0.024, p = 0.896$); infarct side ($z = 0.176, p = 0.345$)).

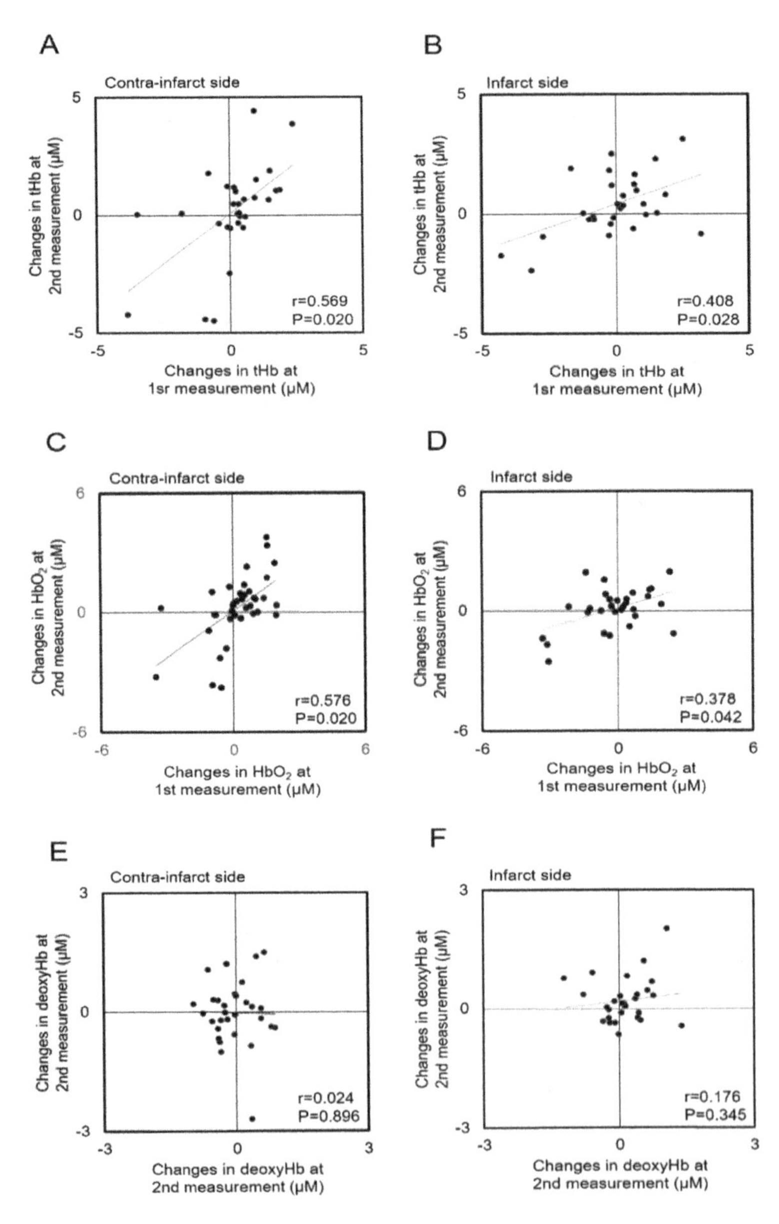

Figure 4. Scatterplots of the changes in total-hemoglobin (tHb) (**A** and **B**), oxygenated-hemoglobin (HbO_2) (**C** and **D**), and deoxygenated-hemoglobin (deoxyHb) (**E** and **F**) concentrations in response to head-of-bed elevation (from 0° to 30°) between the first and second measurements for each hemisphere.

3.5. Correlations of Hemoglobin Concentration Changes with HOB Elevation between Infarct and Contra-Infarct Sides

Figure 5 shows the correlations of ΔtHb, ΔHbO_2, and ΔdeoxyHb in response to HOB elevation between the infarct and contra-infarct sides. At the first measurement, ΔtHb, ΔHbO_2, and ΔdeoxyHb measured on the contra-infarct side did not correlate with those on the infarct side (ΔtHb ($r = 0.114$, $p = 0.539$), ΔHbO_2 ($r = 0.143$, $p = 0.440$); ΔdeoxyHb ($r = 0.227$, $p = 0.221$)) (Figure 5A–C). Notably, the correlation coefficients of ΔtHb, ΔHbO_2, and ΔdeoxyHb values between the infarct and contra-infarct sides at the second measurement were statistically significant, except for ΔdeoxyHb (ΔtHb ($r = 0.491$, $p = 0.008$); ΔHbO_2 ($r = 0.479$, $p = 0.010$); ΔdeoxyHb ($r = 0.358$, $p = 0.054$)) (Figure 5D–F).

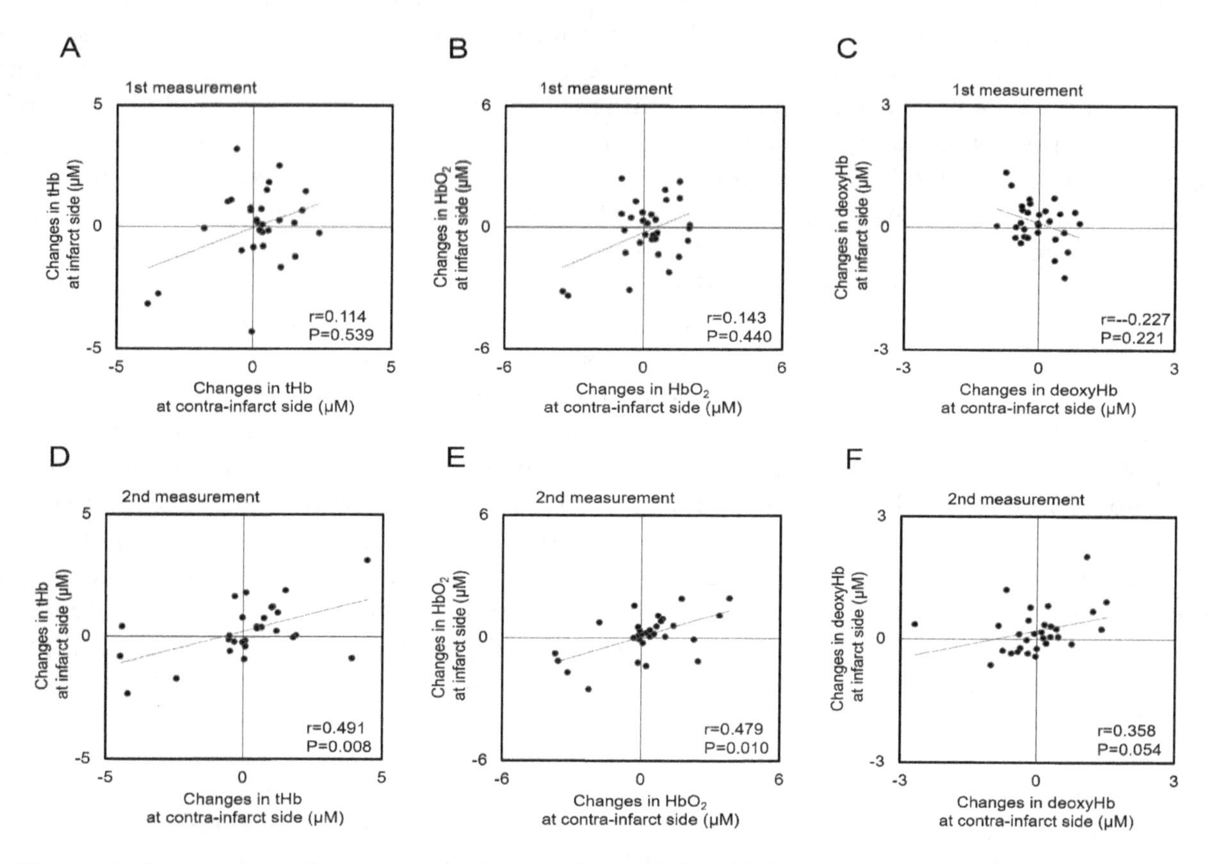

Figure 5. Scatterplots of the changes in total-hemoglobin (tHB), oxygenated-hemoglobin (HbO_2), and deoxygenated-hemoglobin (deoxyHb) concentrations in response to head-of-bed elevation (from 0° to 30°) at the first (**A–C**) and second (**D–F**) measurements for each hemisphere.

4. Discussion

We believe that this is the first study to assess the effect of gradual HOB manipulation (from 0° to 30°) of forehead hemoglobin concentration in AIS patients, revealed by two measurements using NIRS. There were three main findings of this investigation. (1) The HOB elevation from 0° to 30° did not affect systemic blood pressure or heart rate. ΔtHb, ΔHbO_2, and ΔdeoxyHb also did not change in response to HOB elevation, although large interindividual variabilities were observed. (2) ΔtHb and ΔHbO_2 in response to HOB elevation measured within 72 h of AIS onset showed significant correlations with those measured 7–10 days after AIS onset in both hemispheres. (3) Although ΔtHb, ΔHbO_2, and ΔdeoxyHb measured on the infarct side did not correlate with those measured on the contra-infarct side within 72 h of AIS onset, the correlation coefficients of these NIRS parameters were significantly correlated between the hemispheres 7–10 days after AIS onset.

It is known that CBF velocity (CBFV) and the total cerebral Hb concentration are reduced in head-up position of healthy subjects and chronic ischemic stroke patients. Furthermore, decreases in

CBVF and cerebral Hb concentration could be affected by a drop in systemic blood pressure [5,25–27]. In this study, the average blood pressure and heart rate did not change with HOB elevation from 0° to 30°. Neither were there changes in the cohort-averaged tHb, HbO_2, and deoxyHb concentrations for either hemisphere over two measurements. However, as shown in Figures 1–3, changes in tHb, HbO_2, and deoxyHb showed large differences among individuals. Approximately half of our study patients showed increased cerebral hemoglobin concentrations (the so-called paradoxical response) in response to HOB elevation for either hemisphere over the two measurements. This paradoxical response phenomenon was in line with previous reports that evaluated the effect of head-position changes on cerebral oxygenation in AIS patients [7,16,17]. Several previous studies reported that the paradoxical response was also seen in brain-injured patients but not healthy subjects, suggesting that it is pathological [11,28–30]. Although details of the mechanism of the paradoxical response are still unknown, an increasing intracranial pressure, the hemodynamic consequences of heart failure, and an autonomic disturbance have been proposed as causes [17]. Considerably varying individual cerebral oxygenation responses, including the paradoxical response, could explain why the cohort-averaged ΔtHb, ΔHbO_2, and ΔdeoxyHb concentrations did not change in response to HOB elevation.

Correlations of ΔtHb, ΔHbO_2, and ΔdeoxyHb concentrations in response to HOB elevation between the infarct and contra-infarct sides had not been reported prior to this study. Thus, we seem to be the first to show that the ΔtHb and ΔHbO_2 measurements within 72 h of AIS onset significantly correlated with those 7–10 days after AIS onset for either hemisphere. Notably, although the ΔtHb, ΔHbO_2, and ΔdeoxyHb, in response to HOB elevation, did not show a significant correlation between hemispheres within 72 h of AIS onset, correlations of the ΔtHb, ΔHbO_2, and ΔdeoxyHb 7–10 days after onset were statistically significant. Although we could not clarify the mechanism of this alteration, various possible explanations are assumed. Changes in cerebral oxygenation variables in response to HOB manipulation reflected CBF volume change. It could be related with gravitational force acting on passively contacted brain vessels in the ischemic territory [31]. It is also possible that systemic hemodynamics changes affect CBF; however, the HOB elevation from 0° to 30° did not affect systemic blood pressure or heart rate. A previous study, which measured cerebral mean flow velocity by TCD, suggested that the effect of BP change in response to head position change was equivocal [31–33]. In the current study, HOB elevations did not affect SBP, DBP, or HR, and no intraindividual differences in the SBP or heart rate at baseline measurements (HOB 0°) was observed at each measurement session. While cardiac output or stroke volume of the left ventricle was not measured, we thought that the effect of systemic hemodynamics changes could be limited. It is well-recognized that the brain edema is one of the lethal complications for AIS patients, and it causes a decrease in cerebral perfusion pressure through an increased intracranial pressure (ICP) [34]. Although we did not include AIS patients who received surgical decompression for severe brain edema (because of unsuitability of applying a probe to the forehead) and two participants who died before second measurement (suspected brain edema) were excluded from the analyses, the possibility that a raised ICP could affect the changes in ΔtHb, ΔHbO_2, and ΔdeoxyHb on the infarct side in response to HOB elevation could not be denied because we did not monitor the ICP in our participants. Development of collateral circulation also affected the changes in ΔtHb, ΔHbO_2, and ΔdeoxyHb on the infarct side in response to HOB elevation. Our study participants received magnetic resonance angiography (MRA) at the time of admission and 7–10 days after stroke onset. MRA often cannot provide information about the collateral circulation of AIS patients in clinical settings because of motion artifacts and its spatial resolution, whereas recent development of MRA can detect collateral circulation in research settings [35,36]. Furthermore, our study participants did not receive cerebral angiography because they had no indication of thrombolytic therapy at the time of admission. Thus, detailed information of collateral circulation is not available in the current study. Another possible mechanism is the alteration of cerebral autoregulation in AIS patients. Cerebral autoregulation is an inherent process of blood vessels that maintains CBF at a constant level over a wide range of changes in the systemic blood pressure or intracranial pressure. It has been generally accepted that cerebral autoregulation is impaired in patients with AIS [37,38]. Conventionally, TCD has often been used to measure the CBFV to assess cerebral autoregulation [39], and mean flow velocity index of dynamic autoregulation (Mx index) was established as a standard parameter [40,41]. Recent literature; however, has reported that cerebral oxygenation parameters measured by NIRS (e.g., cerebral oxygen saturation, cerebral oxygenation index) are considered surrogates of CBF [42–45]. In addition, it was reported that the NIRS-derived tHb signal reflects regional changes in cerebral blood volume (CBV), and HbO_2 correlates with cerebral capillary oxygen saturation [20,46–48]. Steiner, L. A. and colleagues demonstrated that tissue oxygen index of dynamic autoregulation (Tox) measured by NIRS (NIRO 200, Hamamatsu Photonics K.K.) significantly correlated with the Mx index [41]. Although NIRS is useful for cerebral autoregulation assessment, we could not make mention of the relationship between our results and cerebral autoregulation. We could not calculate the Tox index because we did not measure continuous blood pressure, and TRS-10 could not directly measure the tissue oxygen index. The literature suggests that AIS severity could influence the degree of spatiotemporal compromise of cerebral autoregulation [21,24,49]. Tutaj et al. reported that cerebral autoregulation was transiently impaired at an infarct hemisphere 1.3 ± 0.5 days after the onset of a large-vessel AIS, recovered at 9.75 ± 2.2 days—which could be in line with our findings [21]. Thus, we speculated the possibility that our findings might have been caused, at least in part, by transient changes in cerebral autoregulation. We need to conduct further studies to clarify whether current findings are induced by transient impairment of cerebral autoregulation.

This study has several limitations. The monitored systemic blood pressure and heart rate were not beat-to-beat measurements. Thus, we could not detect a transient drop in blood pressure in response to HOB manipulation. Lam et al. reported that the blood pressure may show a steep drop in response to gradual changes in head position (supine to 30°), although a blood pressure decline was observed in the head-up state [50]. Furthermore, the CBV paralleled blood pressure in the head-up position. These results supported our findings that neither blood pressure nor cerebral oxygenation parameters changed in response to HOB manipulation, at least according to the cohort-averaged assessment. Second, two consecutive NIRS measurements were needed for each participant because the TRS-10 system had only a single channel. Thus, we could not evaluate the cerebral oxygenation changes on the infarct and contra-infarct sides simultaneously. Furthermore, we could investigate forehead blood volume only within a narrow range of the prefrontal cortex. Multi-channel NIRS is currently in mainstream use and should be adopted in future studies to understand fluctuations in cerebral oxygenation in the entire brain in response to postural change. Third, we did not measure either endotidal carbon dioxide tension ($EtCO_2$) or partial pressure of carbon dioxide (pCO_2). It is known that CBF is influenced by CO_2, and hypercapnia dilates cerebral arteries and arterioles and increased blood flow, whereas hypocapnia causes vasoconstriction and decreased blood flow [51,52]. Indeed, Kim, Y.S. et al. reported that orthostatic manipulation decreases $EtCO_2$ from 40 mmHg to 35 mg in elder subjects [26]. Therefore, we cannot exclude that pCO_2 could also affect NIRS metrics. Fourth, we did not assess cerebral autoregulation or differences in the CBV responses among NIRS and other modalities (e.g., TCD, PET). Thus, we could not offer reasons why a statistically significant correlation of changes in cerebral oxygenation parameters between each hemisphere in response to HOB manipulation was found at 7–10 days after AIS onset but not within 72 h.

5. Conclusions

HOB manipulation from 0° to 30° did not affect cohort-averaged hemodynamic parameters. The cohort-averaged cerebral oxygenation parameters also did not change in response to HOB elevation, although large interindividual cerebral oxygenation changes were seen. Although changes in cerebral oxygenation in response to HOB elevation had a laterality difference between the hemispheres within 72 h of AIS onset, the difference decreased, at least partially, 7–10 days after AIS onset, and this could have suggested a sign of cerebral blood flow recovery. These findings suggest that HOB 30° within 72 h might not always be a preferred head position in AIS patients. Further studies are needed to establish the safety and efficacy of NIRS-guided neurological rehabilitation in AIS in the future.

Author Contributions: Conceptualization, N.K., K.O and A.H.; formal analysis, N.K.; investigation, N.K.; methodology, N.K. and K.O.; project administration, K.O.; resources, H.W.; supervision, N.I., K.Y. and H.W.; visualization, N.K.; writing—original draft preparation N.K.; writing—review and editing. K.O. and H.W.

Acknowledgments: We thank Nancy Schatken, BS, MT(ASCP), from Edanz Group (www.edanzediting.com/ac), for editing a draft of this manuscript.

References

1. Murray, C.J.; Vos, T.; Lozano, R.; Naghavi, M.; Flaxman, A.D.; Michaud, C.; Ezzati, M.; Shibuya, K.; Salomon, J.A.; Abdalla, S.; et al. Disability-adjusted life years (dalys) for 291 diseases and injuries in 21 regions, 1990-2010: A systematic analysis for the global burden of disease study 2010. *Lancet* **2012**, *380*, 2197–2223. [CrossRef]
2. Powers, W.J.; Rabinstein, A.A.; Ackerson, T.; Adeoye, O.M.; Bambakidis, N.C.; Becker, K.; Biller, J.; Brown, M.; Demaerschalk, B.M.; Hoh, B.; et al. 2018 guidelines for the early management of patients with acute ischemic stroke: A guideline for healthcare professionals from the american heart association/american stroke association. *Stroke* **2018**, *49*, e46–e110. [CrossRef] [PubMed]
3. Winstein, C.J.; Stein, J.; Arena, R.; Bates, B.; Cherney, L.R.; Cramer, S.C.; Deruyter, F.; Eng, J.J.; Fisher, B.; Harvey, R.L.; et al. Guidelines for adult stroke rehabilitation and recovery: A guideline for healthcare professionals from the american heart association/american stroke association. *Stroke* **2016**, *47*, e98–e169. [CrossRef] [PubMed]
4. AVERT Trial Collaboration group. Efficacy and safety of very early mobilisation within 24 h of stroke onset (avert): A randomised controlled trial. *Lancet* **2015**, *386*, 46–55.
5. Mehagnoul-Schipper, D.J.; Vloet, L.C.; Colier, W.N.; Hoefnagels, W.H.; Jansen, R.W. Cerebral oxygenation declines in healthy elderly subjects in response to assuming the upright position. *Stroke* **2000**, *31*, 1615–1620. [CrossRef]
6. Tyson, S.F.; Nightingale, P. The effects of position on oxygen saturation in acute stroke: A systematic review. *Clin. Rehabil.* **2004**, *18*, 863–871. [CrossRef]
7. Hargroves, D.; Tallis, R.; Pomeroy, V.; Bhalla, A. The influence of positioning upon cerebral oxygenation after acute stroke: A pilot study. *Age ageing* **2008**, *37*, 581–585. [CrossRef]
8. Olavarria, V.V.; Arima, H.; Anderson, C.S.; Brunser, A.M.; Munoz-Venturelli, P.; Heritier, S.; Lavados, P.M. Head position and cerebral blood flow velocity in acute ischemic stroke: A systematic review and meta-analysis. *Cerebrovasc. Dis.* **2014**, *37*, 401–408. [CrossRef]
9. Anderson, C.S.; Arima, H.; Lavados, P.; Billot, L.; Hackett, M.L.; Olavarria, V.V.; Munoz Venturelli, P.; Brunser, A.; Peng, B.; Cui, L.; et al. Cluster-randomized, crossover trial of head positioning in acute stroke. *N. Engl. J. Med.* **2017**, *376*, 2437–2447. [CrossRef]
10. Herold, F.; Wiegel, P.; Scholkmann, F.; Muller, N.G. Applications of functional near-infrared spectroscopy (fnirs) neuroimaging in exercise(-)cognition science: A systematic, methodology-focused review. *J. Clin. Med.* **2018**. [CrossRef]
11. Kim, M.N.; Edlow, B.L.; Durduran, T.; Frangos, S.; Mesquita, R.C.; Levine, J.M.; Greenberg, J.H.; Yodh, A.G.; Detre, J.A. Continuous optical monitoring of cerebral hemodynamics during head-of-bed manipulation in brain-injured adults. *Neurocrit. Care* **2014**, *20*, 443–453. [CrossRef] [PubMed]
12. Harrer, M.; Waldenberger, F.R.; Weiss, G.; Folkmann, S.; Gorlitzer, M.; Moidl, R.; Grabenwoeger, M. Aortic arch surgery using bilateral antegrade selective cerebral perfusion in combination with near-infrared spectroscopy. *Eur. J. Cardiothorac. Surg.* **2010**, *38*, 561–567. [CrossRef] [PubMed]
13. Ogino, H.; Ueda, Y.; Sugita, T.; Morioka, K.; Sakakibara, Y.; Matsubayashi, K.; Nomoto, T. Monitoring of regional cerebral oxygenation by near-infrared spectroscopy during continuous retrograde cerebral perfusion for aortic arch surgery. *Eur. J. Cardiothorac. Surg.* **1998**, *14*, 415–418. [CrossRef]
14. Weindling, A.M. Peripheral oxygenation and management in the perinatal period. *Semin. Fetal Neonatal. Med.* **2010**, *15*, 208–215. [CrossRef]

15. Aries, M.J.; Elting, J.W.; Stewart, R.; De Keyser, J.; Kremer, B.; Vroomen, P. Cerebral blood flow velocity changes during upright positioning in bed after acute stroke: An observational study. *BMJ Open* **2013**. [CrossRef] [PubMed]
16. Favilla, C.G.; Mesquita, R.C.; Mullen, M.; Durduran, T.; Lu, X.; Kim, M.N.; Minkoff, D.L.; Kasner, S.E.; Greenberg, J.H.; Yodh, A.G.; et al. Optical bedside monitoring of cerebral blood flow in acute ischemic stroke patients during head-of-bed manipulation. *Stroke* **2014**, *45*, 1269–1274. [CrossRef]
17. Durduran, T.; Zhou, C.; Edlow, B.L.; Yu, G.; Choe, R.; Kim, M.N.; Cucchiara, B.L.; Putt, M.E.; Shah, Q.; Kasner, S.E.; et al. Transcranial optical monitoring of cerebrovascular hemodynamics in acute stroke patients. *Opt. express* **2009**, *17*, 3884–3902. [CrossRef]
18. Patterson, M.S.; Chance, B.; Wilson, B.C. Time resolved reflectance and transmittance for the non-invasive measurement of tissue optical properties. *Appl. Opt.* **1989**, *28*, 2331–2336. [CrossRef]
19. Sato, C.; Yamaguchi, T.; Seida, M.; Ota, Y.; Yu, I.; Iguchi, Y.; Nemoto, M.; Hoshi, Y. Intraoperative monitoring of depth-dependent hemoglobin concentration changes during carotid endarterectomy by time-resolved spectroscopy. *Appl. Opt.* **2007**, *46*, 2785–2792. [CrossRef]
20. Ohmae, E.; Ouchi, Y.; Oda, M.; Suzuki, T.; Nobesawa, S.; Kanno, T.; Yoshikawa, E.; Futatsubashi, M.; Ueda, Y.; Okada, H.; et al. Cerebral hemodynamics evaluation by near-infrared time-resolved spectroscopy: Correlation with simultaneous positron emission tomography measurements. *NeuroImage* **2006**, *29*, 697–705. [CrossRef]
21. Tutaj, M.; Miller, M.; Krakowska-Stasiak, M.; Piatek, A.; Hebda, J.; Latka, M.; Strojny, J.; Szczudlik, A.; Slowik, A. Dynamic cerebral autoregulation is compromised in ischaemic stroke of undetermined aetiology only in the non-affected hemisphere. *Neurol. Neurochir. Pol.* **2014**, *48*, 91–97. [CrossRef] [PubMed]
22. Petersen, N.H.; Ortega-Gutierrez, S.; Reccius, A.; Masurkar, A.; Huang, A.; Marshall, R.S. Dynamic cerebral autoregulation is transiently impaired for one week after large-vessel acute ischemic stroke. *Cerebrovasc. Dis.* **2015**, *39*, 144–150. [CrossRef] [PubMed]
23. Panerai, R.B.; Jara, J.L.; Saeed, N.P.; Horsfield, M.A.; Robinson, T.G. Dynamic cerebral autoregulation following acute ischaemic stroke: Comparison of transcranial doppler and magnetic resonance imaging techniques. *J. Cereb. Blood Flow Metab.* **2016**, *36*, 2194–2202. [CrossRef] [PubMed]
24. Ma, H.; Guo, Z.N.; Jin, H.; Yan, X.; Liu, J.; Lv, S.; Zhang, P.; Sun, X.; Yang, Y. Preliminary study of dynamic cerebral autoregulation in acute ischemic stroke: Association with clinical factors. *Front Neurol.* **2018**, *9*, 1006. [CrossRef] [PubMed]
25. Novak, V.; Hu, K.; Desrochers, L.; Novak, P.; Caplan, L.; Lipsitz, L.; Selim, M. Cerebral flow velocities during daily activities depend on blood pressure in patients with chronic ischemic infarctions. *Stroke* **2010**, *41*, 61–66. [CrossRef] [PubMed]
26. Kim, Y.S.; Bogert, L.W.; Immink, R.V.; Harms, M.P.; Colier, W.N.; van Lieshout, J.J. Effects of aging on the cerebrovascular orthostatic response. *Neurobiol. Aging* **2011**, *32*, 344–353. [CrossRef] [PubMed]
27. Mehagnoul-Schipper, D.J.; Colier, W.N.; Jansen, R.W. Reproducibility of orthostatic changes in cerebral oxygenation in healthy subjects aged 70 years or older. *Clin. Physiol.* **2001**, *21*, 77–84. [CrossRef]
28. Chieregato, A.; Tanfani, A.; Compagnone, C.; Pascarella, R.; Targa, L.; Fainardi, E. Cerebral blood flow in traumatic contusions is predominantly reduced after an induced acute elevation of cerebral perfusion pressure. *Neurosurgery* **2007**, *60*, 115–123. [CrossRef]
29. Jaeger, M.; Schuhmann, M.U.; Soehle, M.; Nagel, C.; Meixensberger, J. Continuous monitoring of cerebrovascular autoregulation after subarachnoid hemorrhage by brain tissue oxygen pressure reactivity and its relation to delayed cerebral infarction. *Stroke* **2007**, *38*, 981–986. [CrossRef]
30. Gatto, R.; Hoffman, W.; Paisansathan, C.; Mantulin, W.; Gratton, E.; Charbel, F.T. Effect of age on brain oxygenation regulation during changes in position. *J. Neurosci. Methods* **2007**, *164*, 308–311. [CrossRef]
31. Wojner-Alexander, A.W.; Garami, Z.; Chernyshev, O.Y.; Alexandrov, A.V. Heads down: Flat positioning improves blood flow velocity in acute ischemic stroke. *Neurology* **2005**, *64*, 1354–1357. [CrossRef] [PubMed]
32. Wojner, A.W.; El-Mitwalli, A.; Alexandrov, A.V. Effect of head positioning on intracranial blood flow velocities in acute ischemic stroke: A pilot study. *Crit. Care Nurs. Q.* **2002**, *24*, 57–66. [CrossRef] [PubMed]
33. Hunter, A.J.; Snodgrass, S.J.; Quain, D.; Parsons, M.W.; Levi, C.R. Hoboe (head-of-bed optimization of elevation) study: Association of higher angle with reduced cerebral blood flow velocity in acute ischemic stroke. *Phys. Ther.* **2011**, *91*, 1503–1512. [CrossRef] [PubMed]

34. Bevers, M.B.; Kimberly, W.T. Critical care management of acute ischemic stroke. *Curr. Treat. Options Cardiovasc. Med.* **2017**, *19*, 41. [CrossRef]
35. Boujan, T.; Neuberger, U.; Pfaff, J.; Nagel, S.; Herweh, C.; Bendszus, M.; Mohlenbruch, M.A. Value of contrast-enhanced mra versus time-of-flight mra in acute ischemic stroke mri. *AJNR Am. J. Neuroradiol.* **2018**, *39*, 1710–1716. [CrossRef]
36. Bang, O.Y.; Goyal, M.; Liebeskind, D.S. Collateral circulation in ischemic stroke: Assessment tools and therapeutic strategies. *Stroke* **2015**, *46*, 3302–3309. [CrossRef]
37. Markus, H.S. Cerebral perfusion and stroke. *J. Neurol. Neurosurg. Psychiatry* **2004**, *75*, 353–361. [CrossRef]
38. Dohmen, C.; Bosche, B.; Graf, R.; Reithmeier, T.; Ernestus, R.I.; Brinker, G.; Sobesky, J.; Heiss, W.D. Identification and clinical impact of impaired cerebrovascular autoregulation in patients with malignant middle cerebral artery infarction. *Stroke* **2007**, *38*, 56–61. [CrossRef]
39. Aaslid, R.; Lindegaard, K.F.; Sorteberg, W.; Nornes, H. Cerebral autoregulation dynamics in humans. *Stroke* **1989**, *20*, 45–52. [CrossRef]
40. Czosnyka, M.; Smielewski, P.; Kirkpatrick, P.; Menon, D.K.; Pickard, J.D. Monitoring of cerebral autoregulation in head-injured patients. *Stroke* **1996**, *27*, 1829–1834. [CrossRef]
41. Steiner, L.A.; Pfister, D.; Strebel, S.P.; Radolovich, D.; Smielewski, P.; Czosnyka, M. Near-infrared spectroscopy can monitor dynamic cerebral autoregulation in adults. *Neurocrit. Care* **2009**, *10*, 122–128. [CrossRef] [PubMed]
42. Brady, K.M.; Lee, J.K.; Kibler, K.K.; Smielewski, P.; Czosnyka, M.; Easley, R.B.; Koehler, R.C.; Shaffner, D.H. Continuous time-domain analysis of cerebrovascular autoregulation using near-infrared spectroscopy. *Stroke* **2007**, *38*, 2818–2825. [CrossRef] [PubMed]
43. Brady, K.; Joshi, B.; Zweifel, C.; Smielewski, P.; Czosnyka, M.; Easley, R.B.; Hogue, C.W., Jr. Real-time continuous monitoring of cerebral blood flow autoregulation using near-infrared spectroscopy in patients undergoing cardiopulmonary bypass. *Stroke* **2010**, *41*, 1951–1956. [CrossRef]
44. Moerman, A.; De Hert, S. Recent advances in cerebral oximetry. Assessment of cerebral autoregulation with near-infrared spectroscopy: Myth or reality? *F1000Res* **2017**, *6*, 1615. [CrossRef]
45. Rivera-Lara, L.; Geocadin, R.; Zorrilla-Vaca, A.; Healy, R.; Radzik, B.R.; Palmisano, C.; Mirski, M.; Ziai, W.C.; Hogue, C. Validation of near-infrared spectroscopy for monitoring cerebral autoregulation in comatose patients. *Neurocrit. Care* **2017**, *27*, 362–369. [CrossRef] [PubMed]
46. Rostrup, E.; Law, I.; Pott, F.; Ide, K.; Knudsen, G.M. Cerebral hemodynamics measured with simultaneous pet and near-infrared spectroscopy in humans. *Brain Res.* **2002**, *954*, 183–193. [CrossRef]
47. Claassen, J.A.; Colier, W.N.; Jansen, R.W. Reproducibility of cerebral blood volume measurements by near infrared spectroscopy in 16 healthy elderly subjects. *Physiol. Meas.* **2006**, *27*, 255–264. [CrossRef]
48. Rasmussen, P.; Dawson, E.A.; Nybo, L.; van Lieshout, J.J.; Secher, N.H.; Gjedde, A. Capillary-oxygenation-level-dependent near-infrared spectrometry in frontal lobe of humans. *J. Cereb. Blood Flow Metab.* **2007**, *27*, 1082–1093. [CrossRef]
49. Xiong, L.; Tian, G.; Lin, W.; Wang, W.; Wang, L.; Leung, T.; Mok, V.; Liu, J.; Chen, X.; Wong, K.S. Is dynamic cerebral autoregulation bilaterally impaired after unilateral acute ischemic stroke? *J. Stroke Cerebrovasc. Dis.* **2017**, *26*, 1081–1087. [CrossRef]
50. Lam, M.Y.; Haunton, V.J.; Robinson, T.G.; Panerai, R.B. Does gradual change in head positioning affect cerebrovascular physiology? *Physiol. Rep.* **2018**. [CrossRef]
51. Kety, S.S.; Schmidt, C.F. The effects of altered arterial tensions of carbon dioxide and oxygen on cerebral blood flow and cerebral oxygen consumption of normal young men. *J. Clin. Invest.* **1948**, *27*, 484–492. [CrossRef] [PubMed]
52. Reivich, M. Arterial pco2 and cerebral hemodynamics. *Am. J. Physiol.* **1964**, *206*, 25–35. [CrossRef] [PubMed]

6

A Mechanistic and Pathophysiological Approach for Stroke Associated with Drugs of Abuse

Aristides Tsatsakis [1,†], Anca Oana Docea [2,*,†], Daniela Calina [3,*,†], Konstantinos Tsarouhas [4,†], Laura-Maria Zamfira [3], Radu Mitrut [5,6], Javad Sharifi-Rad [7], Leda Kovatsi [8], Vasileios Siokas [9], Efthimios Dardiotis [9], Nikolaos Drakoulis [10], George Lazopoulos [11], Christina Tsitsimpikou [12], Panayiotis Mitsias [13,14] and Monica Neagu [15,16,*]

1 Center of Toxicology Science & Research, Medical School, University of Crete, 71003 Heraklion, Crete, Greece
2 Department of Toxicology, University of Medicine and Pharmacy of Craiova, 200349 Craiova, Romania
3 Department of Clinical Pharmacy, University of Medicine and Pharmacy of Craiova, 200349 Craiova, Romania
4 Department of Cardiology, University Hospital of Larissa, 41221 Larissa, Greece
5 Department of Pathology, University of Medicine and Pharmacy of Craiova, 200349 Craiova, Romania
6 Department of Cardiology, University and Emergency Hospital, 050098 Bucharest, Romania
7 Zabol Medicinal Plants Research Center, Zabol University of Medical Sciences, Zabol 61615-585, Iran
8 Laboratory of Forensic Medicine and Toxicology, School of Medicine, Aristotle University of Thessaloniki, 54248 Thessaloniki, Greece
9 Department of Neurology, Stroke Unit, University of Thessaly, University Hospital of Larissa, 41221 Larissa, Greece
10 Research Group of Clinical Pharmacology and Pharmacogenomics, Faculty of Pharmacy, School of Health Sciences, National and Kapodistrian University of Athens, 15771 Athens, Greece
11 Department of Cardiothoracic Surgery, University General Hospital of Heraklion, University of Crete, Medical School, 71003 Heraklion, Crete, Greece
12 Department of Hazardous Substances, Mixtures and Articles, General Chemical State Laboratory of Greece, 10431 Athens, Greece
13 Department of Neurology, School of Medicine, University of Crete, 71003 Heraklion, Greece
14 Comprehensive Stroke Center and Department of Neurology, Henry Ford Hospital, Detroit, MI 48202, USA
15 Department of Immunology, Victor Babes National Institute of Pathology, 050096 Bucharest, Romania
16 Department of Pathology, Colentina Clinical Hospital, 021183 Bucharest, Romania
* Correspondence: ancadocea@gmail.com (A.O.D.); calinadaniela@gmail.com (D.C.); neagu.monica@gmail.com (M.N.)
† These authors contributed to this paper equally.

Abstract: Drugs of abuse are associated with stroke, especially in young individuals. The major classes of drugs linked to stroke are cocaine, amphetamines, heroin, morphine, cannabis, and new synthetic cannabinoids, along with androgenic anabolic steroids (AASs). Both ischemic and hemorrhagic stroke have been reported due to drug abuse. Several common mechanisms have been identified, such as arrhythmias and cardioembolism, hypoxia, vascular toxicity, vascular spasm and effects on the thrombotic mechanism, as causes for ischemic stroke. For hemorrhagic stroke, acute hypertension, aneurysm formation/rupture and angiitis-like changes have been implicated. In AAS abuse, the effect of blood pressure is rather substance specific, whereas increased erythropoiesis usually leads to thromboembolism. Transient vasospasm, caused by synthetic cannabinoids, could lead to ischemic stroke. Opiates often cause infective endocarditis, resulting in ischemic stroke and hypereosinophilia accompanied by pyogenic arthritis, provoking hemorrhagic stroke. Genetic variants are linked to increased risk for stroke in cocaine abuse. The fact that case reports on cannabis-induced stroke usually refer to the young population is very alarming.

Keywords: stroke; amphetamines; cocaine; cannabis; morphine; heroin; synthetic cannabinoids; anabolic androgenic steroids

1. Introduction

1.1. Stroke Definitions

According to the World Health Organization, a stroke is defined as 'a clinical syndrome consisting of rapidly developing clinical signs of focal (or global in case of coma) disturbance of cerebral function lasting more than 24 h or leading to death with no apparent cause other than a vascular origin'. On the other hand, a transient ischemic attack (TIA) presents the signs and symptoms of a stroke, but without tissue damage and the symptoms usually resolve within 24 h [1,2]. A stroke can be defined as a rupture or blockage of an artery of the brain, which results in bleeding into the brain parenchyma or in decreased blood supply and ischemic damage to specific brain areas respectively [3].

1.2. Epidemiology of Illicit Drugs of Abuse Use and Stroke

The use of psychoactive substances has been known for thousands of years: From the ingestion of plant derivatives, such as the mushroom *Psilocybe hispanica* used in religious rituals performed 6000 years ago, to the abuse of synthetic drugs, such as heroin that was first synthesized in 1874 by C. R. Alder Wright, an English chemist working at St. Mary's Hospital Medical School in London. Nowadays, substance abuse constitutes a major social and medical problem. According to the World Drug Report 2017, issued by the United Nations Office on Drugs and Crime, the number of estimated drug users worldwide has increased by 23% in 11 years, reaching 255 million individuals in 2015. At the same time, drug users with various health disorders, such as lung or heart disease, mental health diseases, infectious diseases, stroke and cancer, reached 29.5 million in 2015, with an increase of 13.5% compared to 2006. The number of deaths attributed to drug abuse has also significantly increased. Out of the total registered deaths due to drug abuse, 67.5% are attributed to amphetamine use, 49.7% to cocaine, 29.6% to opioids and the remaining 23% to other drugs [4].

Stroke is the second leading cause of death in the world, responsible for 5.7 million deaths every year, which is expected to reach approximately 7.8 million by 2030 [5–8]. Moreover, stroke is the leading cause of major disability. A timely diagnosis by computed tomography (CT) and, depending on the circumstances, by CT angiography and CT perfusion is necessary to assure effective management [3,7].

1.3. Classic Concept of Stroke Pathophysiology

A stroke occurs when blood circulation of the brain is disturbed. There are two types of strokes: Ischemic stroke/transient ischemic attack (TIA) and hemorrhagic stroke. Brain tissue destruction is caused by different mechanisms with multifactorial character in the two types of strokes.

Ischemic stroke represents the loss of brain function caused by a decreased blood flow and consequently reduced oxygen supply to the affected brain tissue [9].

The knowledge of the latest physiopathological mechanisms in ischemic stroke is important for the development of new pharmacotherapies. Recent experimental studies in mice with transient middle cerebral artery occlusion (tMCAO) have shown the involvement of the Von Willebrandt factor (vWF) which interacts with and binds to the GPI platelet glycoprotein and the collagen receptor GP VI [10]. This vWF–GPIb axis combined with activated coagulation factor XII triggers the thrombo-inflammatory cascade in acute ischemic stroke [10,11]. In this thrombo-inflammatory process, platelets interact with T cells, which aggravate ischemia-reperfusion injury after recanalization [10,11]. However, targeting stroke-related neuroinflammation with anti-inflammatory drugs may be used with caution in order to detect any potential adverse effects to be avoided [11].

Numerous other pathophysiological studies performed on patients with ischemic stroke demonstrated hemostatic abnormalities such as low serum levels of coagulation factor VII, FVII-activated antithrombin complex, tissue factor and increased serum levels of tissue factor-bearing microparticles (MPs-TF) [12,13].

In hemorrhagic stroke the neuronal injury is supplemented by the compressive effect exerted by the hematoma, the systemic inflammatory response, the neuronal toxicity of the hemoglobin and the effect thrombolysis inside the intracerebral thrombus [14,15].

A key role in controlling stroke mortality lies in controlling the so-called modifiable stroke risk factors [3]. There are several risk factors for stroke including age, gender, hypertension, diabetes mellitus, dyslipidemia, atheromatosis, thrombophilia, atrial fibrillation, sick sinus syndrome, patent foramen ovale or family history of cardiovascular events, hyperhomocysteinemia as well as lifestyle habits, such as low physical activity, obesity, tobacco smoking, poor diet, and alcohol consumption [3,5,6,8,16–18]. Controlling blood pressure and blood glucose levels, using statins for elevated blood lipid levels and reducing the use of oral contraceptives, along with lifestyle changes, can drastically reduce the risk for stroke [5].

Drugs of abuse are also associated with stroke, especially in younger individuals. It has been shown that drug users, between 15 and 44 years old, were 6.5 times more likely to have a stroke compared with non-users [19]. The major classes of drugs linked to stroke are cocaine, amphetamines, heroin, morphine, cannabis, and the new synthetic cannabinoids, along with androgenic anabolic steroids, which are widely used both by professional and recreational athletes but also by the general public.

This article aims to review epidemiological evidence related to drug abuse-associated stroke and elucidate the possible underlying mechanisms of stroke induced by different classes of drugs of abuse.

2. Stroke Linked to Illicit Drugs of Abuse

In general, drugs of abuse can provoke stroke either by causing direct damage to cerebral vessels or indirectly, by affecting other organs, such as the liver (affecting blood coagulation pathways) or the heart, thus negatively affecting cerebral circulation [20,21]. There are substance-specific mechanisms involved. For example, stimulants such as amphetamines, cocaine and their derivatives are associated with both types of stroke, acute ischemic (cerebral infarcts) and hemorrhagic (intracerebral hemorrhages, subarachnoid hemorrhages), where the involved mechanisms differ [21,22].

The increase in blood pressure, caused by stimulants, could lead to a cerebral vessel rupture or aneurysm rupture and a subsequent hemorrhagic stroke. On the other hand, acute ischemic stroke can be attributed to stimulant-induced cerebral vasoconstriction, which reduces blood flow, promotes platelet aggregation and accelerates atherosclerosis and cardiac disturbances [21].

The pathophysiology of stroke, related to drugs of abuse, will be discussed hereafter separately for each class identified.

2.1. *Amphetamines and Amphetamine Derivatives*

Amphetamines are weak bases, chemically similar to natural neurotransmitters, adrenaline, and dopamine. They are synthetic sympathomimetics, which are used as mental stimulants. Their use has increased significantly, mainly because of the euphoria they induce [23]. Amphetamine derivatives include 3,4-methylenedioxymeth-amphetamine (MDMA), N-ethyl-3,4-methylenedioxyamphetamine (MDEA), 3,4-methylenedioxy-amphetamine (MDA) and methylenedioxymethylpropyl-amphetamine (MDMPA).

2.1.1. Mechanisms of Actions of Amphetamines and Amphetamine Derivatives

All amphetamines are rapidly absorbed when taken orally and even faster when they are smoked, chewed or injected [24]. Tolerance develops to standard and designer amphetamines, leading to the need to increase the dose by the consumer. Classical amphetamines, dextroamphetamine, methamphetamine and methylphenidate produce their primary effects through the release of catecholamines, especially dopamine, in the brain [24,25].

These effects are particularly strong in the brain areas associated with pleasure, especially in the cerebral cortex and limbic system. The effect of this pathway is probably responsible for the amphetamine addiction [24]. Catecholamines are similar to natural body compounds and act as neurotransmitters in the central nervous system [25]. Dopamine, an intermediate derived from epinephrine and norepinephrine biosynthesis is one of these compounds [26]. "Designer amphetamines", especially Ecstasy, cause the release of catecholamines, dopamine and norepinephrine, in addition to serotonin, a neurotransmitter that produces hallucinogens effects [27].

The main effects of amphetamines are euphoria, increased productivity and motor movements and decreased appetite. In chronic users, amphetamines create tolerance, addiction, and craving [28].

2.1.2. Influence of Amphetamines and Amphetamine Derivatives on Stroke

Amphetamines, which were initially used to increase intellectual performance and weight loss, are associated with both types of stroke [29–31].

There is also limited evidence that links a delayed ischemic stroke with amphetamine use, such as the case of a 19-year-old woman who developed right occipital infarction 3 months after methamphetamine use [32]. The mechanism involved in triggering delayed ischemic stroke remains unknown but it seems to be associated with chronic vasculitis [32,33].

Intracranial hemorrhage, following amphetamine abuse, is associated with a transient increase in blood pressure [34]. High blood pressure and vasoconstriction may also occur after consuming the so-called "diet pills" containing the amphetamine-like substance [31,35].

An in vivo study on mice revealed that even a single, acute exposure to methamphetamine can induce a biphasic effect in cerebral blood flow: An initial transient increase, followed by a prolonged decrease, 30 min after exposure, that induces vasoconstriction of pial arterioles [36]. Moreover, stroke may be attributed to the direct toxic effect of amphetamines on cerebral vessels, causing necrotizing vasculitis [37]. Many studies report intracranial hemorrhage following the use of amphetamines [38,39]. Figure 1 summarizes the main pathophysiological mechanisms of stroke associated with amphetamines and amphetamine derivative abuse.

2.1.3. Clinical Studies, Case Reports and Epidemiology of Stroke Related to Amphetamines and Amphetamine Derivatives abuse

Amphetamines were first used during World War II by soldiers in order to suppress fatigue. In the 1950s, the legal prescription of amphetamines in the US increased. Worldwide, there are over 35 million people who abuse amphetamines, compared to 15 million cocaine users [28]. The route of administration can be intravenous, oral, intranasal and by inhalation (smoking) [40]. The half-life is between 10 and 30 h and they are metabolized through the liver. Studies have shown that adolescents who use amphetamines have a 5-fold higher risk of stroke than those who do not use these drugs [24,41].

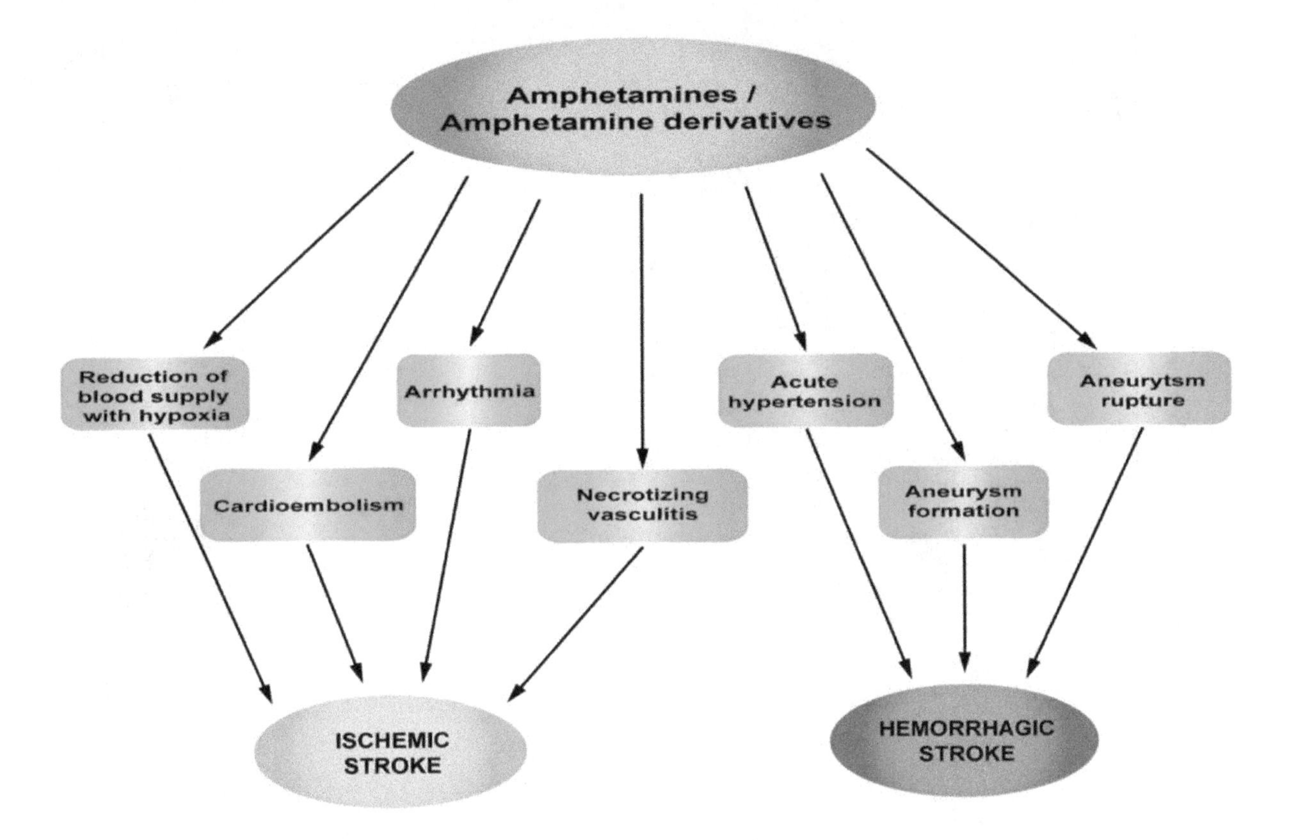

Figure 1. Pathophysiological mechanisms of stroke associated with amphetamines and amphetamine derivative abuse.

Apart from thrombosis and cerebrovascular pathology, several other side effects of amphetamines and amphetamine derivatives have been reported, including cardiomyopathy and arrhythmias, liver failure, renal failure, suicide, confusion, memory loss, psychosis and premature mortality [40]. The risk of stroke is four times higher in amphetamine users than in nonusers and the hemorrhagic stroke may occur twice as often, as in the case of cocaine users [29]. Although it is less frequent compared to amphetamine-associated hemorrhagic stroke, amphetamine-associated ischemic stroke is also described in the literature (Table 1). De Silva reported the case of a 30-year-old woman who developed acute left middle cerebral artery infarction after acute intake of amphetamine [33]. Christensen et al. reported the case of a 33-year-old Caucasian male addicted to amphetamines who died due to bilateral cerebral infarction [42]. In the past, it was believed that amphetamine derivatives were a safer option compared with other stimulants, because it was thought that intracranial hemorrhages occurred only in combination with other stimulant drugs [39]. However, it was later shown that a clear association exists between intracerebral hemorrhage in young people, without comorbidities, and amphetamine, methamphetamine or their derivative intake [43–45]. The most interesting and recent studies that report amphetamine-associated hemorrhagic stroke and amphetamine-associated ischemic stroke are summarized in Table 1.

Table 1. Characteristic case reports that associate amphetamines and amphetamine derivatives abuse with stroke.

Subject/Age	Substance Exposure	Symptoms	Diagnostic Approach	Diagnosis	Intervention	Evolution	Reference
Female, 23, no previous medical history	Took 4-fluoroamphetamine 4 h before, concomitant use of cannabis 7 h before	Collapsed at a dance event, no neurological deficits, sleepy and headache, decreased consciousness 1.5 h later, weakness of the right arm and leg	Plain computed tomography scan (computed tomography (CT) scan); CT angiography	Intracerebral hemorrhage in the left hemisphere; dilated non-responsive right pupil (false localizing sign)	Acute neurosurgical intervention: Hematoma evacuation, removal of the bone flap due to persistent intraoperative brain swelling	Right-sided hemiparalysis and severe aphasia. Replacement of the autologous bone graft after 4 months without complications. Able to talk in her native language and walk with supportive measures	[44]
Female,23, no medical history	Took 110 mg 4-fluoroamphetamine the night before, concomitant use of four units of alcohol	Severe headache, nausea, followed by vomiting 5 h after the intake, dizziness, photophobia	CT scan	Small subarachnoid hemorrhage at the right frontal side	Discharged after 24 h	Headache for weeks that gradually declined cognitive problems. Inability to work for several months	[44]
Female, 29, progressive headache and diplopia for 2 weeks, no medical history	Intravenous methamphetamine use	A 2-day history of left-sided hemiparesis and dysarthria	Cranial nerve examination, CT brain imaging without contrast medium, magnetic resonance imaging (MRI), angiogram	A 25 × 25 × 20-mm hyperdense lesion within the right cerebellopontine angle Initially thought to represent an extra-axial mass (meningioma), confirmed to be a large brainstem hemorrhage, extended from the inferior midbrain to the pontomedullary junction	Transferred to rehabilitation	Deterioration of left hemiparesis, dysarthria and dysphagia after 1 month. No underlying vascular abnormality observed	[45]
Male, Caucasian, 53, history of head and neck squamous cell carcinoma post-surgery and radiation (13 years before), hypothyroidism, hyperlipidemia, gastrointestinal reflux disease	Treatment for Attention Deficit Hyperactivity Disorder (ADHD) with mixed amphetamine salts, starting 5 mg/day to 15 mg/day over 4 months	Posterior headache with left-face numbness, diplopia 2.5 months after last dosing scheme	Head CT without contrast agent; MRI; transthoracic echocardiogram	Right posterior paramedian midbrain hematoma with cerebral aqueduct effacement and mild ventriculomegaly. No hypertension, arteriovenous malformation, cavernous malformation, or aneurysms	-	-	[46]
Male, 31	Amphetamine abuse	-	Transcranial color-coded Doppler sonography; angiography	Intracerebral hemorrhage, diffuse cerebral vasospasm	Surgical removal of intracerebral hemorrhage, pharmaceutical treatment	-	[47]

Table 1. *Cont.*

Subject/Age	Substance Exposure	Symptoms	Diagnostic Approach	Diagnosis	Intervention	Evolution	Reference
Male, African-American, 20	Took 3,4-methylenedioxymeth-amphetamine (MDMA), concomitant use of marijuana and beer	Non-verbal, vomiting and aphasic upon presentation, no sign of trauma, 18 h after ingestion developed right-sided weakness, left-sided facial droop and bilateral hyperreflexia in the lower extremities	MRI; carotid ultrasound; magnetic resonance angiogram of the brain	Left middle cerebral artery complete infarction, no significant stenosis, mild to moderate stenosis observed on the distal left internal carotid artery	Transferred to rehabilitation	-	[48]
Female, 36, history of migraine	Methamphetamine use, concomitant use of oral contraceptives	Sudden onset of speech difficulty and right-sided weakness	Head CT; MRI of the brain; MR angiography	Small infarct in the left frontal lobe, focal narrowing in the left internal carotid artery	Pharmaceutical treatment: IV heparin, discharged on warfarin 5 days after stroke; after 8 months, warfarin was replaced with aspirin 81 mg/day	Recovered after 4 months with only mild expressive aphasia	[49]
Female, 29	History of methamphetamine use for 10 years	Sudden right-sided weakness and speech difficulty 4 days after last use of methamphetamine	Head CT, MRI, MR angiography	Large left middle cerebral artery (MCA) infarct, MCA infarct with hemorrhagic transformation	Discharged after 4 days on aspirin treatment, on day 5th showed worsening deficit, hospitalized; stent-assisted transformation applied	Recovered only with moderate expression aphasia and mild right-hand weakness within 4 months	[49]
Male,31	Methamphetamine ingestion approximately 0.25 and 0.5 g Urine screen positive also for tetrahydrocannabinol (THC)	Severe headache, nausea, vomiting, left-side of the body felt numb, slurred speech, died the next day	Autopsy	Cerebral edema, subarachnoid hemorrhage over the cerebral convexities bilaterally, intracerebral hemorrhage lateral to the basal ganglia extending to involve the lateral aspect of the putamen, external capsule claustrum, insula, and superior longitudinal fasciculus of the right cerebral hemisphere (3.5 cm by 4.5 cm) No evidence of inflammation or vasculitis		Death	[38]

Table 1. *Cont.*

Subject/Age	Substance Exposure	Symptoms	Diagnostic Approach	Diagnosis	Intervention	Evolution	Reference
Male, Caucasian, 33, amphetamine addict	Amphetamine and methamphetamine ingestion. Low concentrations of methadone and codeine in the blood	Bilateral cerebral infarction associated with multi-organ failure	CT scan, autopsy	Extensive infarction of both cerebral hemispheres; symmetrical necrosis of the white matter of both cerebral hemispheres in the autopsy		Died 19 days after hospital admission	[42]
Female, 30, no significant medical history, non-smoker, very light alcohol consumer	Ecstasy ingestion one night before the presentation	Right-sided weakness, global aphasia, right neglect, and right hemiparesis	Brain CT scan; ultrasound of the extracranial carotid arteries; transcranial color-coded Doppler (TCCD); MRI	Left parietal hypodensity consistent with left middle cerebral artery (MCA) infarction; irregularity of the left MCA	Aspirin 100 mg/day	TCCD studies showed normal velocities in the MCA 3 months after onset	[33]
Female, 19, duodenal ulcer at 16, no other medical history, no family history of stroke	Methamphetamine intravenously four times over 2 months, wash-out for 3 months, concomitant use of cigarettes and alcohol	Severe right-sided headache, blurred vision on the left side and numbness of the left arm and leg upon admission, severe headache every time associated with use	Brain CT, MRI and magnetic resonance angiography	Right occipital infarction, segmental narrowing of the right posterior cerebral artery with characteristics of vasculitis	Discharged one week after admission	The right occipital infarction faded with mild atrophy, left superior quadrant hemianopia remained and had persistent headaches 4 months later	[32]

2.2. Cocaine

Cocaine, also known as benzoylmethylecgonine, is extracted from the leaves of the *Erythroxylum coca* shrub, which usually grows in Peru, Bolivia, and Ecuador [50]. In the past, the leaves of this plant were chewed or sucked in order to decrease hunger or obtain euphoric effect. Its use increased after the 1970s. After 2007, cocaine has become one of the most abused drugs, regularly used by five million Americans [50]. Cocaine has two chemical forms: Cocaine hydrochloride and alkaloidal cocaine [50]. Cocaine hydrochloride is water soluble and is readily absorbed after nasal administration [50]. Alkaloidal cocaine is lipid soluble and is a free base. It is synthesized by mixing cocaine hydrochloride with water and ammonia. Another form is produced by mixing cocaine hydrochloride with sodium bicarbonate, known as 'crack cocaine' in street language.

2.2.1. The Mechanism of Action of Cocaine

The main mechanism of action of cocaine is the blockage of noradrenaline reuptake [51]. The side effect is increased norepinephrine release. These effects act synergistically to increase the level of norepinephrine in the nerve endings. Cocaine also causes moderate release and blocking the reuptake of serotonin and dopamine [51]. It is a local anesthetic with effects caused by the blocking of the sodium channels, which determines the inhibition of nerve conduction by decreasing the amplitude of the action potential of the membranes but increasing its duration. Cocaine also blocks the potassium channels and, in some cells, it also blocks the sodium–calcium pump [52]. The drug is soluble in lipids and, therefore, crosses the blood–brain barrier. Cocaine stimulates the central nervous system, especially the limbic system where it potentiates dopaminergic transmission in the basal ventral nuclei, producing the sensation of pleasure, which has led to its widespread use [52]. Cocaine substitutes dopamine, the neurotransmitter involved in mood management [53]. Cocaine use is associated with myocardial infarction, vasoconstriction, chronic uncontrolled hypertension, nervous system stimulation and stroke [53]. Cocaine is associated with vascular toxicity. Various mechanisms are involved, such as hypertension, disturbance of platelet aggregation and homeostasis, effects on cerebral blood flow, and thromboembolism [54].

2.2.2. Influence of Cocaine on Stroke

The risk of stroke is twice as high in cocaine users, compared to age-matched non-users [29,54].

Ischemic stroke related to cocaine is associated with large vessel atherosclerosis, advanced atherosclerosis of intracranial vessels, increased platelet activation and arrhythmias, especially bradyarrhythmias, which can be explained by the ability of cocaine to depress sinus node automaticity and to block the atrioventricular node conduction [53,55].

Although it is well documented that cocaine can cause cerebral ischemia, researchers could not explain the exact mechanism. Cerebral vasospasm is attributed to the sympathomimetic effect of cocaine and the increase in circulating endothelin-1 [56]. Endothelin-1 is a vasoconstrictor protein produced by vascular endothelial cells. When elevated, it leads to nitric oxide decrease and vasoconstriction. In addition, cocaine effects on vasoconstriction are also related to elevated calcium in the vessels [57]. Other causes of stroke, related to acute cocaine use, cervicocephalic or intracranial arterial dissection are additional causes of stroke related to acute cocaine use [53]. A study by You et al. revealed that cocaine can cause a stroke by reducing blood flow to the brain. The researchers visualized exactly what happens in the brain when it is exposed to cocaine. Using quantitative laser-based visualization, it was possible to see exactly how cocaine affects small blood vessels in the brains of mice. Following 30 days of exposure to cocaine (by injection), or even after several injections performed at different time points with short intervals between them, a drastic reduction in blood circulation could be demonstrated. It was shown that in some vessels, cocaine induced micro-ischemia, a state in which blood flow to the brain is not adequate and cerebral hypoxia and ischemic stroke occur. These findings could help physicians to improve neurosurgical techniques and develop more effective methods for treating cocaine users [58].

In a large cohort study on cocaine-related stroke, during a period of 10 years, atherosclerosis of large vessels was found to be the common mechanism of stroke [59]. Cocaine use creates an elevated immune system inflammatory state. Various basal anti-inflammatory markers, like interleukin-10 (IL 10) have been found to be decreased, while pro-inflammatory cytokines (tumor necrosis factor alpha, Interleukin 1β) are increased, thus contributing to vascular disease [60,61].

Acute cocaine use induces acute hypertension, which is implicated in the occurrence of hemorrhagic stroke in users. The implication of cocaine in aneurysm formation and rupture is supported by the high incidence of aneurysmal subarachnoid hemorrhage (SAH) in cocaine users. Only less than half of them have a family history of hypertension [59].

Figure 2 summarizes the main pathophysiological mechanisms of stroke associated with cocaine abuse.

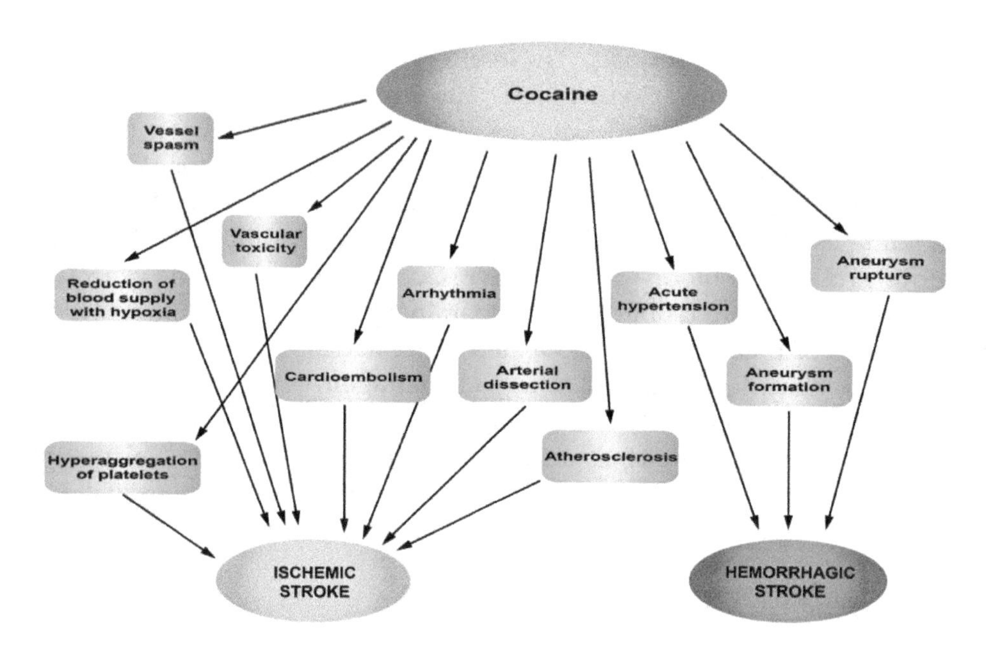

Figure 2. Pathophysiological mechanisms of stroke associated with cocaine abuse.

2.2.3. Clinical Studies, Case Reports and Epidemiology of Stroke Related to Cocaine Abuse

In order to evaluate the net effect of cocaine abuse on stroke risk, co-triggers, predictors, and co-morbidities of stroke (and other vascular diseases) should be taken into account [62]. Factors such as infections with human immunodeficiency virus type 1 (HIV-1) and hepatitis C virus (HCV) are of great importance [63,64]. So far, studies have supported the fact that cocaine use is prevalent in individuals infected with HIV and/or HCV, and vice versa [63–65]. Moreover, a few clinical studies suggested that cocaine abuse may increase HIV-1 viral load, and thus increase acquired immune deficiency syndrome (AIDS)-related mortality, even among patients under antiretroviral therapy (ART) [65]. In a study by Lucas et al. (2015), HIV and HCV infection were associated with carotid plaque progression. Furthermore, cocaine use was associated with higher odds of carotid plaque at baseline, suggesting that it is a risk factor for stroke [62].

Genetic variants are linked to increased risk for stroke in cocaine users. However, their precise impact on stroke risk remains unknown, as the association of the identified variants is considered relatively weak [66]. One of these genetic factors is the histone deacetylase 9 (*HDAC9*) gene, which has been associated with large vessel stroke [66,67]. *HDAC9* belongs to the family of epigenetic molecules, known as the histone deacetylases (HDACs), which are involved in the regulation of maladaptive behavioral changes induced by cocaine use [68,69]. There is evidence that overexpression of *HDAC4* (another member of this family) in the nucleus accumbens of the brain can modulate cocaine reward [69]. Moreover, the single nucleotide polymorphism (SNP) rs3791398 on *HDAC4* is associated with carotid intima–media thickness [70]. Based on the above, it is possible that carriers of particular variants on HDACs are more prone to cocaine abuse and have an inherent susceptibility for stroke.

Among 584,115 patients with stroke, identified from the data of the National Inpatient Sample of the Healthcare Cost and Utilization Project, in-hospital outcomes, mortality and comorbidities between patients with stroke following cocaine use and patients with stroke without cocaine use were compared. The results showed that in the users group, cardiovascular incidences were higher than in the non-users group, including valvular disorders (13.2% versus 9.7%, $p < 0.001$), venous thromboembolism (3.5% versus 2.6%, $p < 0.03$), vasculitis (0.9% versus 0.4%, $p < 0.003$), and sudden cardiac death (0.4% versus 0.2%, $p < 0.02$). In the users group, the incidence of epilepsy and major depression was also higher. In the non-users group, the incidence of certain risk factors for stroke (atherosclerosis, elevated cholesterol, hypertension, cardiac circulatory anomalies, diabetes, family history of stroke, paralysis, transient ischemic attack, coagulopathy, deficiency anemia, and disorders of fluid and electrolytes) was higher. Users also presented higher in-hospital mortality, while venous thromboembolism or vasospasm seemed to be connected to cocaine administration. The chronic use of cocaine seems to make users more vulnerable to stroke, but further research is necessary in order to assess cocaine-induced stroke [71].

The frequency and the route of administration seem to play an important role, when assessing the link between cocaine use and the risk of stroke. Following the acute use of cocaine, a 6.4-fold higher incidence of stroke within 24 h for users is reported, compared to those who had never used cocaine. Furthermore, acute cocaine use has also proven more detrimental compared to chronic use. In addition, smoking cocaine presents the highest risk for stroke. In 26 patients, suffering from stroke following acute cocaine use, the prominent route of administration was smoking ("crack"), while in all cases, typical risk factors for stroke, such as hypertension, myocardial infarction, hyperlipidemia, diabetes mellitus, and tobacco use, co-existed. Some patients were multidrug users (heroin and marijuana) [72]. It is rather likely that stroke can occur following cocaine use, even without other risk factors [73].

Neurovascular implications are rather common among cocaine abusers. Among 96 active or former cocaine users, 45 cases of ischemic stroke/TIA were reported, while intracerebral hemorrhage (ICH) and SAH occurred with a similar prevalence of approximately 25%. ICH and SAH were associated with active cocaine use, while ischemic stroke/TIA was more likely to occur in former cocaine users. Regarding the different forms of cocaine, crack is implicated equally in both types of strokes, while cocaine is implicated more in hemorrhagic stroke [59]. In a paper published by Martin-Schild et al., the authors compared the location, demographics, and outcome of patients with ICH. Out of 3241 patients with stroke, 132 (4.1%) were cocaine users, according to the urine drug screen, and 45 had ICH. Six of the 45 cocaine users with ICH were also using other illicit drugs (such as marijuana and amphetamines). The control group consisted of 105 non-users with ICH. The study showed that cocaine users with ICH had a male predominance and were less likely to be Hispanic (11% vs. 28%; $p = 0.022$) and more likely to be African-American (69% vs. 44%). Cocaine users had a higher median diastolic blood pressure (121 (100–126) vs. 110 (107–141)); $p = 0.024$). Furthermore, cocaine users had more severe ICH, compared to the control group. In addition, cocaine use seems to correlate with the emergence of intraventricular hemorrhage (IVH). This study also showed that cocaine users are more likely to die during their hospitalization, compared to the control group [74]. One study investigated the outcome of strokes related to cocaine abuse, compared with strokes that are not related to cocaine. They concluded that younger age and cardiac arrhythmias are associated with cocaine-related strokes. Regarding other traditional cerebrovascular risk factors, no differences were found between cocaine and non-cocaine related strokes [55].

There are several case reports on hemorrhagic or ischemic stroke after cocaine use and the most recent and interesting are presented in Table 2.

Table 2. Characteristic case reports studies that associate cocaine abuse and stroke.

Subject/Age	Substance Exposure	Symptoms	Diagnostic Approach	Diagnosis	Intervention	Evolution	Reference
Male, African American, 65, diabetes, heart diseases, hepatitis C	Smoking crack cocaine before symptom onset, admitted to intermittent cocaine abuse	Left arm pain described as feeling like "jumping out of the window"	Head CT scan; carotid ultrasound; CT angiography of head and neck	Acute 2.2-cm intraparenchymal hemorrhage that presented in the posterior right parietal lobe vasogenic edema	Send to the rehabilitation unit	Left arm pain resolved after 24 h	[75]
Female, African-American, 66, multi-substance abuser, hepatitis C, heart diseases	Urine samples positive for cocaine	Somnolent a day prior to admission, confused in the day of admission, short-term memory loss, unable to perform usual daily activities	Brain CT; CT angiogram of the head and neck; MRI of the brain associated with MR venogram	Infarction in bilateral posterior inferior cerebellar artery and hippocamp showing multifocal punctate infarcts in the basal ganglia and bilateral posterior cerebral artery secondary to severe vasoconstriction	Neurosurgery consult for possible external ventricular drain placement and posterior fossa decompression	Mental status improved during hospitalization; discharged to a rehabilitation center after 7 days with persistent problems of memory and inability to recognize faces	[76]
Male,22, hypertension and cocaine abuser	Positive for cocaine and tetrahydrocannabinol	Right hemiplegia associated with motor and sensitive aphasia	CT scan	The ischemic region in the left medial cerebral artery region with increased cerebral edema and cerebral midline displacement of 9 mm on the subfalcine region	Not suitable for surgery due to complications	Died in the hospital	[77]
Female, 39, smoker, no other risk factors for stroke	Urine screening positive for cocaine	Global aphasia, left-side total gaze paresis, 7th cranial nerve right-side partial paresis and right hemiplegia	Non-contrast brain CT	Left ischemic stroke—hyperdensity in the left middle cerebral artery (MCA); occlusion in the left and right MCA and an irregular profile of the left internal carotid artery (ICA)	Endovascular treatment, intra-arterial administration of 40 mg of recombinant tissue plasminogen activator (rtPA) associated with a self-expandable and retrievable stent	After 3 months from the event, ischemia at the left basal ganglia	[78]
Male, 31, no medical history	Positive urine screening for cocaine and negative for other drugs	Found unresponsive 6 h after excessive alcohol and intranasal cocaine abuse	MRI; intra- and extracranial CT angiography	Globus pallidus and the vascular watershed zones presents acute bilateral ischemia	-	Consciousness improved progressively; clinical improvements, but mental slowing, executive dysfunction, hypophonia, and verbal fluency deficit persisted	[79]
Female, 31, no medical history, occasional alcohol consumer and smoker	First time snorted cocaine hydrochloride associated with 500 mL of vodka	Acute onset of right hemiplegia and left hemiparesis evolving into quadriplegia	MRI	Thickened pons with focus localized in his central part on the left side (20 mm) (ischemic change)	After 17 days of hospitalization, transferred to rehabilitation	The movements of the left side of the body improved slowly and the rehabilitation continues in ambulatory	[80]

2.3. Cannabis

Cannabis is extracted from the plant *Cannabis sativa* and its varieties, *Cannabis Americana* and *Cannabis Indica*, and has two principal preparations, marijuana and hashish, which can be smoked, ingested or inhaled. Delta 9-tetrahydrocannabinol (THC) is the psychoactive cannabinoid in cannabis. Based on the THC content, potency varies in the preparations of cannabis and it is usually higher in hashish than in marijuana [81]. Cannabis substitutes anandamide, a neurotransmitter involved in mechanisms of appetite regulation, memory, reproduction and cell proliferation (the basis of tumor development).

2.3.1. The Mechanism of Action of Cannabis

The mechanism of action of THC has also been controversial. At first, it was thought that, due to the lipophilic nature, it causes the disruption of the membranes of the cell components. In the 1990s, researchers discovered cannabinoid receptors located in the brain and in the cells of the body, responsible for many of the effects of THC [82]. The molecular mechanism was initially considered nonspecific, of an anesthetic type, for which the lack of stereospecificity of the activity of delta-9-THC and also its lipophilicity was advocated [82]. The first evidence for the specific action of cannabinoids was brought by Howlett, who showed that delta-9-THC inhibits adenylate-cyclase activity in N18TG2 neuroblastoma cells cultured in vitro, and the use of a radiolabeled analogue allowed the detection of cannabinoid sites, specific in the brain [82,83].

There are two types of cannabinoid receptors (CB): CB_1 in the central nervous system and CB_2 in the immune system cells [82,84]. High densities of cannabinoid receptors are found in the frontal cortex, basal ganglia, cerebellum, and hippocampus. They are absent in the brain nuclei. The stimulation of these receptors causes the release of neurotransmitters [82]. The main effects of cannabis are relaxation, euphoria and increased self-confidence. Its side effects include cardiovascular complications, peripheral events (such as kidney infarction or peripheral arteritis) and neurological complications [82,84].

2.3.2. The Influence of Cannabis on Stroke

Cannabis causes transient cerebral ischemic attacks (TIAs) and ischemic strokes.

The possible mechanisms through which cannabis can induce stroke include cerebral vasoconstriction, hypotension, vasospasm, impaired cerebral vasomotor function and fluctuations in blood pressure [81,85]. It is possible that all the above could be attributed to the potential of cannabis to induce sympathetic stimulation and decrease parasympathetic activity [8,86]. There is currently increasing scientific interest towards the determination of the dose and duration of cannabis abuse that would lead to a stroke. In a study conducted on the National Inpatient Sample database from USA, a significant increase in symptomatic cerebral vasospasm was observed in marijuana users [87]. In a case of basal ganglia hemorrhage, reported after an increased intake of cannabis, the proposed mechanism for the pathogenesis of intracerebral hemorrhage was the capacity of cannabis to impair autoregulation and to induce transient arterial hypertension [88,89].

Regarding the mechanism by which cannabis induces thrombotic events, one should consider the fact that platelets synthesize endogenous cannabinoids, mainly the Δ 9-tetrahydrocannabinol (THC) metabolite [90]. Via CB1 and CB2 receptors, the platelet membranes are targets for exogenous cannabinoids, resulting in aggregation, which is nonreversible, at high cannabinoid levels [90,91]. Moreover, cannabinoids lead to the increased reactivation of factor VII and elevated ADP-induced aggregation in platelet-rich plasma [91]. An additional procoagulatory effect appears to be the elevated expression of glycoprotein IIb-IIIa and P selectin on the surfaces of the platelets by THC, dependent though by concentration [90]. The stimulation of the sympathetic system and the inhibition of the parasympathetic system, and the inflammatory processes at the level of at the arterial wall, have been described as other possible THC mechanisms of action, resulting to thrombus formation and endothelial erosion at both cerebral and coronary arteries [92–94]. Finally, cannabinoids can also lead to the activation, adhesion and aggregation of platelets, as a result of the decreased availability of nitric oxide, due to oxidative stress (which is induced by cannabinoids [90,91]. Figure 3 summarizes the main pathophysiological mechanisms of stroke associated with cannabis abuse.

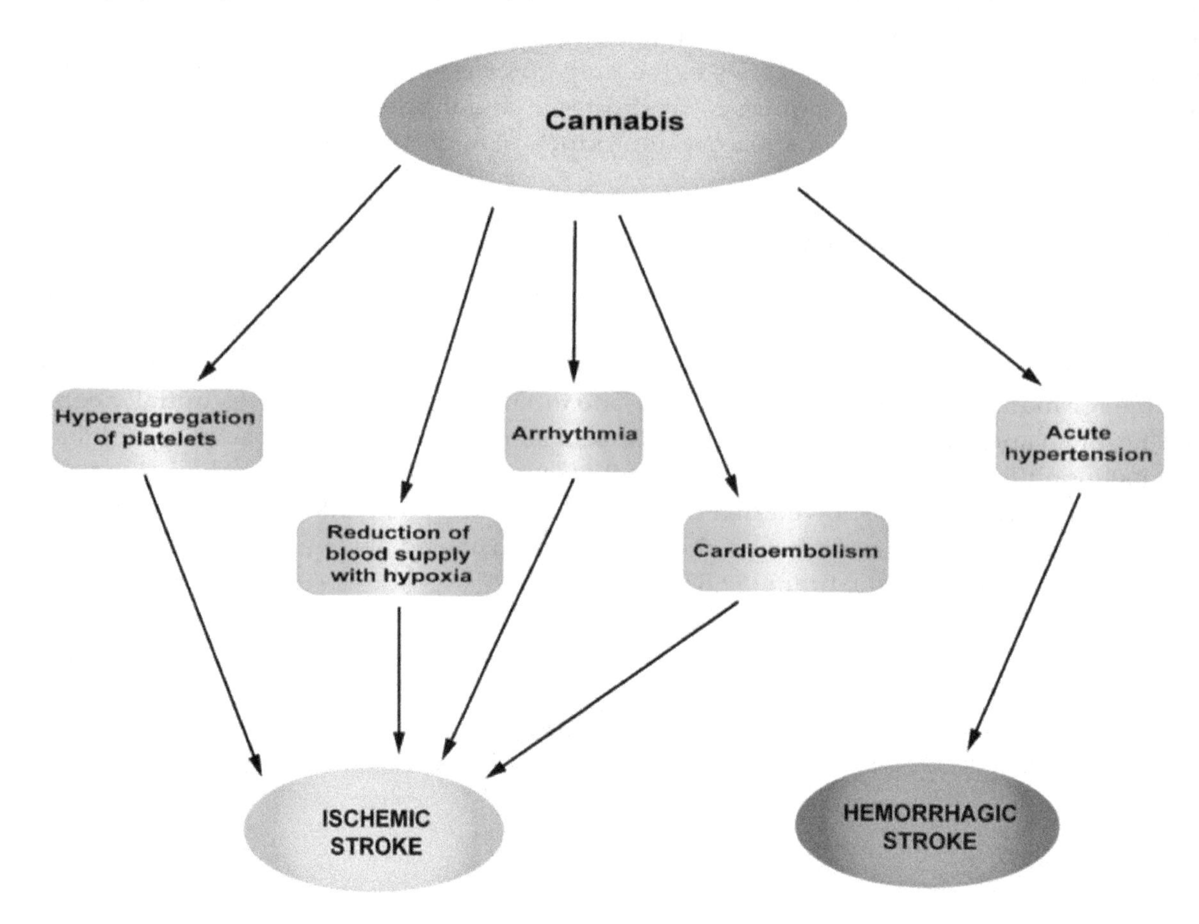

Figure 3. Main pathophysiological mechanisms of stroke associated with cannabis abuse.

2.3.3. Clinical Studies, Case Reports and Epidemiology of Stroke Related to Cannabis

The most widely used psychoactive substance in the world is cannabis, with almost 180 million annual consumers [8]. Most users believe that cannabis is a safe recreational drug. Furthermore, because of its therapeutic applications, 15 states of the US have approved it for medical use [81]. In Europe, countries such as Cyprus, Finland, Germany, Greece, Italy, Israel, Norway, Netherlands, Croatia, Czech Republic, Denmark, Georgia, Luxembourg, Malta, Poland, Portugal, San Marino, Switzerland, United Kingdom have already legalized the use of cannabis for medical purposes and other countries are in the process of legalizing it [95].

Following the chronic use of cannabis, psychological and physical dependence are encountered and the withdrawal syndrome includes sleep difficulties and anxiety [81].

In recent years, there have been several case reports, case series and studies that show a link between cerebrovascular events and cannabis use [96–98]. It seems that cannabis users are more likely to present with neurological conditions, such as multifocal intracranial arterial stenosis, reversible cerebral vasoconstriction syndrome and chronic use of cannabis can lead to increased cerebrovascular resistance. There seems to be a link between cannabis use and stroke/TIA (odds ratio, 2.30; 95% confidence intervals, 1.08–5.08) [96].

In 48 patients (under 45 years of age) admitted to hospital for ischemic stroke, cardiovascular investigations, blood tests and urine screens for cannabinoids were performed, in order to study stroke in young adults. Urine tests were positive for cannabis in 13 patients. Out of these 13 patients, 21% had a distinctive form of multifocal intracranial stenosis (MIS) and suffered from a severe headache.

In seven patients, ischemic stroke was located in the vertebrobasilar territory; in nine patients, MIS was in the posterior cerebral arteries; and in seven patients, it was located in the superior cerebellar arteries. The link between MIS and cannabis was statistically significant (odds ratio, 113 (9–5047); $p < 0.001$) [99].

Studies showed that cannabis can be related to stroke, especially in smokers. Interestingly, in a large cohort of 49,321 Swedish men, born between 1949 and 1951, who had been in the military service between 1969 and 1970, alcohol consumption, cannabis use or tobacco smoking and their association with stroke were studied. Among men who have had a stroke before 60 years of age, the risk factors were often common and included a family history of cardiovascular disease, obesity, high alcohol consumption, and tobacco smoking.

Cannabis use was associated with elevated blood pressure and was more prevalent in stroke at a younger age (< 45 years), but cannabis use alone was not reported as a risk factor for stroke in individuals younger than 45 years old [8]. Rumalla et al., conducted a study on patients between 15 and 54 years old, with a primary diagnosis of acute ischemic stroke (AIS). Data were obtained from the Nationwide Inpatient Sample, the largest inpatient database in the US.

The purpose of this study was to evaluate the correlation between marijuana use and hospitalization for AIS. The researchers identified an increased incidence of AIS in the marijuana cohort, especially in young patients, who were African American males. Multivariable analysis was applied to investigate the risk factor for the occurrence of AIS involving marijuana use alone or in combination with other risk factors. The analysis showed that marijuana use represented a significant risk factor for AIS hospitalization [87].

Cannabis use has been mainly associated with ischemic stroke. Nevertheless, more recent studies show an association between cannabis use and hemorrhagic stroke. Several recent case reports on cannabis-associated stroke are presented in Table 3. A very interesting case is that reported by Atchaneeyasakul et al., It refers to a 27-year-old man who presented right basal ganglia intracerebral hemorrhage (ICH) following the ingestion of cannabis. No vascular abnormality was observed on digital subtraction angiography (DSA) of the cerebral vasculature, CT angiography of the head, and magnetic resonance imaging (MRI) of the brain.

The toxicological tests were positive for cannabinoids, with a serum level of 9-carboxy tetrahydrocannabinol of 222 ng/mL. The patient was not diagnosed with secondary hypertension. The fact that no other risk factor for the basal ganglia hemorrhage was identified in this case supports the role of cannabis in the risk of stroke with robustness [88].

Table 3. Characteristic case reports that associate cannabis abuse with stroke.

Subject/Age	Substance Exposure	Symptoms	Diagnostic Approach	Diagnosis	Intervention	Evolution	Reference
Female, 51, asthma	Long-term cannabis user, positive urine screening for cannabis, a large amount of cannabis was consumed prior to the onset of symptoms	Left-side upper and lower extremities weakness	Head CT scan	Acute right cerebral infarct; after 30 min from arrival, developed in the left pons new hemorrhage associated with decompression on the lateral and left ventricles	Pharmaceutical treatment: Labetalol, recombinant tissue plasminogen activator	Died	[100]
Male, 27, without any known medical history	Single raw cannabis consumption (confirmed by a blood test) just before symptom onset	Sudden progressive left-sided weakness, degradation in mentation, nausea, and vomiting	Brain CT without contrast media; CT angiography; MRI of the brain	Right basal ganglia ICH measuring 32 × 24 mm with extension into the ventricles with mild hydrocephalus, no vasculature abnormality	Intubation and placement of an external ventricular drain, treatment on recombinant tissue plasminogen activator	Improvement of motor function, left hemiparesis	[88]
Female, 14, no remarkable medical history	Toxicological screening positive for cannabis 2-year history of daily cannabis use	Generalized tonic–clonic seizures	Head CT, electroencephalography (EEG); MRI	Multiple ischemic infarcts located in basal ganglia, left frontal lobe, and genu of corpus callosum, which had both chronic and acute features	After stabilization, transferred to rehabilitation	Complained of chronic headache, learning disabilities	[101]
Male, 25	Cannabis ingestion one night before Concomitant ingestion of alcohol	Drowsy, talking irrelevantly and the state degraded	Non-contrast CT of the brain; Coronary CT angiogram	Acute infarct in the right frontoparietal region	After hospitalization was discharged in a stable condition	Left-sided weakness improved	[102]
Male	Marijuana History of smoking marijuana from the age of 1	Presented with weakness of leg, arm and face associated with slurred speech 90 min after smoking marijuana Recurrence of the symptoms twice	Brain CT scan, CT angiogram and MRI	Right lentiform nucleus presents subtle hypodensity; no evidence of vasospasm, thrombus or dissection	Heparin treatment after a recurrent episode of focal neurological deficits	After 2 months, he presented residual weakness in the left arm and leg, left facial droop and spastic tone	[103]
Male, 33, smoker	Urine toxicologic screening positive for cannabis Heavy user of cannabis for 15 years	Transient left hemiparesis and dysarthria, no altered consciousness, chest pain one day before	Brain MRI and CT angiography	The presence of multi focal acute infarctions in the bilateral watershed zones between middle and anterior cerebral artery territories and the right middle cerebral artery territory. Cardioembolic stroke produced by acute myocardial infarction (likely related to cannabis use)	-	No recurrence in the following 6 months of cardiac or neurologic symptoms	[104]
Male, Caucasian French, 24, no medical history	Urine toxicology positive for cannabis; heavy cannabis use one night before admission Regular cannabis smoker for four years	Non-reactive state, with seizures	Cerebral CT scan, EEG, MRI, Doppler examination, magnetic resonance angiography, and angiography	Infarcts in the insular mantle and the lenticular and caudate nuclear structures exclude all other causes of stroke in young people	Treated in the hospital until recovery and transferred to the psychiatric department to be treated for behavioral disorders	In the following 1 and a half years, he returned on seven occasions for generalized tonic–clonic seizures	[98]
Male, 36, with no history of migraine or other known vascular risk factors	Urine toxicological screening positive for cannabis Heavy hashish consumption and alcohol before the symptoms Sporadically hashish user	An acute episode of isolated aphasia, followed by convulsive seizures	Cranial MRI and MR angiography	Had 2 acute ischemic infarcts, one on the left temporal lobe and another area of silent ischemia in the right parietal lobe	Treatment with ticlopidine	After 1 year, a new episode of aphasia and right hemiparesis immediately after hashish smoking and a new episode after 1 and a half years again after hashish use Between the two episodes, he denied consumption	[93]

2.4. *Synthetic Cannabinoids*

Synthetic cannabinoids are a new class of psychoactive chemicals, similar in pharmacological action with THC, the active component of *Cannabis sativa* [105]. Synthetic cannabinoids are not derived from cannabis. They are synthetized in the laboratory and they manifest a full agonist activity on cannabinoid receptors, in contrast to THC which is only a partial agonist [105]. They are metabolized to active metabolites that give them a higher potency compared to THC [106]. Although they are labeled "not for human consumption", they are available in the market as herbal mixtures sprayed with synthetic cannabinoids, in street language known as "spice", "K2", "herbal incense". They are used for recreational purposes and they are called "legal drugs" [106]. Their use has increased in the last years, along with concerns regarding their safety. The market of synthetic cannabinoids is growing very fast and a new compound is synthetized as soon as the previous one is classified as illegal by legislation.

2.4.1. The Mechanism of Action of the Synthetic Cannabinoids

Synthetic cannabinoids act as CB1 and CB2 cannabinoid receptor agonists, similar to tetrahydrocannabinol (THC) but they have a different chemical structure [107]. They cause agitation, anxiety, paranoia, hypertension, rarely myocardial infarction or renal failure [107].

2.4.2. The Influence of Synthetic Cannabinoids on Stroke

Synthetic cannabinoids have been associated with ischemic stroke through various case reports. Unfortunately, epidemiological studies are hard to conduct because these substances are not detected in routine toxicological screen tests [106]. Their increased potency on cannabinoid receptors, their active metabolites, and their cross-reactivity with other receptors induce a strong prothrombotic state, which, in combination with other minor risk factors for stroke, can lead to ischemic stroke [108]. Two case reports that associate AIS with synthetic cannabinoids, support the embolic etiology of stroke which is in agreement with previous reports on severe adverse cardiac events following spice use [109]. In some cases of AIS attributed to synthetic cannabinoid use, past use of cannabis was also reported. In these cases, one could question whether acute synthetic cannabinoid overdose is the actual cause of stroke, or whether chronic cannabis use is also implicated. This theory could be supported by the similarity in the structure of THC and synthetic cannabinoids, which could lead to the same mechanism of cardiovascular injury [106]. Further studies are needed to elucidate the exact mechanism.

The reported cases of hemorrhagic strokes following acute use of synthetic cannabinoids can be explained by the transient vasospasm observed immediately after use [110]. The capacity of synthetic cannabinoids to alter neurotransmitter release from nerve terminals can lead to activation of smooth muscle cells which are associated with disruption of endothelial cell function and can, therefore, lead to ischemia or hemorrhage [111].

Figure 4 summarizes the main pathophysiological mechanisms of strokes associated with synthetic cannabinoid abuse.

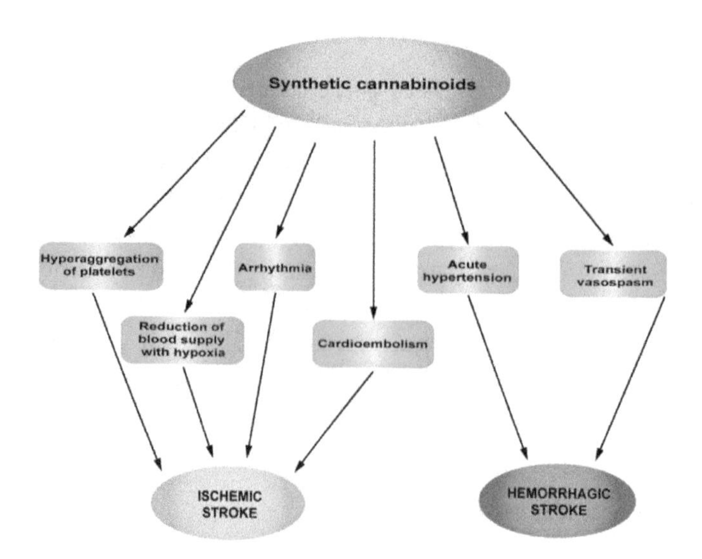

Figure 4. Main pathophysiological mechanisms of strokes associated with synthetic cannabinoid abuse.

2.4.3. Clinical Studies, Case Reports and Epidemiology of Stroke Related to Synthetic Cannabinoid Abuse

To date, only a few studies have investigated the toxic effects of synthetic cannabinoids. Case reports correlate their use with severe adverse and toxic effects, different from those observed after marijuana use. Even deaths have been reported [112].

The association of synthetic cannabinoid consumption and ischemic stroke/TIA was first reported by Bernson-Leung et al.. The group has published two cases of ischemic stroke in young people, pathologies that occurred within hours after a first-time exposure to synthetic cannabinoids. One patient was a 22-year-old woman who developed right middle cerebral artery AIS a few hours after smoking "K2" and the other patient was a 26-year-old woman who developed middle cerebral artery territory infarction after smoking "Peak Extreme". In both cases, the tests for serum vascular risk factors and hypercoagulability were negative. Both cases presented other minor risk factors for stroke: The 22-year-old woman was taking oral contraceptives and the 26-year-old woman had migraine with aura, took oral contraceptives, was an active smoker and had a family history of superficial thrombophlebitis. Even so, both were young and healthy and, most importantly, AIS occurred within a few hours after the first use of synthetic cannabinoids [113]. Another study reported two cases of middle cerebral artery location of AIS in a 26-year-old man and a 19-year-old woman immediately after smoking "spice". Both had positive urine tests for cannabinoids and they confirmed the use of synthetic cannabinoids in the past but not in the days that preceded stroke. The synthetic cannabinoid JWH-018 was found in their urine [109]. Faroqui et al. described a case of a 36-year-old African American man, without a medical history with risk factors for stroke, who showed extensive left cervical and intracranial internal carotid artery occlusion AIS after smoking "K2". He also reported smoking marijuana in the past, but not recently [114].

Only recently, there have been reports linking synthetic cannabinoids to hemorrhagic stroke. Rose et al. reported two cases of SAH after smoking "spice": A 31-year-old man, for whom the consumption of XLR-11((1-(5-fluoropentyl)-1H-indol-3-yl) (2,2,3,3-tetramethylcyclo-propyl) methanone) was confirmed, and a 25-year-old woman [110]. A summary of the main studies is presented in Table 4.

It is interesting to note that case reports on cannabis-associated stroke increased after the appearance of synthetic cannabinoids on the market. Based on the fact that synthetic cannabinoids are usually used together with cannabis and that they cannot be detected in urine through standard screening tests, further studies are needed to elucidate if cannabis is the real cause of these strokes, or whether a synergistic effect is caused by the concurrent use of cannabis and synthetic cannabinoids.

Table 4. Characteristic case reports that associate synthetic cannabinoid use with stroke.

Subject/Age	Substance Exposure	Symptoms	Diagnostic Approach	Diagnosis	Intervention	Evolution	Reference
Male, African American, 36, no history of stroke or coagulopathy or blood disorders	Reported taking K2 on the night before symptom onsetConcomitant use of marijuana in the past	Had a 1-day history of aphasia and weakness in the right side of the body	Non-contrast CT of the head; computed tomography angiography (CTA); MRI; MR angiography	A thrombotic event that lead to an acute ischemic infarct with left MCA distribution characterized by hypodensity in the left basal ganglia and a left hyperdense MCA; a large filling defect observed from the origin of the left ICA into the intracranial portions of the ICA	Aspirin, clopidogrel and enoxaparin	After 10 days, the patient was discharged for short-term rehabilitation after gradual improvement	[114]
Female, 22, in treatment with atomoxetine and estrogen-containing oral contraceptive	Smoked K2; concomitant use of THC, benzodiazepine and salicylates as they were positive at urine toxicological test	While smoking K2 presented dyspnea, palpitations and angor animi. Few hours later after smoking K2, developed dysarthria and difficulty standing	Head CT, MRI, and CT angiogram	Right middle cerebral artery AIS; proximal right M1 occlusion with distal reconstruction	Aspirin	In follow-up, presented limited ambulation and no use of her spastic left arm	[113]
Female, 26, smoker, used estrogen-containing oral contraceptive, suffering from migraine with aura	Smoked 'Peak Extreme'	The next morning after smoking drugs, presented with felt-sided numbness, left facial weakness and dysfluency	CT angiogram, MRI, and head CT	Near occlusion of the right M1 segment with extensive infarction in the middle cerebral artery territory	Warfarin	Improved speech and comprehension	[113]
Male, 33, no medical history	Smoked two "joints" of synthetic cannabinoid product 10 min prior to the onset of symptoms; urine positive also for opiates; synthetic cannabinoid XLR-11-1-(5-fl uoropentyl)-1H-indol-3-yl) (2,2,3,3-tetramethylcyclopropyl) methanone was confirmed in the product used	Right-sided weakness and aphasia	Non-contrast head CT, and electrocardiography	Acute infarction located in the left insular cortex	Aspirin	The neurological problems were completely resolved in 3 days in the hospital; no return to follow-up	[115]
Male, 26, no family history of any stroke risk factors, non-smoker, non-alcohol consumer	Smoked spice "a few hours prior" to his symptom onset; concomitant use of marijuana in the past but not recent	Weakness of right side of face and arm, dysarthria, expressive aphasia that occur suddenly	Non-contrast head CT; CT perfusion; CT angiography; MRI	Hyperdense left middle cerebral artery (MCA); a large area of penumbra without core infarction; left MCA clot	Received IV tissue plasminogen activator (t-PA)	Improved clinically and did not return to follow-up	[109]
Female, 19, smoker, anxiety disorder and panic attacks	Smoked spice; urine drug screening positive for cannabinoids and confirmed for JWH-018	A few minutes after smoking spice, the patient lost consciousness and started vomiting; mental status was persistently altered for several hours; presented with "shaking movements" of the legs and arms according to witnesses	CT angiogram and MRI	Infarctions in the left MCA with large distribution associated with punctate infarcts localized in the right cerebral hemisphere	-	She stabilized neurologically, but right hemiparesis and expressive aphasia remained at a follow-up office visit	[109]

Table 4. *Cont.*

Subject/Age	Substance Exposure	Symptoms	Diagnostic Approach	Diagnosis	Intervention	Evolution	Reference
Male, 31	Smoked spice; toxicological tests confirmed XLR-11	Generalized seizure	Head CT and digital subtraction angiography (DSA)	Hemorrhage in the bifrontal subarachnoid associated with left frontal and right parieto-occipital intraparenchymal hemorrhage	Intra-arterial verapamil	After 10 days from the event the paralysis of left leg, left homonymous hemianopsia and mentation improved	[110]
Female, 25, preeclampsia	Smoked synthetic marijuana; concomitant use of marijuana	Seizure after smoking synthetic and nonsynthetic marijuana; left leg monoplegia	CT, MRI, and DSA	SAH in the bilateral Sylvian fissures and interpeduncular and prepontine cisterns; restricted diffusion localized in the right frontal lobe, left cerebellum, left temporal lobe and bilateral parietal and occipital lobes, which is consistent with the diagnosis of multifocal AIS	Intra-arterial verapamil	Follow-up DSA showed worsening vertebrobasilar vasospasm	[110]

2.5. Opiates/Heroin

The most well-known substances belonging to the class of narcotic analgesics are morphine and heroin. Morphine is a natural substance extracted from some poppy species grown in South-East and South-West Asia, Mexico and Colombia [116]. Heroin (diacetylmorphine) is a semi-synthetic opioid drug, obtained by a chemical reaction between morphine and acetic anhydride [117]. Originally conceived as a substitute for morphine, heroin has been used in the past for the amelioration of withdrawal symptoms in alcohol-addicted individuals. Unfortunately, the synthetic drug is extremely addictive, causing both physical and psychological dependence [117].

2.5.1. The Mechanism of Action of Opiates/Heroin

Narcotic analgesics have a direct action on the vasomotor center and augment parasympathetic activity, reduce sympathetic activity and induce histamine release from mast cells [118]. These effects cause bradycardia, stimulating cardiac automatism, triggering atrial ectopic, atrial fibrillation, idioventricular rhythm or malignant ventricular arrhythmias. A complication of intravenous use is deep venous thrombosis, originating in the deep or superficial femoral vein, with the consequent risk of massive pulmonary embolism and stroke [9,119].

Morphine is rapidly absorbed and metabolized in the liver, and the main active metabolite is 6-glucuronide-morphine. It has a 2-fold increased potency compared to morphine. At the cerebral level, this metabolite has a 100-fold increased potency compared to morphine [116]. The metabolite 6-glucuronide-morphine is responsible for the analgesic action. Morphine has a plasma half-life of 2–3 h with rapid hepatic metabolism. Urinary excretion of metabolites can be detected in urine for up to 48 h (for occasional users) and for up to a few days (for chronic users) [120]. Due to the fact that heroin is more lipid soluble than morphine, it has an increased mode of action [121].

2.5.2. The Influence of Opiates/Heroin on Stroke

A proposed mechanism for heroin-associated ischemic stroke is cardioembolism.

This can occur secondary to infectious endocarditis (which is common in intravenous users), or due to other adulterants found in drugs [122]. The cardiogenic embolic effect of infectious endocarditis is further reinforced by the direct toxic effect of heroin on cerebral arteries [123]. Furthermore, post-anoxic encephalopathy and global hypoperfusion of the brain, due to heroin-induced hypotension, bradycardia, cardiopulmonary arrest, and hypoxia, can also be a possible mechanism [122,124]. Recent reports indicate that heroin-induced hypereosinophilia could be the cause of heroin-induced cerebral infarction. Heroin is known to induce hypereosinophilia in chronic users. Bolz et al. describe the case of a 29-year-old man who admitted sniffing heroin for seven years. He was diagnosed with heroin-induced hypereosinophilia and presented with multiple cerebral infarctions, without having any other cardiovascular risk factors [125]. The mechanism involved in cerebral ischemia could be associated with focal damage of the endothelium of the endocardium and of both small and larger arteries, determined by eosinophilic-associated proteins. This can be associated with increased blood clotting and local hypercoagulation, determined by components of eosinophilic granule [126]. In a study conducted in 2009, Hamzei Moqaddam et al. report that opioid dependence may be considered as an independent risk factor for stroke. The suggested underlying mechanism was that opioid dependence may increase plasma fibrinogen levels, which are known to represent a risk factor for the development of atherosclerosis in the coronary arteries, as well as in peripheral and cerebral vessels, and may, therefore, lead to heart infarctions or stroke [127].

Hemorrhagic stroke induced by heroin has also been reported. The possible pathogenic

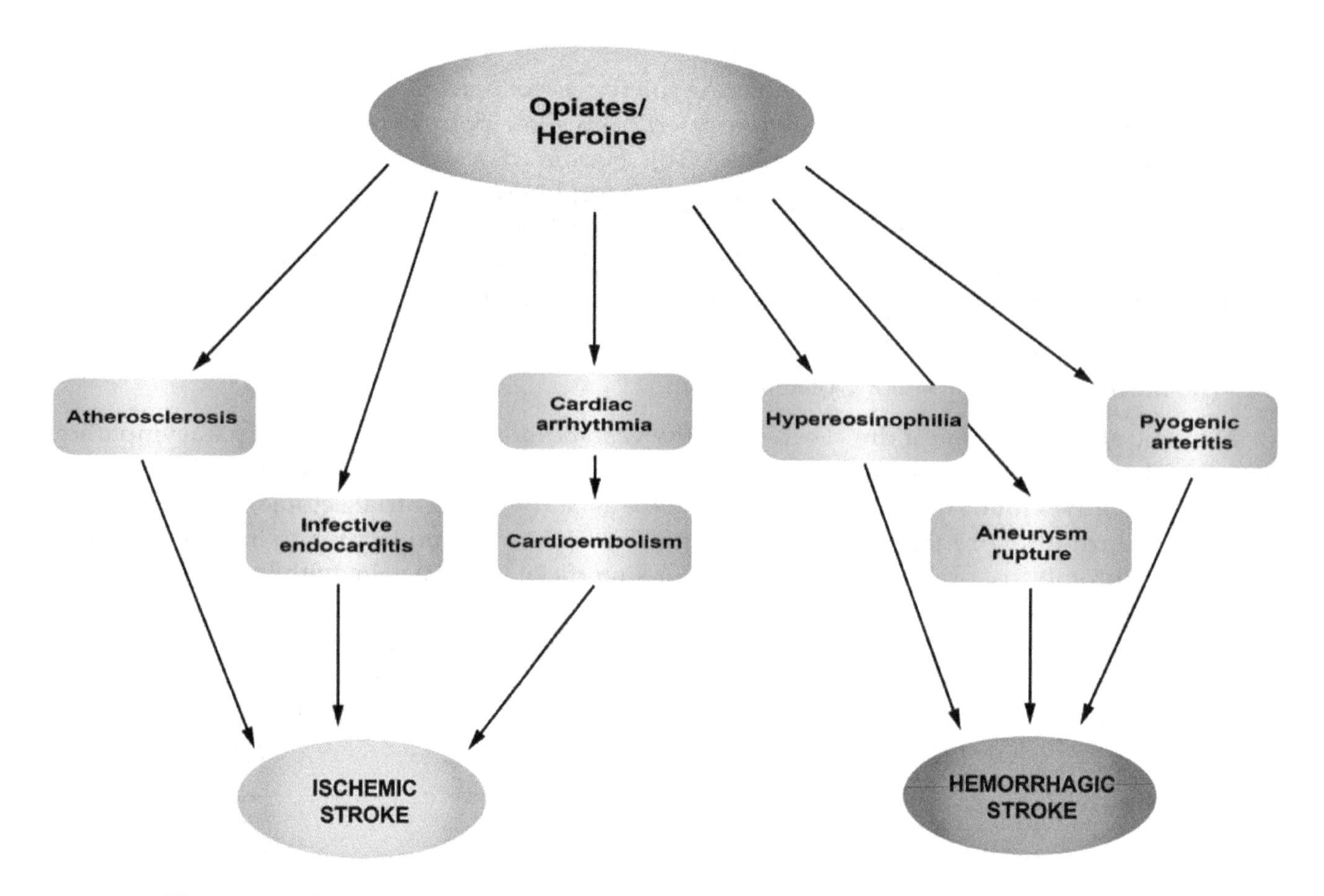

Figure 5. Pathophysiological mechanisms of stroke associated with opiate/heroin abuse.

mechanisms could be: a) the hemorrhagic transformation of ischemic infarction or a hemorrhage determined by pyogenic arteritis and b) the rupture of a mycotic aneurysm [124,128].

Figure 5 summarizes the main pathophysiological mechanisms of strokes associated with opiate/heroin abuse.

2.5.3. Clinical Studies, Case Reports and Epidemiology of Stroke Related to Opiates/Heroin Abuse

Heroin-associated stroke has rarely been reported, but intranasal administration can lead to ischemic lesions of globus pallidus [129]. The ischemic pathology of heroin-associated stroke is more common than hemorrhagic forms [130]. Kumar et al. described a case of a 28-year-old woman who admitted using heroin and presented with intraparenchymal hemorrhage in the left frontal lobe without cardioembolic, vasculitic or other etiologies for stroke [128]. In the literature, there are only a couple of other cases of hemorrhagic stroke in young people who use heroin: A 42-year-old man who presented with massive left intracerebral hemorrhage and a 45-year-old man who presented with right basal ganglia hemorrhage [131]. Chronic morphine treatment may be associated with an increased incidence of stroke in patients with malignancies. A higher correlation is encountered in prostate cancer patients, as shown in a 2013 study in Taiwan [132].

Opiate-addicted individuals have a higher risk of stroke than the general population [133]. In Table 5, the most recent case reports that associate narcotic analgesic use and stroke are presented.

Table 5. Case reports that associate narcotic analgesic use with stroke.

Subject/Age	Substance Exposure	Symptoms	Diagnostic Approach	Diagnosis	Intervention	Evolution	Reference
Female, 28	Admitted to using heroin	Altered mental status	Head CT	A large 5.1 × 5-cm intraparenchymal hemorrhage in the left frontal lobe, vasogenic edema, and a 5-mm midline shift	Surgical intervention was unnecessary. After discharge, was transferred to rehabilitation	Improvement in cognitive function was mild; the patient continue to be confused and presented significant memory loss	[128]
Male, 29, without cardiovascular risk factors	Sniffed heroin with regularity in the last seven years	Left-sided hemihypesthesia and gait disturbance	MRI and MR angiography	Multiple cerebral and cerebellar areas of diffusion restriction in different territories; heroin-induced eosinophilia	Steroid pulse treatment (methylprednisolone 250 mg IV) in the first three days followed by another 21 days of oral prednisolone (60 mg)—for eosinophilia and antiplatelet therapy with aspirin	A slight improvement in his sensorium and gait but only incomplete recovery	[125]
Male, 33	Heroin inhalation	Amnesia 48 h after first heroin inhalation	MRI	Cortical laminar necrosis of the left hippocampus without vascular abnormality	-	Impaired performance on the verbal and visual level	[134]
Male, 33	Used heroin for 13 years Concomitant use of methamphetamine. For 6 months, started methadone treatment to quit heroin	Found unconsciousness	Brain CT and MRI	Acute ischemic strokes localized in bilateral fronto-parieto-temporal white matter and in bilateral corona radiate. Damage was noted in the bilateral globus pallidus and left cerebral peduncle; rhabdomyolysis	Active treatment in the intensive care unit	-	[135]

2.6. *Androgenic Anabolic Steroids*

Anabolic androgenic steroids (AASs) are either endogenous (e.g., testosterone) or synthetic, exogenous substances (e.g., nandrolone and stanozolol), acting through specific androgen receptors. AASs are used for the treatment of several disorders, such as hypogonadism, cachexia of various etiologies, hypercalcemia, hypercalciuria, and along with other chronic diseases also in oncology as a supportive treatment [136].

2.6.1. The Mechanism of Action of AASs

The mechanism is complex and is associated with several parameters. More specifically, changes in the lipid profile have also been observed, both at chronic therapeutic doses and during short term treatment, with the reduction in high-density lipoprotein (HDL) cholesterol being the most profound change. Interestingly, molecular biology tests revealed that a concomitant increase in total cholesterol was accompanied by increased mRNA and protein expression of HMG-CoA reductase, a key enzyme in the formation of cholesterol by the liver [137]. The decrease in HDL cholesterol may reach 20% and, similarly, the increase in low-density lipoprotein (LDL) cholesterol may reach 20%, possibly as a result of the lipoproteins' lipolytic degradation and their subtraction by receptors due to the modification of apolipoprotein A-I and B synthesis [138]. Apolipoprotein B has been connected to atherosclerosis, via the interaction between the arterial wall and LDL cholesterol [139]. Abnormalities in lipoprotein expand the hazard of coronary artery disease by 3–6 fold and it may occur within 9 weeks of AAS use. In addition to its atherogenic effects, the excess of LDL-C may be oxidized at the arterial endothelium leading to impaired endothelium-dependent arterial relaxation via inhibition of nitric oxide production. This could predispose to the development of coronary vasospasm [140]. Fortunately, the effects of lipids appear to be reversible [141].

The effects of anabolic steroids on blood pressure remain conflicting. A few studies have reported elevated blood pressure levels in anabolic steroid users [142], which might be maintained even 5 to 12 months after discontinuation [143]. The mechanism involved could be the ability of AASs to increase the activity of the sympathetic nervous system activity, to baroreflex control and to endothelial dysfunction as well [144]. The mode of action seems to be substance specific. For example, nandrolone has no effects on blood pressure, while the cardiac hypertrophy caused by nandrolone administration was not associated with the systemic renin–angiotensin system but with its effects at a local level. Unfortunately, data so far are not sufficient to settle on whether the prolonged AAS use can lead to irreversible elevated levels of blood pressure [145].

2.6.2. The Influence of AASs on Stroke

Atherothrombosis or embolization could lead to thromboembolic ischemic strokes. Peripheral vascular disease can occur through the same mechanisms. The main action of AASs is anabolism. It is involved in growth-promoting effects on cardiac tissue, following AAS administration and causes hypertrophic cardiomyopathy. Probably as a counteracting effect, apoptotic cell death has also been observed—a process that is mediated by membrane receptor second messenger cascades that increase intracellular Ca^{2+} influx and mobilization, leading to the release of apoptogenic factors [146–148]. In vitro studies performed in isolated human myocytes have shown that AASs bind to androgen receptors. Therefore, it is possible that hypertrophy may be induced directly, via tissue upregulation of the renin–angiotensin system [149]. Supporting evidence lies in the fact that the AT1 receptor antagonist prevented similar effects induced by nandrolone administration [150]. Moreover, nandrolone treatment, in combination with swimming training, increased left ventricular angiotensin-converting enzyme (LV-ACE) activity and CYP11B2 expression, implying an elevation in both angiotensin II and aldosterone and the promotion of cardiac dysfunction [151].

Sex hormone-related mechanisms also seem to be involved in the pathogenesis of various cardiovascular disorders, with ischemic stroke included, particularly for men. However, these findings are not specifically informative about endogenous testosterone or testosterone supplementation [152]. Testosterone supplementation for therapeutic purposes has not been conclusively linked with a high thrombotic risk. In a cohort of 3422 male US military service members, aged 40–64 years, treated with testosterone for low testosterone levels, there was no difference in event-free survival with regard to thromboembolism, compared to an appropriately matched control group [153]. On the other hand, elevated testosterone was independently associated with an increased risk for both ischemic stroke (odds ratio 3.9) and cerebral venous thrombosis (odds ratio 5.5) [154]. Nevertheless, the Guidelines of the Endocrine Society suggest that testosterone therapy should be avoided in patients with, among other clinical conditions, elevated hematocrit, myocardial infarction or stroke within the last 6 months or thrombophilia. Furthermore, measuring serum testosterone concentrations and hematocrit is highly recommended [155].

The effect of AASs on the hemostatic system may lead to a prothrombotic profile, depending on the dose and the duration of AAS administration. Low doses decrease platelet threshold activation to collagen. In addition, androgens reduce plasminogen activator inhibitor-1 (PAI-1) levels and increase fibrinolytic activity via high tissue plasminogen activator (t-PA) levels. Both the release of t-PA from endothelial cells into the circulation and the amount of t-PA inhibitor (PAI-1) that is present in the circulation regulate fibrinolytic activity [156,157]. Possible vascular thrombosis due to increased fibrinolytic activity as a result of decreased PAI-1 levels can consequently be speculated [158]. Higher doses have been associated with the elevated aggregation of platelets and possibly affect the activity of vascular cyclooxygenase enzyme, which may lead to a procoagulant state [159]. Several AASs appear to be involved in procoagulatory pathways, by increasing plasma levels of factor VIII and IX [160]. They also increase the aggregation of platelets and the formation of thrombus formation via increased platelet production of thromboxane A2, and via decreased production of prostacyclin and increased fibrinogen levels [139]. At the same time, as animal experiments have shown, extracellular matrix, nitric oxide production and the arachidonic metabolism of endothelial cells and platelets are also influenced [161]. Moreover, both exogenous and endogenous AASs can provoke polycythemia and consequent ischemic cardiovascular events through the reduction of hepcidin and the stimulation of erythropoiesis, by recalibrating the erythropoietin set point [162,163]. Testosterone has also been shown to stabilize telomeres in bone marrow progenitors, which may play a role in increased red cell production [164].

Figure 6 summarizes the main pathophysiological mechanisms of stroke associated with anabolic androgenic steroid abuse.

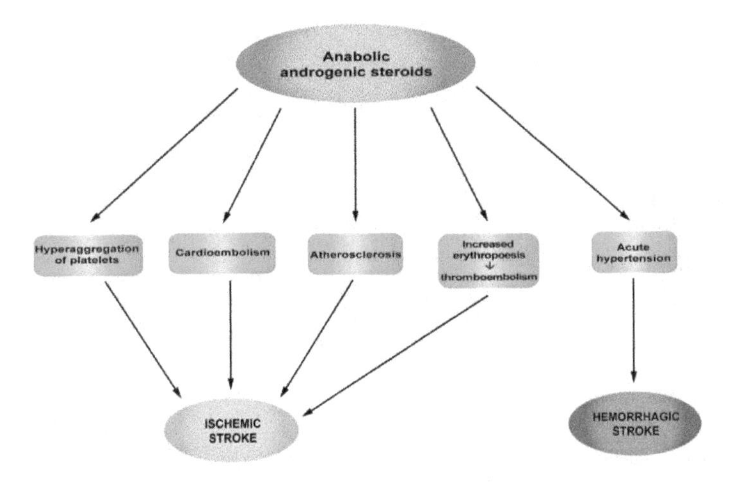

Figure 6. Pathophysiological mechanisms of strokes associated with anabolic androgenic steroid abuse.

2.6.3. Clinical Studies, Case Reports and Epidemiology of Stroke Related to AAS Abuse

Since the early 1930s, AASs have been extensively used by amateur or professional athletes and the general public for the improvement of physical conditions and athletic performance [165–168]. When used for ergogenic or recreational purposes, the doses are usually 5–15 times higher than the recommended therapeutic ones [145,167,169]. At such high levels, AASs can cause a number of serious side effects, including liver dysfunction, renal disorders, cardiotoxicity and potentially stroke [136].

Indeed, athletes abusing AASs for years have a high probability to develop atherothrombotic phenomena (cardiovascular and cerebrovascular disorders, such as cerebral ischemia, i.e., transitory ischemic attacks resulting in stroke, peripheral artery occlusive disease and venous thromboembolism) [143]. These phenomena can be attributed to arterial hypertension, lipid metabolism disorders, increased vascular tone and increased platelet counts and hematocrit [139,145,170]. The reversibility of such myocardial and vascular effects after discontinuation is still controversial [171]. Several case reports describe stroke in AAS abusers, and the most interesting ones are summarized in Table 6.

Table 6. Case reports that associate androgenic anabolic steroid (AAS) abuse with stroke.

Subject/Age	Substance Exposure	Symptoms	Diagnostic Approach	Diagnosis	Reference
Male, 27, with an American father and a mother who was half Japanese, no known stroke risk factors, regularly training, AAS user	Methasterone, prostanozol for the past 6 months	Sudden right hemiparalysis, homonymous hemianopia, dysarthria, tinnitus, and double vision in the middle of muscle training	MRI with and without gadolinium enhancement, MR angiography, three-dimensional CT angiography, carotid ultrasonography, transcranial Doppler and transesophageal echocardiography, and duplex ultrasonography	Cardiogenic embolism and atrial septal aneurysm and large patent foramen ovule, suspected deep vein thrombosis	[170]
Male, 37, no history of alcohol or any other substance abuse, negative medical and family histories	Methandienone, methenolone acetate for the past 2 years	Acute right-sided hemiparesis (grade 3) with right-sided facial weakness, associated with a confused state followed a first-ever experience of generalized tonic–clonic seizure	Brain CT and MRI, ECG, chest X-ray, abdominal ultrasound, and echocardiography	Chronic infarction in the left frontal lobe and subacute left temporoparietal infarction Dilated cardiomyopathy and multiple thrombi in the left ventricle Hepatomegaly, mild ascites and bilateral pleural effusion in addition to a grade I nephropathy	[140]
Male, 16, healthy bodybuilder (weight 87 kg and height 181 cm), unremarkable past medical record	Concomitant use of cannabis (up to 1.5 g/day) and methandrostenolone (40 mg/day) for the past 5 months	Sudden dizziness and right hemiparesis	Cerebral CT, MRI, conventional and magnetic resonance angiography, transesophageal echocardiography, cervical Doppler duplex ultrasound, transcranial Doppler, and ECG	Acute ischemic stroke	[156]
Male, 39, bodybuilder, 3 months earlier sudden loss of vision in the left eye, weakness and numbness in the left upper and lower limbs, lasting less than 1 h, refused admission to hospital	Intramuscular injections of nandrolone twice weekly for the past three years	Dizziness and expressive aphasia for the last 6 h	Brain CT and MRI, ECG, chest X-ray, echocardiography, and magnetic resonance angiography	Dilated cardiomyopathy with LV thrombus formation; embolic stroke and peripheral vascular disease as a complication of the former	[141]
Male, 31, kickboxer	Nandrolone, testosterone clenbuterol since the age of 16; cocaine, ecstasy and alcohol abuser for three years	Patient disoriented in space, mild dysarthria without aphasic elements, oculocephalic preference to right, left homonymous hemianopsia, paresis (3/5), hemicorporal anesthesia on the left side and somatoagnosia	Cranial CT, cerebral arteriography, transesophageal and transthoracic echocardiography, and magnetic resonance angiography	Acute ischemic stroke: Cerebral infarction due to occlusion of the artery cerebral media of unknown etiology	[172]
Male	Injectable (nandrolone decanoate) and oral (methandrostenolone/ danabol) three months prior to the incidence Previous intravenous (heroin), and inhaled (marijuana) drug use	Visual disturbances and left-sided weakness commencing 24 h prior to presentation Homonymous hemianopia, mild left-sided weakness in his upper limbs and ataxia in his left upper limb, and high hemoglobin (200 g/L)	Brain magnetic resonance, magnetic resonance angiography, transthoracic echocardiogram, and 24-h Holter monitoring, extensive hematological screening, and thrombophilia screening	Cerebral infarction: Extensive region of acute infarction in the right posterior cerebral artery territory and ongoing occlusion in his right posterior cerebral artery Polycythemia	[173]

Table 7 summarizes the association between the different classes of drugs of abuse with different types of stroke.

Table 7. The incidence of ischemic stroke and hemorrhagic stroke in different classes of drugs of abuse.

Drugs of Abuse		Ischemic Stroke	Hemorrhagic Stroke
Amphetamines		**+**	**+++**
Amphetamine derivatives		+	+++ Risk in young people without comorbidities
Cocaine	Cocaine	In those with a history of use	In active users
	Hydrochloride	+	+++
	Crack	++	++
Cannabis		++	+ In recent case reports
Synthetic cannabinoids		++	+In recent case reports
Opiates/Heroin		++	+In recent case reports
Anabolic androgenic steroids		++	

+ mild evidence. ++ medium evidence. +++ high evidence.

3. Management

Stroke can occur either in minutes/hours following illicit drug use or later as a consequence of complications, such as vasculitis or endocarditis, resulting in septic emboli [45,174].

Acute stroke is a medical emergency. Patients should be transported by ambulance to a medical facility that is organized and equipped to manage acute stroke as soon as possible after symptom onset and capable of offering emergency treatments such as intravenous thrombolysis and endovascular thrombectomy—organized acute stroke unit management. These treatments are typically offered in departments of neurology with organized stroke centers [40].

The outcome of ICH depends on the hematoma location and volume, the promptness of treatment, and the management of associated diseases. The mortality of ICH remains very high. For those who survive, recovery is difficult and long lasting, with a negative impact on quality of life. Risk factors, such as high blood pressure, smoking, obesity and drug use, play an important role. Prevention plays a central role and can be favorably influenced by changing lifestyle and taking therapeutic measures, especially for hypertension control.

4. Conclusions

Drug abuse represents a major social and public health problem, with huge financial implications. Epidemiological studies and case reports have shown that drug abuse is a risk factor for both hemorrhagic and ischemic stroke. Stimulants, such as amphetamines, amphetamine derivatives, and cocaine have been associated with both types of stroke—more so of the hemorrhagic type. "Crack" cocaine can cause both acute ischemic stroke and hemorrhagic strokes, while cocaine hydrochloride is more likely to cause hemorrhagic strokes. Stroke can emerge after cocaine use, even in the absence of other traditional stroke risk factors. The association between cannabis, synthetic cannabinoids, or opioid/heroin use and stroke has not been entirely proven by epidemiological studies that offer contradictory findings. New case reports describe the correlation between cannabinoids and synthetic cannabinoids and hemorrhagic stroke. Anabolic androgenic steroids are associated with cardiotoxicity and atherothrombotic phenomena which can lead to ischemic stroke. Given the epidemic of illicit drug use, we recommend that every hospitalized stroke patient, and especially those who are young for stroke, is subjected to toxicological screening.

Author Contributions: All the authors contributed equally to conceiving and designing the manuscript. A.O.D., D.C., L.-M.Z. and C.T. searched the literature for inclusion in the study that was then checked and reviewed by A.T., K.T., R.M., L.K., J.S.R., P.D.M. and N.D. D.C., A.O.D., G.L., C.T. and M.N. drafted and wrote the manuscript. A.T., P.D.M., L.K., V.S., E.D. critically revised the manuscript. A.O.D., D.C., J.S.-R. and L.M.D. designed the figures. A.O.D., C.T. and R.M. designed the tables. All the authors have read and approved the final version of the manuscript.

Acknowledgments: This paper and APC was supported by Grants PN-III-P1-1.2-PCCDI-2017-0341/2018, PN 19.29.01.01 and by the Ministry of Research and Innovation in Romania under Program 1: The Improvement of the National System of Research and Development, Subprogram 1.2: Institutional Excellence—Projects of Excellence Funding in RDI, Contract No. 7PFE/16.10.2018.

References

1. Easton, J.D.; Saver, J.L.; Albers, G.W.; Alberts, M.J.; Chaturvedi, S.; Feldmann, E.; Hatsukami, T.S.; Higashida, R.T.; Johnston, S.C.; Kidwell, C.S.; et al. Definition and evaluation of transient ischemic attack: A scientific statement for healthcare professionals from the American Heart Association/American Stroke Association Stroke Council; Council on Cardiovascular Surgery and Anesthesia; Council on Cardiovascular Radiology and Intervention; Council on Cardiovascular Nursing; and the Interdisciplinary Council on Peripheral Vascular Disease. The American Academy of Neurology affirms the value of this statement as an educational tool for neurologists. *Stroke* **2009**, *40*, 2276–2293. [CrossRef] [PubMed]
2. National Collaborating Centre for Chronic Conditions. National Collaborating Centre for Chronic Conditions. National Institute for Health and Clinical Excellence: Guidance. In *Stroke: National Clinical Guideline for Diagnosis and Initial Management of Acute Stroke and Transient Ischaemic Attack (TIA)*; Royal College of Physicians (UK) Royal College of Physicians of London: London, UK, 2008.
3. Johnson, W.; Onuma, O.; Owolabi, M.; Sachdev, S. Stroke: A global response is needed. *Bull. World Health Organ.* **2016**, *94*. [CrossRef] [PubMed]
4. United Nations Oddice on Drugs and Crime. World Drug Report 2017. Available online: https://www.unodc.org/wdr2017/field/WDR_2017_presentation_lauch_version.pdf (accessed on 26 February 2019).
5. Smajlovic, D. Strokes in young adults: Epidemiology and prevention. *Vasc. Health Risk Manag.* **2015**, *11*, 157–164. [CrossRef] [PubMed]
6. Mendis, S. Stroke disability and rehabilitation of stroke: World Health Organization perspective. *Int. J. Stroke* **2013**, *8*, 3–4. [CrossRef] [PubMed]
7. Jivan, K.; Ranchod, K.; Modi, G. Management of ischaemic stroke in the acute setting: Review of the current status. *Cardiovasc. J. Afr.* **2013**, *24*, 86–92. [CrossRef] [PubMed]
8. Falkstedt, D.; Wolff, V.; Allebeck, P.; Hemmingsson, T.; Danielsson, A.K. Cannabis, Tobacco, Alcohol Use, and the Risk of Early Stroke: A Population-Based Cohort Study of 45,000 Swedish Men. *Stroke* **2017**, *48*, 265–270. [CrossRef] [PubMed]
9. Sloan, M.A. Illicit drug use/abuse and stroke. *Handb. Clin. Neurol.* **2009**, *93*, 823–840. [CrossRef] [PubMed]
10. Nieswandt, B.; Kleinschnitz, C.; Stoll, G. Ischaemic stroke: A thrombo-inflammatory disease? *J. Physiol.* **2011**, *589*, 4115–4123. [CrossRef]
11. Stoll, G.; Nieswandt, B. Thrombo-inflammation in acute ischaemic stroke—Implications for treatment. *Nat. Rev. Neurol.* **2019**, *15*, 473–481. [CrossRef]
12. Slomka, A.; Switonska, M.; Sinkiewicz, W.; Zekanowska, E. Assessing Circulating Factor VIIa-Antithrombin Complexes in Acute Ischemic Stroke: A Pilot Study. *Clin. Appl. Thromb. Hemost.* **2017**, *23*, 351–359. [CrossRef]
13. Switonska, M.; Slomka, A.; Sinkiewicz, W.; Zekanowska, E. Tissue-factor-bearing microparticles (MPs-TF) in patients with acute ischaemic stroke: The influence of stroke treatment on MPs-TF generation. *Eur. J. Neurol.* **2015**, *22*, e328–e399. [CrossRef] [PubMed]
14. Brouwers, H.B.; Greenberg, S.M. Hematoma expansion following acute intracerebral hemorrhage. *Cerebrovasc. Dis.* **2013**, *35*, 195–201. [CrossRef] [PubMed]
15. Sonni, S.; Lioutas, V.A.; Selim, M.H. New avenues for treatment of intracranial hemorrhage. *Curr. Treat. Options Cardiovasc. Med.* **2014**, *16*, 277. [CrossRef] [PubMed]

16. Dardiotis, E.; Aloizou, A.M.; Markoula, S.; Siokas, V.; Tsarouhas, K.; Tzanakakis, G.; Libra, M.; Kyritsis, A.P.; Brotis, A.G.; Aschner, M.; et al. Cancer-associated stroke: Pathophysiology, detection and management (Review). *Int. J. Oncol.* **2019**, *54*, 779–796. [CrossRef]
17. Teodoro, M.; Briguglio, G.; Fenga, C.; Costa, C. Genetic polymorphisms as determinants of pesticide toxicity: Recent advances. *Toxicol. Rep.* **2019**. [CrossRef] [PubMed]
18. Kaye, S.; Darke, S.; Duflou, J.; McKetin, R. Methamphetamine-related fatalities in Australia: Demographics, circumstances, toxicology and major organ pathology. *Addiction* **2008**, *103*, 1353–1360. [CrossRef]
19. Kaku, D.A.; Lowenstein, D.H. Emergence of recreational drug abuse as a major risk factor for stroke in young adults. *Ann. Intern. Med.* **1990**, *113*, 821–827. [CrossRef]
20. Ho, E.L.; Josephson, S.A.; Lee, H.S.; Smith, W.S. Cerebrovascular complications of methamphetamine abuse. *Neurocrit. Care* **2009**, *10*, 295–305. [CrossRef]
21. Buttner, A. Review: The neuropathology of drug abuse. *Neuropathol. Appl. Neurobiol.* **2011**, *37*, 118–134. [CrossRef]
22. Sloan, M.A.; Kittner, S.J.; Rigamonti, D.; Price, T.R. Occurrence of stroke associated with use/abuse of drugs. *Neurology* **1991**, *41*, 1358–1364. [CrossRef]
23. Parrott, A.C.; Milani, R.M.; Gouzoulis-Mayfrank, E.; Daumann, J. Cannabis and Ecstasy/MDMA (3,4-methylenedioxymethamphetamine): An analysis of their neuropsychobiological interactions in recreational users. *J. Neural Transm. (Vienna, Austria: 1996)* **2007**, *114*, 959–968. [CrossRef] [PubMed]
24. Heal, D.J.; Smith, S.L.; Gosden, J.; Nutt, D.J. Amphetamine, past and present—A pharmacological and clinical perspective. *J. Psychopharmacol. (Oxford, UK)* **2013**, *27*, 479–496. [CrossRef] [PubMed]
25. Walker-Batson, D.; Mehta, J.; Smith, P.; Johnson, M. Amphetamine and other pharmacological agents in human and animal studies of recovery from stroke. *Prog. Neuropsychopharmacol. Biol. Psychiatry* **2016**, *64*, 225–230. [CrossRef] [PubMed]
26. Calipari, E.S.; Ferris, M.J. Amphetamine mechanisms and actions at the dopamine terminal revisited. *J. Neurosci.* **2013**, *33*, 8923–8925. [CrossRef] [PubMed]
27. Christophersen, A.S. Amphetamine designer drugs—An overview and epidemiology. *Toxicol. Lett.* **2000**, *112–113*, 127–131. [CrossRef]
28. Albertson, T.E.; Derlet, R.W.; Van Hoozen, B.E. Methamphetamine and the expanding complications of amphetamines. *West. J. Med.* **1999**, *170*, 214–219. [PubMed]
29. Westover, A.N.; McBride, S.; Haley, R.W. Stroke in young adults who abuse amphetamines or cocaine: A population-based study of hospitalized patients. *Arch. Gen. Psychiatry* **2007**, *64*, 495–502. [CrossRef]
30. Phillips, M.C.; Leyden, J.M.; Chong, W.K.; Kleinig, T.; Czapran, P.; Lee, A.; Koblar, S.A.; Jannes, J. Ischaemic stroke among young people aged 15 to 50 years in Adelaide, South Australia. *Med. J. Aust.* **2011**, *195*, 610–614. [CrossRef]
31. Indave, B.I.; Sordo, L.; Bravo, M.J.; Sarasa-Renedo, A.; Fernandez-Balbuena, S.; De la Fuente, L.; Sonego, M. Risk of stroke in prescription and other amphetamine-type stimulants use: A systematic review. *Drug Alcohol Rev.* **2018**, *37*, 56–69. [CrossRef]
32. Ohta, K.; Mori, M.; Yoritaka, A.; Okamoto, K.; Kishida, S. Delayed ischemic stroke associated with methamphetamine use. *J. Emerg. Med.* **2005**, *28*, 165–167. [CrossRef]
33. De Silva, D.A.; Wong, M.C.; Lee, M.P.; Chen, C.L.; Chang, H.M. Amphetamine-associated ischemic stroke: Clinical presentation and proposed pathogenesis. *J. Stroke Cerebrovasc. Dis.* **2007**, *16*, 185–186. [CrossRef] [PubMed]
34. Weiss, S.R.; Raskind, R.; Morganstern, N.L.; Pytlyk, P.J.; Baiz, T.C. Intracerebral and subarachnoid hemorrhage following use of methamphetamine ("speed"). *Int. J. Surg.* **1970**, *53*, 123–127.
35. Yakoot, M. Phenylpropanolamine and the hemorrhagic stroke: A new search for the culprit. *J. Pharmacol. Pharmacother.* **2012**, *3*, 4–6. [CrossRef] [PubMed]
36. Polesskaya, O.; Silva, J.; Sanfilippo, C.; Desrosiers, T.; Sun, A.; Shen, J.; Feng, C.; Polesskiy, A.; Deane, R.; Zlokovic, B.; et al. Methamphetamine causes sustained depression in cerebral blood flow. *Brain Res.* **2011**, *1373*, 91–100. [CrossRef] [PubMed]
37. Berlit, P. Diagnosis and treatment of cerebral vasculitis. *Ther. Adv. Neurol. Disord.* **2010**, *3*, 29–42. [CrossRef] [PubMed]

38. McGee, S.M.; McGee, D.N.; McGee, M.B. Spontaneous intracerebral hemorrhage related to methamphetamine abuse: Autopsy findings and clinical correlation. *Am. J. Forensic Med. Pathol.* **2004**, *25*, 334–337. [CrossRef] [PubMed]
39. Pilgrim, J.L.; Gerostamoulos, D.; Drummer, O.H.; Bollmann, M. Involvement of amphetamines in sudden and unexpected death. *J. Forensic Sci.* **2009**, *54*, 478–485. [CrossRef] [PubMed]
40. Lappin, J.M.; Darke, S.; Farrell, M. Stroke and methamphetamine use in young adults: A review. *J. Neurol. Neurosurg. Psychiatry* **2017**, *88*, 1079–1091. [CrossRef]
41. Huang, M.C.; Yang, S.Y.; Lin, S.K.; Chen, K.Y.; Chen, Y.Y.; Kuo, C.J.; Hung, Y.N. Risk of Cardiovascular Diseases and Stroke Events in Methamphetamine Users: A 10-Year Follow-Up Study. *J. Clin. Psychiatry* **2016**, *77*, 1396–1403. [CrossRef]
42. Christensen, M.R.; Lesnikova, I.; Madsen, L.B.; Rosendal, I.; Banner, J. Drug-induced bilateral ischemic infarction in an amphetamine addict. *Forensic Sci. Med. Pathol.* **2013**, *9*, 458–461. [CrossRef]
43. Kahn, D.E.; Ferraro, N.; Benveniste, R.J. 3 cases of primary intracranial hemorrhage associated with "Molly", a purified form of 3,4-methylenedioxymethamphetamine (MDMA). *J. Neurol. Sci.* **2012**, *323*, 257–260. [CrossRef] [PubMed]
44. Wijers, C.H.W.; Visser, M.C.; van Litsenburg, R.T.H.; Niesink, R.J.M.; Willemse, R.B.; Croes, E.A. Haemorrhagic stroke related to the use of 4-fluoroamphetamine. *J. Neurol.* **2018**, *265*, 1607–1611. [CrossRef] [PubMed]
45. Chiu, Z.K.; Bennett, I.E.; Chan, P.; Rosenfeld, J.V. Methamphetamine-related brainstem haemorrhage. *J. Clin. Neurosci.* **2016**, *32*, 137–139. [CrossRef] [PubMed]
46. Kapetanovic, S.; Kim, M.A. Hemorrhagic stroke in a patient recently started on mixed amphetamine salts. *Am. J. Psychiatry* **2010**, *167*, 1277–1278. [CrossRef] [PubMed]
47. Lyson, T.; Kochanowicz, J.; Rutkowski, R.; Turek, G.; Lewko, J. Cerebral vasospasm in patient with hemorrhagic stroke after amphetamine intake—Case report. *Pol. Merkur. Lek. Organ Pol. Tow. Lek.* **2008**, *24*, 265–267.
48. Muntan, C.D.; Tuckler, V. Cerebrovascular accident following MDMA ingestion. *J. Med. Toxicol.* **2006**, *2*, 16–18. [CrossRef] [PubMed]
49. McIntosh, A.; Hungs, M.; Kostanian, V.; Yu, W. Carotid artery dissection and middle cerebral artery stroke following methamphetamine use. *Neurology* **2006**, *67*, 2259–2260. [CrossRef]
50. Treadwell, S.D.; Robinson, T.G. Cocaine use and stroke. *Postgrad. Med. J.* **2007**, *83*, 389–394. [CrossRef]
51. Kishi, T.; Matsuda, Y.; Iwata, N.; Correll, C.U. Antipsychotics for cocaine or psychostimulant dependence: Systematic review and meta-analysis of randomized, placebo-controlled trials. *J. Clin. Psychiatry* **2013**, *74*, e1169–e1180. [CrossRef]
52. Riezzo, I.; Fiore, C.; De Carlo, D.; Pascale, N.; Neri, M.; Turillazzi, E.; Fineschi, V. Side effects of cocaine abuse: Multiorgan toxicity and pathological consequences. *Curr. Med. Chem.* **2012**, *19*, 5624–5646. [CrossRef]
53. Bachi, K.; Mani, V.; Jeyachandran, D.; Fayad, Z.A.; Goldstein, R.Z.; Alia-Klein, N. Vascular disease in cocaine addiction. *Atherosclerosis* **2017**, *262*, 154–162. [CrossRef] [PubMed]
54. Sordo, L.; Indave, B.I.; Barrio, G.; Degenhardt, L.; de la Fuente, L.; Bravo, M.J. Cocaine use and risk of stroke: A systematic review. *Drug Alcohol Depend.* **2014**, *142*, 1–13. [CrossRef] [PubMed]
55. Bhattacharya, P.; Taraman, S.; Shankar, L.; Chaturvedi, S.; Madhavan, R. Clinical Profiles, Complications, and Disability in Cocaine-Related Ischemic Stroke. *J. Stroke Cerebrovasc. Dis.* **2011**, *20*, 443–449. [CrossRef] [PubMed]
56. Pradhan, L.; Mondal, D.; Chandra, S.; Ali, M.; Agrawal, K.C. Molecular analysis of cocaine-induced endothelial dysfunction: Role of endothelin-1 and nitric oxide. *Cardiovasc. Toxicol.* **2008**, *8*, 161–171. [CrossRef] [PubMed]
57. He, G.Q.; Zhang, A.; Altura, B.T.; Altura, B.M. Cocaine-induced cerebrovasospasm and its possible mechanism of action. *J. Pharmacol. Exp. Ther.* **1994**, *268*, 1532–1539. [PubMed]
58. You, J.; Du, C.; Volkow, N.D.; Pan, Y. Optical coherence Doppler tomography for quantitative cerebral blood flow imaging. *Biomed. Opt. Express* **2014**, *5*, 3217–3230. [CrossRef] [PubMed]
59. Toossi, S.; Hess, C.P.; Hills, N.K.; Josephson, S.A. Neurovascular Complications of Cocaine Use at a Tertiary Stroke Center. *J. Stroke Cerebrovasc. Dis.* **2010**, *19*, 273–278. [CrossRef]
60. Narvaez, J.C.; Magalhaes, P.V.; Fries, G.R.; Colpo, G.D.; Czepielewski, L.S.; Vianna, P.; Chies, J.A.; Rosa, A.R.; Von Diemen, L.; Vieta, E.; et al. Peripheral toxicity in crack cocaine use disorders. *Neurosci. Lett.* **2013**, *544*, 80–84. [CrossRef]

61. Fox, H.C.; D'Sa, C.; Kimmerling, A.; Siedlarz, K.M.; Tuit, K.L.; Stowe, R.; Sinha, R. Immune system inflammation in cocaine dependent individuals: Implications for medications development. *Hum. Psychopharmacol.* **2012**, *27*, 156–166. [CrossRef]
62. Lucas, G.M.; Atta, M.G.; Fine, D.M.; McFall, A.M.; Estrella, M.M.; Zook, K.; Stein, J.H. HIV, Cocaine Use, and Hepatitis C Virus: A Triad of Nontraditional Risk Factors for Subclinical Cardiovascular Disease. *Arterioscler. Thromb. Vasc. Biol.* **2016**, *36*, 2100–2107. [CrossRef]
63. Harsch, H.H.; Pankiewicz, J.; Bloom, A.S.; Rainey, C.; Cho, J.K.; Sperry, L.; Stein, E.A. Hepatitis C virus infection in cocaine users—A silent epidemic. *Community Ment. Health J.* **2000**, *36*, 225–233. [CrossRef] [PubMed]
64. Kalichman, S.C.; Washington, C.; Kegler, C.; Grebler, T.; Kalichman, M.O.; Cherry, C.; Eaton, L. Continued Substance Use Among People Living With HIV-Hepatitis-C Co-Infection and Receiving Antiretroviral Therapy. *Subst. Use Misuse* **2015**, *50*, 1536–1543. [CrossRef] [PubMed]
65. Dash, S.; Balasubramaniam, M.; Villalta, F.; Dash, C.; Pandhare, J. Impact of cocaine abuse on HIV pathogenesis. *Front. Microbiol.* **2015**, *6*, 1111. [CrossRef] [PubMed]
66. Boehme, A.K.; Esenwa, C.; Elkind, M.S. Stroke Risk Factors, Genetics, and Prevention. *Circ. Res.* **2017**, *120*, 472–495. [CrossRef] [PubMed]
67. Gretarsdottir, S.; Thorleifsson, G.; Manolescu, A.; Styrkarsdottir, U.; Helgadottir, A.; Gschwendtner, A.; Kostulas, K.; Kuhlenbaumer, G.; Bevan, S.; Jonsdottir, T.; et al. Risk variants for atrial fibrillation on chromosome 4q25 associate with ischemic stroke. *Ann. Neurol.* **2008**, *64*, 402–409. [CrossRef] [PubMed]
68. Kouzarides, T. Histone acetylases and deacetylases in cell proliferation. *Curr. Opin. Genet. Dev.* **1999**, *9*, 40–48. [CrossRef]
69. Penrod, R.D.; Carreira, M.B.; Taniguchi, M.; Kumar, J.; Maddox, S.A.; Cowan, C.W. Novel role and regulation of HDAC4 in cocaine-related behaviors. *Addict. Biol.* **2018**, *23*, 653–664. [CrossRef] [PubMed]
70. Lanktree, M.B.; Hegele, R.A.; Yusuf, S.; Anand, S.S. Multi-ethnic genetic association study of carotid intima-media thickness using a targeted cardiovascular SNP microarray. *Stroke* **2009**, *40*, 3173–3179. [CrossRef]
71. Desai, R.; Patel, U.; Rupareliya, C.; Singh, S.; Shah, M.; Patel, R.S.; Patel, S.; Mahuwala, Z. Impact of Cocaine Use on Acute Ischemic Stroke Patients: Insights from Nationwide Inpatient Sample in the United States. *Cureus* **2017**, *9*, e1536. [CrossRef]
72. Cheng, Y.C.; Ryan, K.A.; Qadwai, S.A.; Shah, J.; Sparks, M.J.; Wozniak, M.A.; Stern, B.J.; Phipps, M.S.; Cronin, C.A.; Magder, L.S.; et al. Cocaine Use and Risk of Ischemic Stroke in Young Adults. *Stroke* **2016**, *47*, 918–922. [CrossRef]
73. Daras, M.; Tuchman, A.J.; Marks, S. Central nervous system infarction related to cocaine abuse. *Stroke* **1991**, *22*, 1320–1325. [CrossRef] [PubMed]
74. Martin-Schild, S.; Albright, K.C.; Hallevi, H.; Barreto, A.D.; Philip, M.; Misra, V.; Grotta, J.C.; Savitz, S.I. Intracerebral hemorrhage in cocaine users. *Stroke* **2010**, *41*, 680–684. [CrossRef] [PubMed]
75. Lucerna, A.; Espinosa, J.; Zaman, T.; Hertz, R.; Stranges, D. Limb Pain as Unusual Presentation of a Parietal Intraparenchymal Bleeding Associated with Crack Cocaine Use: A Case Report. *Case Rep. Neurol. Med.* **2018**, *2018*, 9598675. [CrossRef] [PubMed]
76. Mullaguri, N.; Battineni, A.; Narayan, A.; Guddeti, R. Cocaine Induced Bilateral Posterior Inferior Cerebellar Artery and Hippocampal Infarction. *Cureus* **2018**, *10*, e2576. [CrossRef] [PubMed]
77. Rico-Mesa, J.S.; Rico-Mesa, M.A.; Berrouet, M.C. Ischemic stroke related to acute consumption of cocaine. *CES Medicina* **2017**, *31*, 207–214. [CrossRef]
78. Vidale, S.; Peroni, R.; Di Palma, F.; Sampietro, A.; Gozzi, G.; Arnaboldi, M. Intra-arterial thrombolysis in a young patient with cocaine-associated stroke. *Neurol. Sci.* **2014**, *35*, 1465–1466. [CrossRef] [PubMed]
79. Renard, D.; Brunel, H.; Gaillard, N. Bilateral haemorrhagic infarction of the globus pallidus after cocaine and alcohol intoxication. *Acta Neurol. Belg.* **2009**, *109*, 159–161. [PubMed]
80. Sein Anand, J.; Chodorowski, Z.; Wisniewski, M.; Golska, A. A cocaine-associated quadriplegia and motor aphasia after first use of cocaine. *Przegl. Lek.* **2007**, *64*, 316–317. [PubMed]
81. Wolff, V.; Armspach, J.P.; Lauer, V.; Rouyer, O.; Bataillard, M.; Marescaux, C.; Geny, B. Cannabis-related stroke: Myth or reality? *Stroke* **2013**, *44*, 558–563. [CrossRef]
82. Zou, S.; Kumar, U. Cannabinoid Receptors and the Endocannabinoid System: Signaling and Function in the Central Nervous System. *Int. J. Mol. Sci.* **2018**, *19*, 833. [CrossRef]

83. Howlett, A.C.; Fleming, R.M. Cannabinoid inhibition of adenylate cyclase. Pharmacology of the response in neuroblastoma cell membranes. *Mol. Pharmacol.* **1984**, *26*, 532–538. [PubMed]
84. Pertwee, R.G. The pharmacology of cannabinoid receptors and their ligands: An overview. *Int. J. Obes.* **2006**, *30*, S13–S18. [CrossRef] [PubMed]
85. Wolff, V.; Armspach, J.P.; Lauer, V.; Rouyer, O.; Ducros, A.; Marescaux, C.; Geny, B. Ischaemic strokes with reversible vasoconstriction and without thunderclap headache: A variant of the reversible cerebral vasoconstriction syndrome? *Cerebrovasc. Dis.* **2015**, *39*, 31–38. [CrossRef] [PubMed]
86. Hemachandra, D.; McKetin, R.; Cherbuin, N.; Anstey, K.J. Heavy cannabis users at elevated risk of stroke: Evidence from a general population survey. *Aust. N. Z. J. Public Health* **2016**, *40*, 226–230. [CrossRef] [PubMed]
87. Rumalla, K.; Reddy, A.Y.; Mittal, M.K. Recreational marijuana use and acute ischemic stroke: A population-based analysis of hospitalized patients in the United States. *J. Neurol. Sci.* **2016**, *364*, 191–196. [CrossRef] [PubMed]
88. Atchaneeyasakul, K.; Torres, L.F.; Malik, A.M. Large Amount of Cannabis Ingestion Resulting in Spontaneous Intracerebral Hemorrhage: A Case Report. *J. Stroke Cerebrovasc. Dis.* **2017**, *26*, e138–e139. [CrossRef] [PubMed]
89. Ince, B.; Benbir, G.; Yuksel, O.; Koseoglu, L.; Uluduz, D. Both hemorrhagic and ischemic stroke following high doses of cannabis consumption. *Presse Med.* **2015**, *44*, 106–107. [CrossRef] [PubMed]
90. Deusch, E.; Kress, H.G.; Kraft, B.; Kozek-Langenecker, S.A. The procoagulatory effects of delta-9-tetrahydrocannabinol in human platelets. *Anesth. Analg.* **2004**, *99*, 1127–1130. [CrossRef]
91. Levy, R.; Schurr, A.; Nathan, I.; Dvilanski, A.; Livn, A. Impairment of ADP-Induced Platelet Aggregation by Hashish Components. *Thromb. Haemost.* **1976**, *36*, 634–640. [CrossRef]
92. Thanvi, B.R.; Treadwell, S.D. Cannabis and stroke: Is there a link? *Postgrad. Med. J.* **2009**, *85*, 80–83. [CrossRef]
93. Mateo, I.; Pinedo, A.; Gomez-Beldarrain, M.; Basterretxea, J.M.; Garcia-Monco, J.C. Recurrent stroke associated with cannabis use. *J. Neurol. Neurosurg. Psychiatry* **2005**, *76*, 435–437. [CrossRef] [PubMed]
94. Bailly, C.; Merceron, O.; Hammoudi, N.; Dorent, R.; Michel, P.L. Cannabis induced acute coronary syndrome in a young female. *Int. J. Cardiol.* **2010**, *143*, e4–e6. [CrossRef] [PubMed]
95. EMCDDA. *Medical Use of Cannabis and Cannabinoids: Questions and Answers for Policymaking*; Publications Office of the European Union: Luxembourg, Luxembourg, 2018.
96. Barber, P.A.; Pridmore, H.M.; Krishnamurthy, V.; Roberts, S.; Spriggs, D.A.; Carter, K.N.; Anderson, N.E. Cannabis, ischemic stroke, and transient ischemic attack: A case-control study. *Stroke* **2013**, *44*, 2327–2329. [CrossRef] [PubMed]
97. Jamil, M.; Zafar, A.; Adeel Faizi, S.; Zawar, I. Stroke from Vasospasm due to Marijuana Use: Can Cannabis Synergistically with Other Medications Trigger Cerebral Vasospasm? *Case Rep. Neurol. Med.* **2016**, *2016*, 5313795. [CrossRef] [PubMed]
98. Trojak, B.; Leclerq, S.; Meille, V.; Khoumri, C.; Chauvet-Gelinier, J.C.; Giroud, M.; Bonin, B.; Gisselmann, A. Stroke with neuropsychiatric sequelae after cannabis use in a man: A case report. *J. Med. Case Rep.* **2011**, *5*, 264. [CrossRef]
99. Wolff, V.; Lauer, V.; Rouyer, O.; Sellal, F.; Meyer, N.; Raul, J.S.; Sabourdy, C.; Boujan, F.; Jahn, C.; Beaujeux, R.; et al. Cannabis use, ischemic stroke, and multifocal intracranial vasoconstriction: A prospective study in 48 consecutive young patients. *Stroke* **2011**, *42*, 1778–1780. [CrossRef]
100. Shere, A.; Goyal, H. Cannabis can augment thrombolytic properties of rtPA: Intracranial hemorrhage in a heavy cannabis user. *Am. J. Emerg. Med.* **2017**, *35*, 1988-e1. [CrossRef]
101. Volpon, L.C.; Sousa, C.; Moreira, S.K.K.; Teixeira, S.R.; Carlotti, A. Multiple Cerebral Infarcts in a Young Patient Associated With Marijuana Use. *J. Addict. Med.* **2017**, *11*, 405–407. [CrossRef]
102. Tirkey, N.K.; Gupta, S. Acute Antero-Inferior Wall Ischaemia with Acute Ischaemic Stroke Caused by Oral Ingestion of Cannabis in a Young Male. *J. Assoc. Physicians India* **2016**, *64*, 93–94.
103. Baharnoori, M.; Kassardjian, C.D.; Saposnik, G. Cannabis use associated with capsular warning syndrome and ischemic stroke. *Can. J. Neurol. Sci.* **2014**, *41*, 272–273. [CrossRef]
104. Renard, D.; Taieb, G.; Gras-Combe, G.; Labauge, P. Cannabis-related myocardial infarction and cardioembolic stroke. *J. Stroke Cerebrovasc. Dis.* **2012**, *21*, 82–83. [CrossRef] [PubMed]
105. Castaneto, M.S.; Gorelick, D.A.; Desrosiers, N.A.; Hartman, R.L.; Pirard, S.; Huestis, M.A. Synthetic cannabinoids: Epidemiology, pharmacodynamics, and clinical implications. *Drug Alcohol Depend.* **2014**, *144*, 12–41. [CrossRef] [PubMed]

106. Seely, K.A.; Lapoint, J.; Moran, J.H.; Fattore, L. Spice drugs are more than harmless herbal blends: A review of the pharmacology and toxicology of synthetic cannabinoids. *Prog. Neuropsychopharmacol. Biol. Psychiatry* **2012**, *39*, 234–243. [CrossRef] [PubMed]
107. Tai, S.; Fantegrossi, W.E. Synthetic Cannabinoids: Pharmacology, Behavioral Effects, and Abuse Potential. *Curr. Addict. Rep.* **2014**, *1*, 129–136. [CrossRef] [PubMed]
108. Brents, L.K.; Reichard, E.E.; Zimmerman, S.M.; Moran, J.H.; Fantegrossi, W.E.; Prather, P.L. Phase I hydroxylated metabolites of the K2 synthetic cannabinoid JWH-018 retain in vitro and in vivo cannabinoid 1 receptor affinity and activity. *PLoS ONE* **2011**, *6*, e21917. [CrossRef] [PubMed]
109. Freeman, M.J.; Rose, D.Z.; Myers, M.A.; Gooch, C.L.; Bozeman, A.C.; Burgin, W.S. Ischemic stroke after use of the synthetic marijuana "spice". *Neurology* **2013**, *81*, 2090–2093. [CrossRef] [PubMed]
110. Rose, D.Z.; Guerrero, W.R.; Mokin, M.V.; Gooch, C.L.; Bozeman, A.C.; Pearson, J.M.; Burgin, W.S. Hemorrhagic stroke following use of the synthetic marijuana "spice". *Neurology* **2015**, *85*, 1177–1179. [CrossRef] [PubMed]
111. Hillard, C.J. Endocannabinoids and vascular function. *J. Pharmacol. Exp. Ther.* **2000**, *294*, 27–32. [PubMed]
112. Brents, L.K.; Prather, P.L. The K2/Spice phenomenon: Emergence, identification, legislation and metabolic characterization of synthetic cannabinoids in herbal incense products. *Drug Metab. Rev.* **2014**, *46*, 72–85. [CrossRef] [PubMed]
113. Bernson-Leung, M.E.; Leung, L.Y.; Kumar, S. Synthetic cannabis and acute ischemic stroke. *J. Stroke Cerebrovasc. Dis.* **2014**, *23*, 1239–1241. [CrossRef] [PubMed]
114. Faroqui, R.; Mena, P.; Wolfe, A.R.; Bibawy, J.; Visvikis, G.A.; Mantello, M.T. Acute carotid thrombosis and ischemic stroke following overdose of the synthetic cannabinoid K2 in a previously healthy young adult male. *Radiol. Case Rep.* **2018**, *13*, 747–752. [CrossRef] [PubMed]
115. Takematsu, M.; Hoffman, R.S.; Nelson, L.S.; Schechter, J.M.; Moran, J.H.; Wiener, S.W. A case of acute cerebral ischemia following inhalation of a synthetic cannabinoid. *Clin. Toxicol.* **2014**, *52*, 973–975. [CrossRef] [PubMed]
116. Lachenmeier, D.W.; Sproll, C.; Musshoff, F. Poppy seed foods and opiate drug testing—Where are we today? *Ther. Drug Monit.* **2010**, *32*, 11–18. [CrossRef] [PubMed]
117. Mars, S.G.; Bourgois, P.; Karandinos, G.; Montero, F.; Ciccarone, D. The Textures of Heroin: User Perspectives on "Black Tar" and Powder Heroin in Two U.S. Cities. *J. Psychoact. Drugs* **2016**, *48*, 270–278. [CrossRef] [PubMed]
118. Freye, E.; Levy, J. *Opioids in Medicine—A Comprehensive Review on the Mode of Action and the Use of Analgesics in Different Clinical Pain States*; Springer Science + Business Media BV: Dordrecht, The Netherlands, 2008.
119. Dinis-Oliveira, R.J.; Carvalho, F.; Moreira, R.; Duarte, J.A.; Proenca, J.B.; Santos, A.; Magalhaes, T. Clinical and forensic signs related to opioids abuse. *Curr. Drug Abus. Rev.* **2012**, *5*, 273–290. [CrossRef]
120. Yeh, S.Y. Urinary excretion of morphine and its metabolites in morphine-dependent subjects. *J. Pharmacol. Exp. Ther.* **1975**, *192*, 201–210. [PubMed]
121. Meyer, M.R.; Schutz, A.; Maurer, H.H. Contribution of human esterases to the metabolism of selected drugs of abuse. *Toxicol. Lett.* **2015**, *232*, 159–166. [CrossRef] [PubMed]
122. Fonseca, A.C.; Ferro, J.M. Drug abuse and stroke. *Curr. Neurol. Neurosci. Rep.* **2013**, *13*, 325. [CrossRef]
123. Niehaus, L.; Roricht, S.; Meyer, B.U.; Sander, B. Nuclear magnetic resonance tomography detection of heroin-associated CNS lesions. *Aktuelle Radiol.* **1997**, *7*, 309–311.
124. Enevoldson, T.P. Recreational drugs and their neurological consequences. *J. Neurol. Neurosurg. Psychiatry* **2004**, *75*, iii9–iii15. [CrossRef]
125. Bolz, J.; Meves, S.H.; Kara, K.; Reinacher-Schick, A.; Gold, R.; Krogias, C. Multiple cerebral infarctions in a young patient with heroin-induced hypereosinophilic syndrome. *J. Neurol. Sci.* **2015**, *356*, 193–195. [CrossRef] [PubMed]
126. Prick, J.J.; Gabreels-Festen, A.A.; Korten, J.J.; van der Wiel, T.W. Neurological manifestations of the hypereosinophilic syndrome (HES). *Clin. Neurol. Neurosurg.* **1988**, *90*, 269–273. [CrossRef]
127. Hamzei Moqaddam, A.; Ahmadi Musavi, S.M.R.; Khademizadeh, K. Relationship of opium dependency and stroke. *Addict. Health* **2009**, *1*, 6–10. [PubMed]
128. Kumar, N.; Bhalla, M.C.; Frey, J.A.; Southern, A. Intraparenchymal hemorrhage after heroin use. *Am. J. Emerg. Med.* **2015**, *33*, 1109-e3. [CrossRef] [PubMed]
129. Alquist, C.R.; McGoey, R.; Bastian, F.; Newman, W., 3rd. Bilateral globus pallidus lesions. *J. La. State Med. Soc.* **2012**, *164*, 145–146. [PubMed]

130. Vila, N.; Chamorro, A. Ballistic movements due to ischemic infarcts after intravenous heroin overdose: Report of two cases. *Clin. Neurol. Neurosurg.* **1997**, *99*, 259–262. [CrossRef]
131. Brust, J.C.; Richter, R.W. Stroke associated with addiction to heroin. *J. Neurol. Neurosurg. Psychiatry* **1976**, *39*, 194–199. [CrossRef]
132. Lee, C.W.; Muo, C.H.; Liang, J.A.; Sung, F.C.; Kao, C.H. Association of intensive morphine treatment and increased stroke incidence in prostate cancer patients: A population-based nested case-control study. *Jpn. J. Clin. Oncol.* **2013**, *43*, 776–781. [CrossRef]
133. Hamzei-Moghaddam, A.; Shafa, M.A.; Khanjani, N.; Farahat, R. Frequency of Opium Addiction in Patients with Ischemic Stroke and Comparing their Cerebrovascular Doppler Ultrasound Changes to Non-Addicts. *Addict. Health* **2013**, *5*, 95–101.
134. Benoilid, A.; Collongues, N.; de Seze, J.; Blanc, F. Heroin inhalation-induced unilateral complete hippocampal stroke. *Neurocase* **2013**, *19*, 313–315. [CrossRef]
135. Hsu, W.Y.; Chiu, N.Y.; Liao, Y.C. Rhabdomyolysis and brain ischemic stroke in a heroin-dependent male under methadone maintenance therapy. *Acta Psychiatr. Scand.* **2009**, *120*, 76–79. [CrossRef] [PubMed]
136. Brenu, E.W.; McNaughton, L.; Marshall-Gradisnik, S.M. Is there a potential immune dysfunction with anabolic androgenic steroid use: A review. *Mini Rev. Med. Chem.* **2011**, *11*, 438–445. [CrossRef] [PubMed]
137. Kenna, G.A.; Lewis, D.C. Risk factors for alcohol and other drug use by healthcare professionals. *Subst. Abus. Treat. Prev. Policy* **2008**, *3*, 3. [CrossRef] [PubMed]
138. Hartgens, F.; Rietjens, G.; Keizer, H.A.; Kuipers, H.; Wolffenbuttel, B.H. Effects of androgenic-anabolic steroids on apolipoproteins and lipoprotein (a). *Br. J. Sports Med.* **2004**, *38*, 253–259. [CrossRef] [PubMed]
139. Santamarina, R.D.; Besocke, A.G.; Romano, L.M.; Ioli, P.L.; Gonorazky, S.E. Ischemic stroke related to anabolic abuse. *Clin. Neuropharmacol.* **2008**, *31*, 80–85. [CrossRef] [PubMed]
140. Shamloul, R.M.; Aborayah, A.F.; Hashad, A.; Abd-Allah, F. Anabolic steroids abuse-induced cardiomyopathy and ischaemic stroke in a young male patient. *BMJ Case Rep.* **2014**, *2014*. [CrossRef] [PubMed]
141. Youssef, M.Y.; Alqallaf, A.; Abdella, N. Anabolic androgenic steroid-induced cardiomyopathy, stroke and peripheral vascular disease. *BMJ Case Rep.* **2011**, *2011*. [CrossRef] [PubMed]
142. Pearson, A.C.; Schiff, M.; Mrosek, D.; Labovitz, A.J.; Williams, G.A. Left ventricular diastolic function in weight lifters. *Am. J. Cardiol.* **1986**, *58*, 1254–1259. [CrossRef]
143. Lippi, G.; Banfi, G. Doping and thrombosis in sports. *Semin. Thromb. Hemost.* **2011**, *37*, 918–928. [CrossRef]
144. Beutel, A.; Bergamaschi, C.T.; Campos, R.R. Effects of chronic anabolic steroid treatment on tonic and reflex cardiovascular control in male rats. *J. Steroid Biochem. Mol. Biol.* **2005**, *93*, 43–48. [CrossRef]
145. Santos, M.A.; Oliveira, C.V.; Silva, A.S. Adverse cardiovascular effects from the use of anabolic-androgenic steroids as ergogenic resources. *Subst. Use Misuse* **2014**, *49*, 1132–1137. [CrossRef] [PubMed]
146. Achar, S.; Rostamian, A.; Narayan, S.M. Cardiac and metabolic effects of anabolic-androgenic steroid abuse on lipids, blood pressure, left ventricular dimensions, and rhythm. *Am. J. Cardiol.* **2010**, *106*, 893–901. [CrossRef] [PubMed]
147. D'Ascenzo, S.; Millimaggi, D.; Di Massimo, C.; Saccani-Jotti, G.; Botre, F.; Carta, G.; Tozzi-Ciancarelli, M.G.; Pavan, A.; Dolo, V. Detrimental effects of anabolic steroids on human endothelial cells. *Toxicol. Lett.* **2007**, *169*, 129–136. [CrossRef] [PubMed]
148. Hartgens, F.; Kuipers, H. Effects of androgenic-anabolic steroids in athletes. *Sports Med.* **2004**, *34*, 513–554. [CrossRef] [PubMed]
149. Liu, P.Y.; Death, A.K.; Handelsman, D.J. Androgens and cardiovascular disease. *Endocr. Rev.* **2003**, *24*, 313–340. [CrossRef] [PubMed]
150. Rocha, F.L.; Carmo, E.C.; Roque, F.R.; Hashimoto, N.Y.; Rossoni, L.V.; Frimm, C.; Aneas, I.; Negrao, C.E.; Krieger, J.E.; Oliveira, E.M. Anabolic steroids induce cardiac renin-angiotensin system and impair the beneficial effects of aerobic training in rats. *Am. J. Physiol. Heart Circ. Physiol.* **2007**, *293*, H3575–H3583. [CrossRef] [PubMed]
151. Do Carmo, E.C.; Fernandes, T.; Koike, D.; Da Silva, N.D., Jr.; Mattos, K.C.; Rosa, K.T.; Barretti, D.; Melo, S.F.; Wichi, R.B.; Irigoyen, M.C.; et al. Anabolic steroid associated to physical training induces deleterious cardiac effects. *Med. Sci. Sports Exerc.* **2011**, *43*, 1836–1848. [CrossRef] [PubMed]
152. Schooling, C.M.; Luo, S.; Au Yeung, S.L.; Thompson, D.J.; Karthikeyan, S.; Bolton, T.R.; Mason, A.M.; Ingelsson, E.; Burgess, S. Genetic predictors of testosterone and their associations with cardiovascular disease and risk factors: A Mendelian randomization investigation. *Int. J. Cardiol.* **2018**, *267*, 171–176. [CrossRef] [PubMed]

153. Cole, A.P.; Hanske, J. Impact of testosterone replacement therapy on thromboembolism, heart disease and obstructive sleep apnoea in men. *BJU Int.* **2018**, *121*, 811–818. [CrossRef] [PubMed]
154. Normann, S.; de Veber, G.; Fobker, M.; Langer, C.; Kenet, G.; Bernard, T.J.; Fiedler, B.; Sträter, R.; Goldenberg, N.A.; Nowak-Göttl, U. Role of endogenous testosterone concentration in pediatric stroke. *Ann. Neurol.* **2009**, *66*, 754–758. [CrossRef] [PubMed]
155. Bhasin, S.; Brito, J.P.; Cunningham, G.R.; Hayes, F.J.; Hodis, H.N.; Matsumoto, A.M.; Snyder, P.J.; Swerdloff, R.S.; Wu, F.C.; Yialamas, M.A. Testosterone Therapy in Men With Hypogonadism: An Endocrine Society Clinical Practice Guideline. *J. Clin. Endocrinol. Metab.* **2018**, *103*, 1715–1744. [CrossRef] [PubMed]
156. El Scheich, T.; Weber, A.A.; Klee, D.; Schweiger, D.; Mayatepek, E.; Karenfort, M. Adolescent ischemic stroke associated with anabolic steroid and cannabis abuse. *J. Pediatr. Endocrinol. Metab.* **2013**, *26*, 161–165. [CrossRef] [PubMed]
157. Juhan-Vague, I.; Pyke, S.D.; Alessi, M.C.; Jespersen, J.; Haverkate, F.; Thompson, S.G. Fibrinolytic factors and the risk of myocardial infarction or sudden death in patients with angina pectoris. ECAT Study Group. European Concerted Action on Thrombosis and Disabilities. *Circulation* **1996**, *94*, 2057–2063. [CrossRef] [PubMed]
158. Siokas, V.; Dardiotis, E.; Sokolakis, T.; Kotoula, M.; Tachmitzi, S.V.; Chatzoulis, D.Z.; Almpanidou, P.; Stefanidis, I.; Hadjigeorgiou, G.M.; Tsironi, E.E. Plasminogen Activator Inhibitor Type-1 Tag Single-Nucleotide Polymorphisms in Patients with Diabetes Mellitus Type 2 and Diabetic Retinopathy. *Curr. Eye Res.* **2017**, *42*, 1048–1053. [CrossRef] [PubMed]
159. Winkler, U.H. Effects of androgens on haemostasis. *Maturitas* **1996**, *24*, 147–155. [CrossRef]
160. Nieminen, M.S.; Ramo, M.P.; Viitasalo, M.; Heikkila, P.; Karjalainen, J.; Mantysaari, M.; Heikkila, J. Serious cardiovascular side effects of large doses of anabolic steroids in weight lifters. *Eur. Heart J.* **1996**, *17*, 1576–1583. [CrossRef] [PubMed]
161. Kalin, M.F.; Zumoff, B. Sex hormones and coronary disease: A review of the clinical studies. *Steroids* **1990**, *55*, 330–352. [CrossRef]
162. Bachman, E.; Feng, R.; Travison, T.; Li, M.; Olbina, G.; Ostland, V.; Ulloor, J.; Zhang, A.; Basaria, S.; Ganz, T.; et al. Testosterone suppresses hepcidin in men: A potential mechanism for testosterone-induced erythrocytosis. *J. Clin. Endocrinol. Metab.* **2010**, *95*, 4743–4747. [CrossRef]
163. Bachman, E.; Travison, T.G.; Basaria, S.; Davda, M.N.; Guo, W.; Li, M.; Connor Westfall, J.; Bae, H.; Gordeuk, V.; Bhasin, S. Testosterone induces erythrocytosis via increased erythropoietin and suppressed hepcidin: Evidence for a new erythropoietin/hemoglobin set point. *J. Gerontol. A Biol. Sci. Med. Sci.* **2014**, *69*, 725–735. [CrossRef]
164. Young, N.S. Telomere biology and telomere diseases: Implications for practice and research. *Hematol. Am. Soc. Hematol. Educ. Program* **2010**, *2010*, 30–35. [CrossRef]
165. Tsarouhas, K.; Kioukia-Fougia, N.; Papalexis, P.; Tsatsakis, A.; Kouretas, D.; Bacopoulou, F.; Tsitsimpikou, C. Use of nutritional supplements contaminated with banned doping substances by recreational adolescent athletes in Athens, Greece. *Food Chem. Toxicol. Int. J. Publ. Br. Ind. Biol. Res. Assoc.* **2018**, *115*, 447–450. [CrossRef] [PubMed]
166. Tsitsimpikou, C.; Chrisostomou, N.; Papalexis, P.; Tsarouhas, K.; Tsatsakis, A.; Jamurtas, A. The use of nutritional supplements among recreational athletes in Athens, Greece. *Int. J. Sport Nutr. Exerc. Metab.* **2011**, *21*, 377–384. [CrossRef] [PubMed]
167. Vasilaki, F.; Tsitsimpikou, C.; Tsarouhas, K.; Germanakis, I.; Tzardi, M.; Kavvalakis, M.; Ozcagli, E.; Kouretas, D.; Tsatsakis, A.M. Cardiotoxicity in rabbits after long-term nandrolone decanoate administration. *Toxicol. Lett.* **2016**, *241*, 143–151. [CrossRef] [PubMed]
168. Baggish, A.L.; Weiner, R.B.; Kanayama, G.; Hudson, J.I.; Picard, M.H.; Hutter, A.M., Jr.; Pope, H.G., Jr. Long-term anabolic-androgenic steroid use is associated with left ventricular dysfunction. *Circ. Heart Fail.* **2010**, *3*, 472–476. [CrossRef] [PubMed]
169. Sattler, F.R.; Jaque, S.V.; Schroeder, E.T.; Olson, C.; Dube, M.P.; Martinez, C.; Briggs, W.; Horton, R.; Azen, S. Effects of pharmacological doses of nandrolone decanoate and progressive resistance training in immunodeficient patients infected with human immunodeficiency virus. *J. Clin. Endocrinol. Metab.* **1999**, *84*, 1268–1276. [CrossRef] [PubMed]

170. Shimada, Y.; Yoritaka, A.; Tanaka, Y.; Miyamoto, N.; Ueno, Y.; Hattori, N.; Takao, U. Cerebral Infarction in a Young Man Using High-dose Anabolic Steroids. *J. Stroke Cerebrovasc. Dis.* **2012**, *21*, 906-e9. [CrossRef] [PubMed]
171. D'Andrea, A.; Caso, P.; Salerno, G.; Scarafile, R.; De Corato, G.; Mita, C.; Di Salvo, G.; Severino, S.; Cuomo, S.; Liccardo, B.; et al. Left ventricular early myocardial dysfunction after chronic misuse of anabolic androgenic steroids: A Doppler myocardial and strain imaging analysis. *Br. J. Sports Med.* **2007**, *41*, 149–155. [CrossRef] [PubMed]
172. Garcia-Esperon, C.; Hervas-Garcia, J.V.; Jimenez-Gonzalez, M.; Perez de la Ossa-Herrero, N.; Gomis-Cortina, M.; Dorado-Bouix, L.; Lopez-Cancio Martinez, E.; Castano-Duque, C.H.; Millan-Torne, M.; Davalos, A. [Ingestion of anabolic steroids and ischaemic stroke. A clinical case report and review of the literature]. *Rev. Neurol.* **2013**, *56*, 327–331.
173. Low, M.S.; Vilcassim, S.; Fedele, P.; Grigoriadis, G. Anabolic androgenic steroids, an easily forgotten cause of polycythaemia and cerebral infarction. *Intern. Med. J.* **2016**, *46*, 497–499. [CrossRef]
174. Jouanjus, E.; Lapeyre-Mestre, M.; Micallef, J. Cannabis use: Signal of increasing risk of serious cardiovascular disorders. *J. Am. Heart Assoc.* **2014**, *3*, e000638. [CrossRef]

Increased Citrullinated Histone H3 Levels in the Early Post-Resuscitative Period are Associated with Poor Neurologic Function in Cardiac Arrest Survivors

Lisa-Marie Mauracher [1], Nina Buchtele [1,2], Christian Schörgenhofer [2], Christoph Weiser [3], Harald Herkner [3], Anne Merrelaar [3], Alexander O. Spiel [3], Lena Hell [1], Cihan Ay [1,4], Ingrid Pabinger [1], Bernd Jilma [2] and Michael Schwameis [3,*]

[1] Clinical Division of Hematology and Hemostaseology, Department of Medicine I, Medical University of Vienna, 1090 Vienna, Austria; lisa-marie.mauracher@meduniwien.ac.at (L.-M.M.); nina.buchtele@meduniwien.ac.at (N.B.); lena.hell@meduniwien.ac.at (L.H.); cihan.ay@meduniwien.ac.at (C.A.); ingrid.pabinger@meduniwien.ac.at (I.P.)

[2] Department of Clinical Pharmacology, Medical University of Vienna, 1090 Vienna, Austria; christian.schoergenhofer@meduniwien.ac.at (C.S.); bernd.jilma@meduniwien.ac.at (B.J.)

[3] Department of Emergency Medicine, Medical University of Vienna, 1090 Vienna, Austria; christoph.weiser@meduniwien.ac.at (C.W.); Harald.herkner@meduniwien.ac.at (H.H.); anne.merrelaar@meduniwien.ac.at (A.M.); alexander.spiel@meduniwien.ac.at (A.O.S.)

[4] I.M. Sechenov First Moscow State Medical University (Sechenov University), 119146 Moscow, Russia

* Correspondence: michael.schwameis@meduniwien.ac.at

Abstract: The exact contribution of neutrophils to post-resuscitative brain damage is unknown. We aimed to investigate whether neutrophil extracellular trap (NET) formation in the early phase after return of spontaneous circulation (ROSC) may be associated with poor 30 day neurologic function in cardiac arrest survivors. This study prospectively included adult (≥18 years) out-of-hospital cardiac arrest (OHCA) survivors with cardiac origin, who were subjected to targeted temperature management. Plasma levels of specific (citrullinated histone H3, H3Cit) and putative (cell-free DNA (cfDNA) and nucleosomes) biomarkers of NET formation were assessed at 0 and 12 h after admission. The primary outcome was neurologic function on day 30 after admission, which was assessed using the five-point cerebral performance category (CPC) score, classifying patients into good (CPC 1–2) or poor (CPC 3–5) neurologic function. The main variable of interest was the effect of H3Cit level quintiles at 12 h on 30 day neurologic function, assessed by logistic regression. The first quintile was used as a baseline reference. Results are given as crude odds ratio (OR) with 95% confidence interval (95% CI). Sixty-two patients (79% male, median age: 57 years) were enrolled. The odds of poor neurologic function increased linearly, with 0 h levels of cfNDA (crude OR 1.8, 95% CI: 1.2–2.7, $p = 0.007$) and nucleosomes (crude OR 1.7, 95% CI: 1.0–2.2, $p = 0.049$), as well as with 12 h levels of cfDNA (crude OR 1.6, 95% CI: 1.1–2.4, $p = 0.024$), nucleosomes (crude OR 1.7, 95% CI: 1.1–2.5, $p = 0.020$), and H3Cit (crude OR 1.6, 95% CI: 1.1–2.3, $p = 0.029$). Patients in the fourth (7.9, 95% CI: 1.1–56, $p = 0.039$) and fifth (9.0, 95% CI: 1.3–63, $p = 0.027$) H3Cit quintile had significantly higher odds of poor 30 day neurologic function compared to patients in the first quintile. Increased plasma levels of H3Cit, 12 h after admission, are associated with poor 30 day neurologic function in adult OHCA survivors, which may suggest a contribution of NET formation to post-resuscitative brain damage and therefore provide a therapeutic target in the future.

Keywords: neutrophil extracellular traps; citrullinated histone H3; cardiac arrest; neurologic function

1. Introduction

In cardiac arrest survivors good neurologic outcome remains difficult to achieve [1]. Brain injury does not occur solely during circulatory interruption, but may progress during the reperfusion period after sustained return of spontaneous circulation (ROSC) [2]. Ischemic reperfusion is considered a main trigger of a complex cascade of pro-inflammatory and pro-thrombotic events occurring hours to days after resuscitation, which may impair cerebral microvascular perfusion despite restoration of macrovascular flow [3,4]. Recent data suggest that the response of neutrophils to hypoxia could be an early and critical mediator of ischemic reperfusion injury [5]. This is consistent with previous studies reporting substantial mortality and neurologic morbidity in resuscitated cardiac arrest patients with an elevated number of blood neutrophils in relation to other leukocyte counts [6–8]. The mechanisms by which neutrophils may contribute to post-resuscitative brain damage have, however, not yet been elucidated.

In recent years, neutrophil extracellular traps (NETs) have emerged as a central player in inflammation, thrombogenesis, and cardiovascular disease [9–14]. NETs are chromatin fibers consisting of histones, cell free DNA (cfDNA), and granular proteins, and are released within minutes [15] to hours [16] following activation by various stimuli including ischemia and reperfusion [17]. While NETs have primarily been recognized as mediators of antimicrobial host defense, they may exert detrimental inflammatory and procoagulant effects causing endothelial damage, platelet activation, microvessel occlusions, and ultimately tissue malperfusion [18]. In particular, neutrophil histones and DNA are considered cytotoxic and procoagulant components of NETs [19], and have been implicated in organ damage in various noninfectious conditions [20,21]. Citrullination of histone H3 (H3Cit) by peptidylarginine deiminase 4 (PAD4) is a key signal for chromatin decondensation and NET formation [22]. H3Cit is commonly accepted as a NET biomarker, and has been measured in various studies to investigate NET formation. Despite this, the role of NETs in cardiac arrest has not yet been investigated. Pro-inflammatory and pro-thrombotic properties, however, render them possible mediators of neutrophil-borne brain injury after successful resuscitation.

We hypothesized that neutrophil extracellular trap (NET) formation may be associated with poor neurologic function after cardiac arrest. This study aimed to assess plasma levels of NET biomarkers in the early phase after ROSC and investigate its association with short-term neurologic function in a selected cohort of out-of-hospital cardiac arrest (OHCA) survivors.

2. Methods

This prospective single-center observational cohort study was conducted at the Emergency Department at the Medical University of Vienna. Adult (≥18 years) OHCA survivors with cardiac origin who received in-hospital targeted temperature management (33 ± 0.5 °C) were enrolled. Exclusion criteria included current oral anticoagulation therapy, thrombolytic therapy, intravascular cooling, and application of extracorporeal assist devices (Figure S1). A waiver for written informed consent was obtained from the local ethics committee. The informed consent was permanently waived if the patient did not regain consciousness. Patients who regained consciousness were informed of their participation as soon as they were able to understand the purpose of the study. Post-resuscitation care was performed in accordance with the International Liaison Committee on resuscitation guidelines [23]. The primary outcome was neurologic function on day 30 after admission, which was assessed by independent study fellows blinded to levels of NET-related biomarker measurement. For primary outcome assessment, the five-point cerebral performance category (CPC) score was used, which classifies patients into good (CPC 1–2) and poor neurologic function (CPC 3–5; 3 = severe cerebral disability, 4 = coma or vegetative state, 5 = death) [24].

Resuscitation-related parameters were collected via structured telephone interviews with the dispatch center, the emergency physicians, and paramedics at the scene, as well as the bystander who made the emergency call. These parameters included location of cardiac arrest (home vs. public), initial rhythm (non-shockable vs. shockable), witness status, basic life support, downtime (interval from collapse to ROSC), the amount of epinephrine administered, and the administration of heparin by the emergency medical service (EMS). Demographics and chronic health conditions that existed pre-arrest were collected by review of past medical reports and interviews with relatives and the general practitioner if available.

The study was approved by the ethics committee of the Medical University of Vienna (EC Number 1674/2013) and conducted in accordance with Helsinki declarations.

2.1. Blood Sampling

Whole blood was obtained on admission immediately after vascular access was available and again 12 h later and stored in blood collection tubes containing 3.8% trisodium citrate (Greiner BioOne, Kremsmünster, Austria). Immediately thereafter, samples were centrifuged for 10 min at 3000 *g* and platelet poor plasma was stored at −80 °C until final analysis.

2.2. Laboratory Analysis of NET Related Biomarker

Citrullinated histone H3 (H3Cit), nucleosome, and cell free DNA (cfDNA) levels were obtained from plasma samples as previously described [12]. Briefly, cfDNA was measured using Quant-iT PicoGreen dsDNA Assay Kit (Thermo Fisher Scientific, Waltham, MA, USA) according to the manufacturer's instructions. Nucleosomes were measured using Cell Death Detection ELISAPLUS (Roche Diagnostics, Mannheim, Germany) and the resultant values were compared to a plasma pool from male healthy controls. H3Cit levels were obtained by using a Cell Death Detection ELISA Kit (Sigma Aldrich, St. Louis, MO, USA). After overnight coating with anti-histone antibody at 4 °C, the 96-well plate (Nunc MicroWell 96-well microplates, Thermo Fisher Scientific, Waltham, MA, USA) was blocked with incubation buffer. After washing with phosphate buffered saline (PBS)-Tween, self-made H3Cit standards as well as plasma samples were incubated for 1.5 h at room temperature and washed again. Anti-H3Cit antibody (1:1000 ab5103, Abcam, Cambridge, MA, USA) was applied and incubated for 1.5 h at room temperature. After another washing step, secondary antibody (1:5000 goat anti-rabbit IgG horseradish peroxidase (HRP), Biorad, Hertfordshire, U.K.) was incubated for 1 h at room temperature and washed again. Incubation with TMB (3,3′, 5,5′-tetramethylbenzidine, Sigma Aldrich, St. Louis, MO, USA) for 25 min and the addition of 2% sulfuric acid resulted in a colorimetric change, readable at 450 nm. Measurement of NET biomarkers was performed without an awareness of neurologic assessment outcome. NET-related biomarkers were obtained in duplicate, and the respective mean value was used for the final statistical analysis. Resulted values are given in ng/mL, multiple-of-the-mean (MoM), and ng/mL for cfDNA, nucleosomes, and H3Cit respectively.

2.3. Statistical Methods

Categorical data are presented as absolute count numbers (n) and relative frequencies (%), continuous data as medians and 25–75% interquartile ranges. The patients were analyzed according to their neurologic function on day 30 (CPC 3–5/poor vs. 1–2/good). For between-group comparisons we used the Mann–Whitney U test for continuous variables and the Fisher's exact test for categorical variables. We used a score test to assess a trend of increasing biomarker levels at specific time points for neurologic outcome and logistic regression models, including each relevant co-variable separately, to estimate the effect of NET biomarkers on neurologic function. A subgroup analysis of the effect of H3Cit on the primary outcome included only patients with a CPC of 1–4 on day 30 after admission. The score test is a nonparametric test for a trend across ordered groups as an extension of the Wilcoxon rank-sum test [25]. Results are given as crude odds ratio (OR) with 95% confidence interval (95% CI). NET biomarker levels were categorized into quintiles prior to analysis. The first quintile of each biomarker level distribution was used as a baseline reference. Covariables judged to be clinically plausible included age, sex, location of cardiac arrest (place of residence vs. public place), initial rhythm (non-shockable vs. shockable), witnessed status, basic life support, downtime (interval from collapse to ROSC equaling the sum of no-flow and low-flow time), amount of epinephrine administered, and d-dimer and lactate levels. D-dimer and lactate levels were log transformed to normalize data distribution. The likelihood ratio test was performed to assess deviations from linearity. The Spearman method was used to assess the correlation between plasma levels of cfDNA, nucleosomes, and H3cit. No data-imputation was applied for missing data. We used Stata Statistical Software (Release 14, StataCorp LLC, College Station, TX, USA) for data analysis and GraphPad Prism Version 8.0.2 for Windows (GraphPad Software, La Jolla, CA, USA) to draw figures. Generally, we considered a two-sided p-value < 0.05 as statistically significant.

3. Results

Between January 2014 and January 2017, 62 patients (79% male, median age: 57 years, 46–67) with OHCA who had achieved ROSC on admission were enrolled. In total, 52% of patients ($n = 32$) had a poor 30 day neurologic function. The number of patients with acute coronary syndrome was similar between patients with good and those with poor 30 day neurologic function (77% vs. 66%, $p = 0.338$). The time interval between collapse and study-related blood sampling was longer in patients with poor outcome (65 min vs. 56 min, $p = 0.033$). At 12 h, both the neutrophil count (11.8 vs. 9.9 G/L, $p = 0.051$) and the neutrophil-to-lymphocyte ratio (11.6 vs. 6.8, $p = 0.046$) were higher in patients with poor function compared with those with good neurologic function. The characteristics of the study patients, including median levels of NET-related biomarkers at 0 and 12 h, are shown in Table 1. Across all patients, there was no association between H3Cit and cfDNA (0 h: rho = 0.05, $p = 0.718$; 12 h: rho = 0.18, $p = 0.189$) or nucleosome levels (0 h: rho = 0.06, $p = 0.669$; 12 h: rho = 0.13, $p = 0.328$), neither on admission nor 12 h later. In contrast, cfDNA levels correlated with nucleosome levels at both time points (0 h: rho = 0.64, $p < 0.001$; 12 h: rho = 0.53; $p < 0.001$).

Table 1. Patient characteristics according to neurologic function on day 30. Data are n (%) or median (25–75% interquartile range).

Variable	Total ($n = 62$)	Good Function CPC 1–2 ($n = 30$)	Poor Function CPC 3–5 ($n = 32$)	p-Value
Male sex	49 (79)	25 (83)	24 (75)	0.421
Age, years	57 (46–67)	52 (44–61)	61 (53–70)	0.030 *
Cause of cardiac arrest				0.338
Acute coronary syndrome	44 (71)	23 (77)	21 (66)	
Primary arrhythmia	18 (29)	7 (23)	11 (34)	
PCI with stenting	42 (68)	22 (73)	20 (63)	0.362
Resuscitation characteristics				
CPC prior to cardiac arrest				
CPC 1	61 (98)	30 (100)	31 (95)	1.0
CPC 2	1 (2)	0	1 (5)	
Location of cardiac arrest				
Place of residence	35 (57)	19 (63)	16 (50)	0.290
Public place	27 (43)	11 (37)	16 (50)	
Witnessed	54 (87)	28 (93)	26 (81)	0.258
Basic life support	44 (71)	23 (77)	21 (66)	0.338
Shockable rhythm	46 (77)	27 (93)	19 (61)	0.004 *
Administration of heparin by EMS	28 (45.2)	14 (47)	14 (44)	0.795
Epinephrine, mg	3 (1–4)	1 (0–4)	3 (2–5)	0.004 *
Down time, min	29 (19–47)	23 (11–36)	38 (24–50)	0.011 *
Temp at admission, °C	35.3 (34.8–35.7)	35.4 (35.0–35.6)	35.1 (34.7–36)	0.676
Time from collapse to blood sampling, min	60 (49–72)	65 (52–87)	56 (43–65)	0.033 *
Laboratory values				
Lactate, mmol/L 0 h	7 (5–10)	6 (3–7)	10 (6–12)	0.001 *
D-dimer, µg/mL 0 h	8 (3–17)	4 (2–8)	14 (8–21)	0.003 *
D-dimer, µg/mL 12 h	4 (2–6)	2 (1–4)	6 (3–8)	0.009 *
Aptt, s 0 h	47 (36–121)	48 (33–129)	46 (37–119)	0.444
Aptt, s 12 h	37 (34–42)	37 (34–42)	38 (34–45)	0.487
Prothrombin time, % 0 h	79 (67–61)	79 (64–88)	78 (71–91)	0.418

Table 1. *Cont.*

Variable	Total (n = 62)	Good Function CPC 1–2 (n = 30)	Poor Function CPC 3–5 (n = 32)	p-Value
Prothrombin time, % 12 h	77 (66–87)	80 (68–88)	76 (63–86)	0.549
Fibrinogen, mg/dL 0 h	290 (242–322)	297 (246–317)	283 (240–343)	0.983
Fibrinogen, mg/dL 12 h	297 (258–350)	295 (260–346)	308 (241–359)	0.502
Platelet count, G/L 0 h	204 (163–245)	204 (163–235)	204 (164–251)	0.972
Platelet count, G/L 12h	193 (141–240)	193 (141–239)	193 (150–252)	0.490
CRP, mg/dL 0 h	0.2 (0.1–0.6)	0.2 (0.1–0.4)	0.3 (0.1–0.7)	0.410
CRP, mg/dL 12 h	1.6 (0.7–3.1)	1.0 (0.3–2.8)	1.7 (1.0–3.3)	0.057
Neutrophils 0 h, G/L	8.5 (6.2–12.8)	7.8 (6.0–12.8)	9.6 (6.4–13.2)	0.443
Neutrophils 12 h, G/L	10.9 (8.5–14.6)	9.9 (7.7–12.2)	11.8 (8.8–16)	0.051
NLR 0 h	2.5 (1.4–4.4)	2.6 (1.4–4.7)	2.4 (1.3–3.8)	0.375
NLR 12 h	10.3 (6.1–14.8)	6.8 (5.7–11.5)	11.6 (7–18)	0.046 *
cfDNA 0h, ng/mL	1481 (948–2176)	1197 (835–1544)	1898 (1148–2377)	0.007 *
cfDNA 12 h, ng/mL	555 (436–721)	489 (404–634)	593 (516–807)	0.016 *
Nucleosomes 0 h, MoM	4.4 (2.4–7.1)	3.8 (1.6–4.9)	5.6 (2.8–9.7)	0.032 *
Nucleosomes 12 h, MoM	0.7 (0.3–1.8)	0.4 (0.2–1.1)	1.1 (0.5–2.4)	0.036 *
H3Cit 0 h, ng/mL	447 (228–772)	447 (229–744)	434 (205–899)	0.755
H3Cit 12 h, ng/mL	386 (207–968)	299 (146–789)	667 (300–1201)	0.047 *

cfDNA, cell-free DNA; CPC, cerebral performance category; CRP, C-reactive protein; EMS, emergency medical service; H3Cit, citrullinated histones H3; MoM, multiple-of-the-mean; NLR, neutrophil-to-lymphocyte ratio; PCI, percutaneous coronary intervention; Temp, temperature; TnT, troponin. * indicates significance.

The poor neurologic function group had higher on-admission levels of cfDNA (1898 vs. 1197 ng/mL, $p = 0.007$) and nucleosomes (5.6 vs. 3.8 MoM, $p = 0.032$), but similar levels of H3Cit (434 vs. 447 ng/mL, $p = 0.755$) compared to patients with good neurologic function. While median levels of cfDNA and nucleosomes decreased in both groups from admission to 12 h, median levels of H3Cit increased in patients with poor 30 day neurologic function (Figure 1). At 12 h, all three biomarkers were higher in patients with poor 30 day neurologic function (cfDNA, 589 vs. 493 ng/mL, $p = 0.016$; nucleosomes, 1.1 vs. 0.4 MoM, $p = 0.036$; H3Cit, 667 vs. 299 ng/mL, $p = 0.043$). The score test showed a consistent trend towards poor neurologic function with increasing NET biomarker levels ($p < 0.05$) on admission ($p > 0.85$). This did not apply to H3Cit levels (Table S2).

In crude regression analysis, the odds of poor neurologic function on day 30 increased with increasing levels of NET-related biomarkers at both time points (Figure 2). In this, 0 h levels of cfDNA and nucleosomes were associated with 1.8 (crude OR, 95% CI: 1.2–2.7, $p = 0.007$) and 1.7 (crude OR, 95% CI: 1.0–2.2, $p = 0.049$) times higher odds of poor neurologic function. 12 h levels of cfDNA, nucleosomes, and H3Cit were associated with 1.6 (crude OR, 95% CI: 1.1–2.4, $p = 0.024$), 1.7 (crude OR, 95% CI: 1.1–2.5; $p = 0.02$), and 1.6 (crude OR, 95% CI: 1.1–2.3; $p = 0.029$) times higher odds of poor neurologic function. In patients with a CPC of 1–4 ($n = 50$), the odds of poor neurologic function on day 30 likewise increased with increasing 12 h levels of H3Cit (crude OR 1.7, 95% CI 1.0–3.0). The test for deviation from linearity indicated a linear association for all these biomarkers. The effect remained unchanged after adjustment for covariables (Table S1).

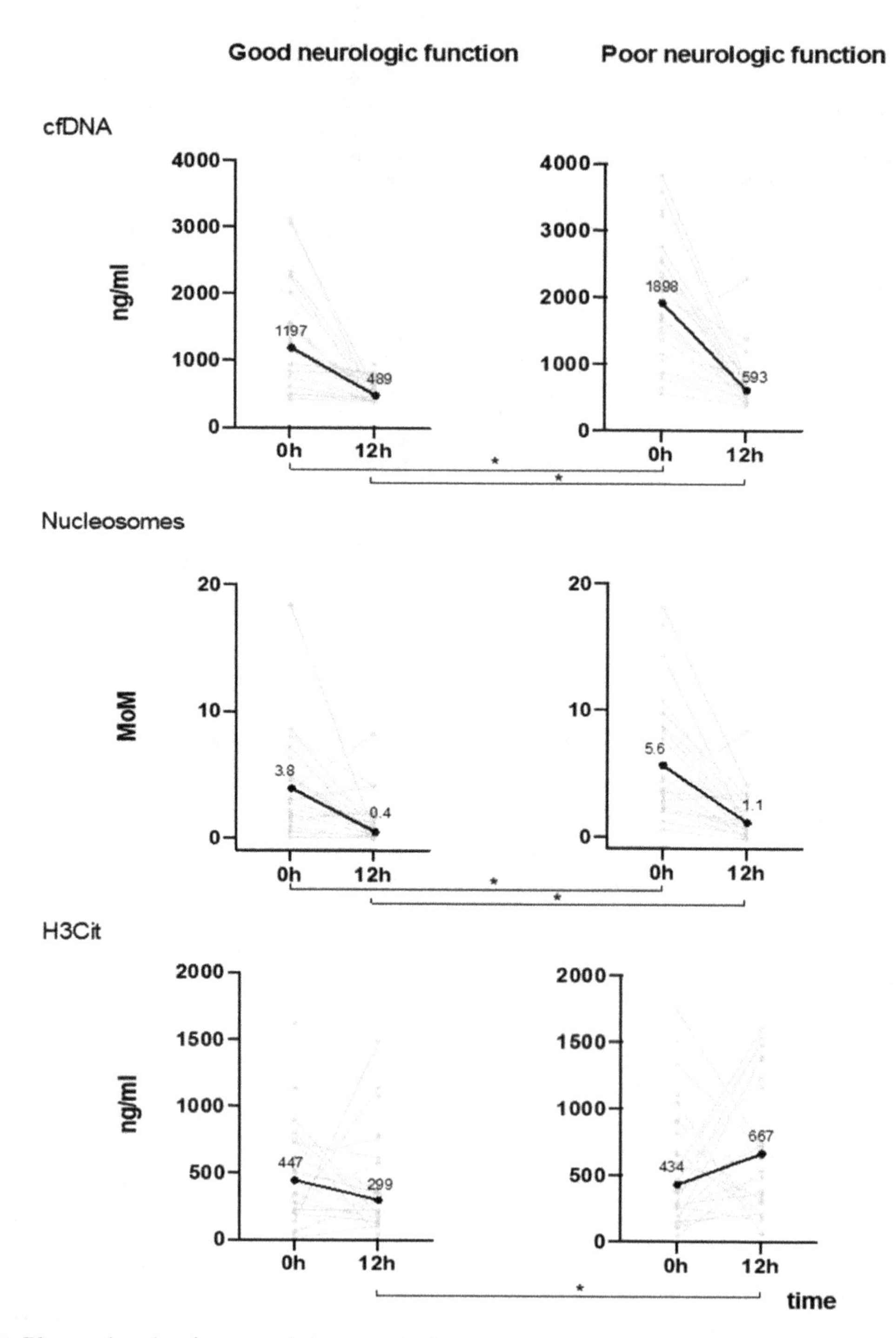

Figure 1. Plasma levels of neutrophil extracellular trap (NET) components (y-axis) on admission (0 h) and at 12 h (x-axis) in patients with good (left) and poor (right) 30 day neurologic function. Median levels of cfDNA and nucleosomes decreased in both groups from 0 to 12 h, while median H3Cit levels increased only in patients with poor 30 day neurologic function. Grey lines indicate individual data points, black lines represent median levels of NET-related biomarkers. * indicates significant difference. Individual and median d-dimer levels at 0 h and 12 h in the poor outcome group are available in the Supplementary Materials (Figure S2).

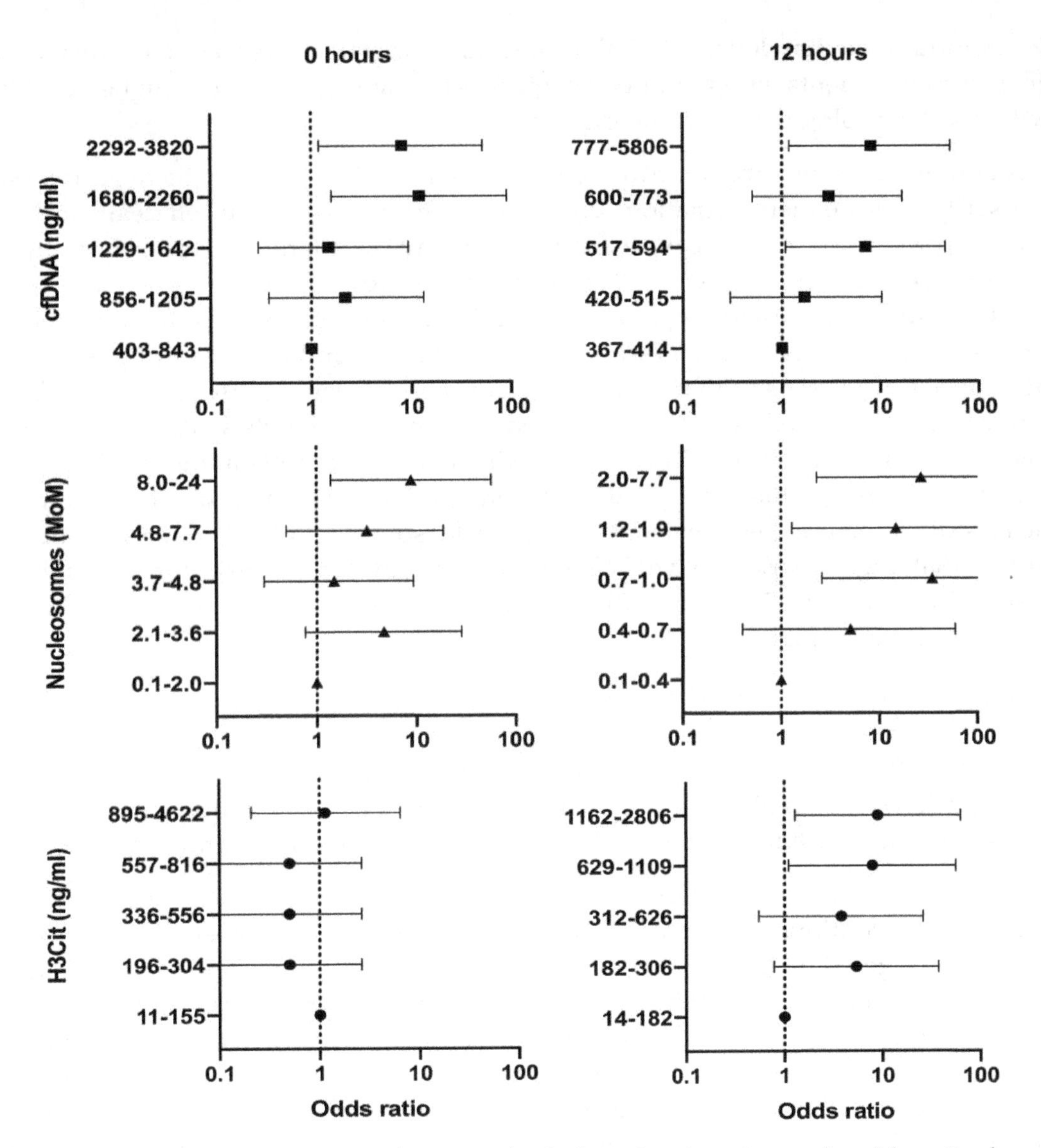

Figure 2. The crude odds of poor 30 day neurologic function (x-axis; crude odds ratio, log scale) according to plasma level quintiles of NET components (y-axis) on admission (left) and at 12 h (right). Confidence bands represent 95% confidence intervals. MoM, multiple-of-the-mean.

4. Discussion

Neurologic disability causes a high degree of morbidity in cardiac arrest survivors. This study investigated whether early plasma NET formation is associated with poor neurologic 30 day function following successful out-of-hospital resuscitation. The study was built on previous data suggesting a possible role of neutrophils in the development of post-resuscitative organ damage and was driven by the hypothesis that excessive NET release upon ischemic reperfusion may contribute to cerebral micro-circulatory compromise and thus neurologic disability in cardiac arrest survivors [5–8].

Previous studies reported increased mortality and neurologic morbidity in resuscitated cardiac arrest patients presenting with markers of neutrophil inflammation or elevated neutrophil counts in proportion to other leucocytes [6–8,26–28]. However, it has not been investigated whether these findings simply reflect stress response or whether neutrophils might be causally involved in the progression of organ injury following successful resuscitation.

This study provides a first indication that components of NETs may be involved in post-resuscitative brain damage. We found that NET-related biomarkers were already markedly elevated in cardiac arrest survivors at the time of admission, with these being even higher than levels measured in patients with cancer [12]. Although median levels of cfDNA and nucleosomes decreased over time, median levels of H3Cit increased in patients with poor neurologic function and were 30-fold higher at 12 h compared to those with good neurologic function on day 30.

cfDNA and nucleosomes are structural components of NETs but may have various sources and do not necessarily indicate their formation. Both are unspecific markers of cell death and cell turnover and may be interpreted as a measure of disease burden, but do not necessarily reflect the mechanism or source of disease. In this context, cfDNA levels have previously been shown to correlate with hospital mortality in cardiac arrest survivors [29]. H3Cit, in contrast, is considered a specific indicator of NET formation. Consistently, in this study, levels of cfDNA and nucleosomes on admission were significantly higher in patients with poor 30 day neurologic function, but decreased after successful resuscitation. In contrast, median H3Cit increased to significant levels at 12 h only in patients with poor 30 day neurologic function. It is likely that H3Cit are not detectable immediately upon admission, but take time to be formed, while less-specific markers originating from ischemic cell damage fall after ROSC. The lack of correlation between cfDNA and nucleosomes and H3Cit levels in our patients may further suggest that the biomarkers have different origins, and this is consistent with previous data on NET formation in patients with cancer [12], in whom H3Cit levels were likewise associated with an increased risk of mortality [30].

Although links in the chain of survival have substantially improved over the past decades, neurologic outcomes remain poor [31]. This is mainly attributable to the fact that several outcome-success factors cannot be influenced, such as witness status or a bystander's capability to provide basic life support. It might, however, highlight the lack of knowledge of the mechanisms driving post-resuscitative organ damage, limiting current post-resuscitation care to targeted temperature management [32].

The potential of post-resuscitation care to improve neurologic outcome is yet to be realized. Timely targeted interventions may offer the opportunity to alleviate or even interrupt early organ damage cascades triggered by ischemic reperfusion. Our data show that NETs may be associated with poor neurologic function 30 days after successful resuscitation. In contrast to previously identified coagulation makers associated with poor outcome after cardiac arrest [33,34], NET components may have the potential to serve as therapeutic target structures. NET-targeting agents administered soon after or even during resuscitation could contribute to preventing secondary brain injury and improving neurologic function. Supporting evidence comes from a recent mouse model study that shows the critical involvement of high mobility group box 1 formation in NET formation [35]. High mobility group box 1 is released by neutrophils [36], and the inhibition of high mobility group box 1 formation upon ischemic reperfusion successfully attenuated post-resuscitative brain injury in a rat model study [37].

However, it remains to be determined which step of NET formation should be targeted for therapy and which component of NETs is most appropriate to serve as a target structure. From our data we are able to infer that the early inhibition of histone H3 citrullination by selective peptidylarginine deiminase 4 (PAD 4) inhibitors might be a promising approach. This has already proven effective in disrupting in vitro NET formation in mouse and human neutrophils as well as in vivo [38,39]. Therapeutic degradation of formed NETs by DNase 1 may be an alternative or additional approach, one that has already been successfully used in mouse models to prevent thromboembolic disease [40]. In septic mice, infusion of DNase 1 resulted in significantly lower quantities of intravascular thrombin activity, reduced platelet aggregation, and ultimately improved microvascular perfusion.

The use of DNase 1 might be particularly beneficial in cardiac arrest patients with myocardial infarction, as coronary DNase activity has been found to negatively correlate with coronary NET burden and also with infarct size [11]. In this study, we analyzed a group of patients who had cardiac arrest of cardiac etiology. These patients commonly receive early antithrombotic and anticoagulant therapy and may thus be prone to experiencing hemorrhagic complications. A possible advantage of PAD 4 inhibitors and DNase 1 may be that both are considered to preserve physiological coagulation and thus should not cause additional bleeding risk [40]. Until advancements are made in human clinical testing, we can only speculate on the safety of these substances in humans. If further studies confirm our results, however, interventional trials investigating the safety and efficacy of NET-targeting agents in resuscitated animals may be warranted.

Limitations

The study was mainly limited by its sample size, resulting in large confidence intervals and the limited outcome events rate. We attempted to compensate for possible confounding by adjustment for clinically plausible covariables. Multivariable analyses including each relevant co-variable separately did not indicate relevant confounding. We included and analyzed a highly selected sample of patients with cardiac arrest of cardiac etiology who had achieved ROSC prior to hospital admission. Appropriate caution needs to be taken when interpreting our results. Furthermore, it must be mentioned that single patients with poor 30 day neurologic function did not show an increase in H3Cit levels from 0 to 12 h, while H3Cit levels did increase in some individuals with good neurologic outcome. Larger sampled studies investigating a more heterogeneous sample of cardiac arrest patients over a prolonged period of time may expand our results and aim at identifying specific patient characteristics, which allow for reliable prediction of NET formation in the individual patient in the early post-resuscitative stage.

Furthermore, a gold standard method for reliable measurement of NET formation in plasma is not available. We assessed three established NET-related biomarkers including H3Cit, which is considered a specific indicator of NET formation in plasma. It is, however, conceivable, that the assessment of additional NET components may gain test specificity and ultimately provide different results. The most reliable measure would perhaps be direct visualization of tissue NET formation, which may be investigated once a validated method becomes available.

Finally, we analyzed NET biomarker levels at only two time points, on admission and 12 h later. A more precise assessment of the time course of NET formation after cardiac arrest, however, may be of interest, because any NET-targeted therapy should likely be administered as early as possible to achieve the maximum beneficial effect.

5. Conclusions

We found that plasma levels of NET biomarkers assessed at an early post-resuscitative stage are associated with poor 30 day neurologic function in successfully resuscitated adults with OHCA. Further studies may assess whether NETs are causally involved in the pathophysiology of post-resuscitative brain damage, as well as discovering which components of NETs may have the potential to serve as therapeutic target structures to improve neurologic outcomes in cardiac arrest survivors in the future.

Author Contributions: Conceptualization, L.-M.M., N.B., B.J. and M.S.; data curation, N.B., C.S., C.W., A.M., A.O.S. and M.S.; formal analysis, L.-M.M., H.H. and M.S.; funding acquisition, I.P. and B.J.; methodology, L.-M.M., L.H., C.A. and I.P.; Writing—Original draft, L.-M.M., N.B. and M.S.; Writing—Review and editing, C.S., C.W, H.H., A.M., A.O.S., L.H., C.A., I.P. and B.J. The manuscript has been seen and approved by all authors, has not been previously published, and is not under consideration for publication in the same or substantially similar form in any other peer-reviewed media.

Acknowledgments: The authors thank Gerhard Ruzicka and study fellows for their valuable support. Open Access Funding by the Austrian Science Fund (Fonds zur Förderung der wissenschaftlichen Forschung, FWF).

References

1. Lilja, G.; Nielsen, N.; Friberg, H.; Horn, J.; Kjaergaard, J.; Nilsson, F.; Pellis, T.; Wetterslev, J.; Wise, M.P.; Bosch, F.; et al. Cognitive function in survivors of out-of-hospital cardiac arrest after target temperature management at 33 degrees C versus 36 degrees C. *Circulation* **2015**, *131*, 1340–1349. [CrossRef] [PubMed]
2. Sugita, A.; Kinoshita, K.; Sakurai, A.; Chiba, N.; Yamaguchi, J.; Kuwana, T.; Sawada, N.; Hori, S. Systemic impact on secondary brain aggravation due to ischemia/reperfusion injury in post-cardiac arrest syndrome: A prospective observational study using high-mobility group box 1 protein. *Crit. Care* **2017**, *21*, 247. [CrossRef] [PubMed]
3. Mongardon, N.; Dumas, F.; Ricome, S.; Grimaldi, D.; Hissem, T.; Pene, F.; Cariou, A. Postcardiac arrest syndrome: From immediate resuscitation to long-term outcome. *Ann. Intensive Care* **2011**, *1*, 45. [CrossRef] [PubMed]
4. Wada, T. Coagulofibrinolytic Changes in Patients with Post-cardiac Arrest Syndrome. *Front. Med. (Lausanne)* **2017**, *4*, 156. [CrossRef]
5. Cho, Y.D.; Park, S.J.; Choi, S.H.; Yoon, Y.H.; Kim, J.Y.; Lee, S.W.; Lim, C.S. The inflammatory response of neutrophils in an in vitro model that approximates the postcardiac arrest state. *Ann. Surg. Treat. Res.* **2017**, *93*, 217–224. [CrossRef]
6. Weiser, C.; Schwameis, M.; Sterz, F.; Herkner, H.; Lang, I.M.; Schwarzinger, I.; Spiel, A.O. Mortality in patients resuscitated from out-of-hospital cardiac arrest based on automated blood cell count and neutrophil lymphocyte ratio at admission. *Resuscitation* **2017**, *116*, 49–55. [CrossRef]
7. Patel, V.H.; Vendittelli, P.; Garg, R.; Szpunar, S.; LaLonde, T.; Lee, J.; Rosman, H.; Mehta, R.H.; Othman, H. Neutrophil-lymphocyte ratio: A prognostic tool in patients with in-hospital cardiac arrest. *World J. Crit. Care Med.* **2019**, *8*, 9–17. [CrossRef]
8. Kim, H.J.; Park, K.N.; Kim, S.H.; Lee, B.K.; Oh, S.H.; Moon, H.K.; Jeung, K.W.; Choi, S.P.; Cho, I.S.; Youn, C.S. Association between the neutrophil-to-lymphocyte ratio and neurological outcomes in patients undergoing targeted temperature management after cardiac arrest. *J. Crit. Care* **2018**, *47*, 227–231. [CrossRef]
9. Boeltz, S.; Amini, P.; Anders, H.J.; Andrade, F.; Bilyy, R.; Chatfield, S.; Cichon, I.; Clancy, D.M.; Desai, J.; Dumych, T.; et al. To NET or not to NET:current opinions and state of the science regarding the formation of neutrophil extracellular traps. *Cell Death Differ.* **2019**, *26*, 395–408. [CrossRef]
10. Kimball, A.S.; Obi, A.T.; Diaz, J.A.; Henke, P.K. The Emerging Role of NETs in Venous Thrombosis and Immunothrombosis. *Front. Immunol.* **2016**, *7*, 236. [CrossRef]
11. Mangold, A.; Alias, S.; Scherz, T.; Hofbauer, T.; Jakowitsch, J.; Panzenbock, A.; Simon, D.; Laimer, D.; Bangert, C.; Kammerlander, A.; et al. Coronary neutrophil extracellular trap burden and deoxyribonuclease activity in ST-elevation acute coronary syndrome are predictors of ST-segment resolution and infarct size. *Circ. Res.* **2015**, *116*, 1182–1192. [CrossRef] [PubMed]
12. Mauracher, L.M.; Posch, F.; Martinod, K.; Grilz, E.; Daullary, T.; Hell, L.; Brostjan, C.; Zielinski, C.; Ay, C.; Wagner, D.D.; et al. Citrullinated histone H3, a biomarker of neutrophil extracellular trap formation, predicts the risk of venous thromboembolism in cancer patients. *J. Thromb. Haemost.* **2018**, *16*, 508–518. [CrossRef] [PubMed]
13. Papayannopoulos, V. Neutrophil extracellular traps in immunity and disease. *Nat. Rev. Immunol.* **2018**, *18*, 134–147. [CrossRef] [PubMed]
14. Pertiwi, K.R.; van der Wal, A.C.; Pabittei, D.R.; Mackaaij, C.; van Leeuwen, M.B.; Li, X.; de Boer, O.J. Neutrophil Extracellular Traps Participate in All Different Types of Thrombotic and Haemorrhagic Complications of Coronary Atherosclerosis. *Thromb. Haemost.* **2018**, *118*, 1078–1087. [CrossRef]
15. Yipp, B.G.; Petri, B.; Salina, D.; Jenne, C.N.; Scott, B.N.; Zbytnuik, L.D.; Pittman, K.; Asaduzzaman, M.; Wu, K.; Meijndert, H.C.; et al. Infection-induced NETosis is a dynamic process involving neutrophil multitasking in vivo. *Nat. Med.* **2012**, *18*, 1386–1393. [CrossRef]
16. Fuchs, T.A.; Abed, U.; Goosmann, C.; Hurwitz, R.; Schulze, I.; Wahn, V.; Weinrauch, Y.; Brinkmann, V.; Zychlinsky, A. Novel cell death program leads to neutrophil extracellular traps. *J. Cell Biol.* **2007**, *176*, 231–241. [CrossRef]
17. Ge, L.; Zhou, X.; Ji, W.J.; Lu, R.Y.; Zhang, Y.; Zhang, Y.D.; Ma, Y.Q.; Zhao, J.H.; Li, Y.M. Neutrophil extracellular traps in ischemia-reperfusion injury-induced myocardial no-reflow: Therapeutic potential of DNase-based reperfusion strategy. *Am. J. Physiol. Heart Circ. Physiol.* **2015**, *308*, H500–H509. [CrossRef]

18. Gould, T.J.; Lysov, Z.; Liaw, P.C. Extracellular DNA and histones: Double-edged swords in immunothrombosis. *J. Thromb. Haemost.* **2015**, *13*, S82–S91. [CrossRef]
19. Noubouossie, D.F.; Whelihan, M.F.; Yu, Y.B.; Sparkenbaugh, E.; Pawlinski, R.; Monroe, D.M.; Key, N.S. In vitro activation of coagulation by human neutrophil DNA and histone proteins but not neutrophil extracellular traps. *Blood* **2017**, *129*, 1021–1029. [CrossRef]
20. Silk, E.; Zhao, H.; Weng, H.; Ma, D. The role of extracellular histone in organ injury. *Cell Death Dis.* **2017**, *8*, e2812. [CrossRef]
21. Jorch, S.K.; Kubes, P. An emerging role for neutrophil extracellular traps in noninfectious disease. *Nat. Med.* **2017**, *23*, 279–287. [CrossRef] [PubMed]
22. Li, P.; Li, M.; Lindberg, M.R.; Kennett, M.J.; Xiong, N.; Wang, Y. PAD4 is essential for antibacterial innate immunity mediated by neutrophil extracellular traps. *J. Exp. Med.* **2010**, *207*, 1853–1862. [CrossRef]
23. Nolan, J.P.; Hazinski, M.F.; Aickin, R.; Bhanji, F.; Billi, J.E.; Callaway, C.W.; Castren, M.; de Caen, A.R.; Ferrer, J.M.; Finn, J.C.; et al. Part 1: Executive summary: 2015 International Consensus on Cardiopulmonary Resuscitation and Emergency Cardiovascular Care Science with Treatment Recommendations. *Resuscitation* **2015**, *95*, e1–e31. [CrossRef]
24. Edgren, E.; Hedstrand, U.; Kelsey, S.; Sutton-Tyrrell, K.; Safar, P. Assessment of neurological prognosis in comatose survivors of cardiac arrest. BRCT I Study Group. *Lancet* **1994**, *343*, 1055–1059. [CrossRef]
25. Cuzick, J. A Wilcoxon-type test for trend. *Stat. Med.* **1985**, *4*, 87–90. [CrossRef]
26. Peberdy, M.A.; Andersen, L.W.; Abbate, A.; Thacker, L.R.; Gaieski, D.; Abella, B.S.; Grossestreuer, A.V.; Rittenberger, J.C.; Clore, J.; Ornato, J.; et al. Inflammatory markers following resuscitation from out-of-hospital cardiac arrest-A prospective multicenter observational study. *Resuscitation* **2016**, *103*, 117–124. [CrossRef] [PubMed]
27. Bro-Jeppesen, J.; Kjaergaard, J.; Wanscher, M.; Nielsen, N.; Friberg, H.; Bjerre, M.; Hassager, C. The inflammatory response after out-of-hospital cardiac arrest is not modified by targeted temperature management at 33 degrees C or 36 degrees C. *Resuscitation* **2014**, *85*, 1480–1487. [CrossRef] [PubMed]
28. Bro-Jeppesen, J.; Kjaergaard, J.; Stammet, P.; Wise, M.P.; Hovdenes, J.; Aneman, A.; Horn, J.; Devaux, Y.; Erlinge, D.; Gasche, Y.; et al. Predictive value of interleukin-6 in post-cardiac arrest patients treated with targeted temperature management at 33 degrees C or 36 degrees C. *Resuscitation* **2016**, *98*, 1–8. [CrossRef]
29. Arnalich, F.; Menendez, M.; Lagos, V.; Ciria, E.; Quesada, A.; Codoceo, R.; Vazquez, J.J.; Lopez-Collazo, E.; Montiel, C. Prognostic value of cell-free plasma DNA in patients with cardiac arrest outside the hospital: An observational cohort study. *Crit. Care* **2010**, *14*, R47. [CrossRef]
30. Grilz, E.; Mauracher, L.M.; Posch, F.; Konigsbrugge, O.; Zochbauer-Muller, S.; Marosi, C.; Lang, I.; Pabinger, I.; Ay, C. Citrullinated histone H3, a biomarker for neutrophil extracellular trap formation, predicts the risk of mortality in patients with cancer. *Br. J. Haematol.* **2019**, *186*, 311–320. [CrossRef] [PubMed]
31. Sulzgruber, P.; Sterz, F.; Schober, A.; Uray, T.; Van Tulder, R.; Hubner, P.; Wallmuller, C.; El-Tattan, D.; Graf, N.; Ruzicka, G.; et al. Editor's Choice-Progress in the chain of survival and its impact on outcomes of patients admitted to a specialized high-volume cardiac arrest center during the past two decades. *Eur. Heart J. Acute Cardiovasc. Care* **2016**, *5*, 3–12. [CrossRef] [PubMed]
32. Arrich, J.; Holzer, M.; Havel, C.; Mullner, M.; Herkner, H. Hypothermia for neuroprotection in adults after cardiopulmonary resuscitation. *Cochrane Database Syst. Rev.* **2016**, *2*, CD004128. [CrossRef] [PubMed]
33. Adrie, C.; Monchi, M.; Laurent, I.; Um, S.; Yan, S.B.; Thuong, M.; Cariou, A.; Charpentier, J.; Dhainaut, J.F. Coagulopathy after successful cardiopulmonary resuscitation following cardiac arrest: Implication of the protein C anticoagulant pathway. *J. Am. Coll. Cardiol.* **2005**, *46*, 21–28. [CrossRef] [PubMed]
34. Buchtele, N.; Schober, A.; Schoergenhofer, C.; Spiel, A.O.; Mauracher, L.; Weiser, C.; Sterz, F.; Jilma, B.; Schwameis, M. Added value of the DIC score and of D-dimer to predict outcome after successfully resuscitated out-of-hospital cardiac arrest. *Eur. J. Intern. Med.* **2018**, *57*, 44–48. [CrossRef]
35. Tadie, J.M.; Bae, H.B.; Jiang, S.; Park, D.W.; Bell, C.P.; Yang, H.; Pittet, J.F.; Tracey, K.; Thannickal, V.J.; Abraham, E.; et al. HMGB1 promotes neutrophil extracellular trap formation through interactions with Toll-like receptor 4. *Am. J. Physiol. Lung Cell. Mol. Physiol.* **2013**, *304*, L342–L349. [CrossRef] [PubMed]
36. Ito, I.; Fukazawa, J.; Yoshida, M. Post-translational methylation of high mobility group box 1 (HMGB1) causes its cytoplasmic localization in neutrophils. *J. Biol. Chem.* **2007**, *282*, 16336–16344. [CrossRef] [PubMed]

37. Shi, X.; Li, M.; Huang, K.; Zhou, S.; Hu, Y.; Pan, S.; Gu, Y. HMGB1 binding heptamer peptide improves survival and ameliorates brain injury in rats after cardiac arrest and cardiopulmonary resuscitation. *Neuroscience* **2017**, *360*, 128–138. [CrossRef]
38. Lewis, H.D.; Liddle, J.; Coote, J.E.; Atkinson, S.J.; Barker, M.D.; Bax, B.D.; Bicker, K.L.; Bingham, R.P.; Campbell, M.; Chen, Y.H.; et al. Inhibition of PAD4 activity is sufficient to disrupt mouse and human NET formation. *Nat. Chem. Biol.* **2015**, *11*, 189–191. [CrossRef]
39. Martinod, K.; Demers, M.; Fuchs, T.A.; Wong, S.L.; Brill, A.; Gallant, M.; Hu, J.; Wang, Y.; Wagner, D.D. Neutrophil histone modification by peptidylarginine deiminase 4 is critical for deep vein thrombosis in mice. *Proc. Natl. Acad. Sci. USA* **2013**, *110*, 8674–8679. [CrossRef]
40. Martinod, K.; Wagner, D.D. Thrombosis: Tangled up in NETs. *Blood* **2014**, *123*, 2768–2776. [CrossRef]

Effects of Fructose or Glucose on Circulating ApoCIII and Triglyceride and Cholesterol Content of Lipoprotein Subfractions in Humans

Bettina Hieronimus [1], Steven C. Griffen [2], Nancy L. Keim [3,4], Andrew A. Bremer [5], Lars Berglund [2], Katsuyuki Nakajima [6,7,8,9], Peter J. Havel [1,4] and Kimber L. Stanhope [1,*]

[1] Department of Molecular Biosciences, School of Veterinary Medicine, University of California, Davis, CA 95616, USA
[2] Department of Internal Medicine, School of Medicine, University of California, Davis, Sacramento, CA 95817, USA
[3] United States Department of Agriculture, Western Human Nutrition Research Center, Davis, CA 95616, USA
[4] Department of Nutrition, University of California, Davis, CA 95616, USA
[5] Department of Pediatrics, School of Medicine, University of California, Davis, Sacramento, CA 95817, USA
[6] Department of Clinical Laboratory Medicine, Gunma University Graduate School of Medicine, Maebashi, Gunma 371-8510, Japan
[7] Hidaka Hospital, Takasaki, Gunma 370-0001, Japan
[8] General Internal Medicine, Kanazawa Medical University, Kanazawa 920-0265, Japan
[9] Laboratory of Clinical Nutrition and Medicine, Kagawa Nutrition University, Tokyo 350-0288, Japan
[*] Correspondence: klstanhope@ucdavis.edu

Abstract: ApoCIII and triglyceride (TG)-rich lipoproteins (TRL), particularly, large TG-rich lipoproteins particles, have been described as important mediators of cardiovascular disease (CVD) risk. The effects of sustained consumption of dietary fructose compared with those of sustained glucose consumption on circulating apoCIII and large TRL particles have not been reported. We measured apoCIII concentrations and the TG and cholesterol content of lipoprotein subfractions separated by size in fasting and postprandial plasma collected from men and women (age: 54 ± 8 years) before and after they consumed glucose- or fructose-sweetened beverages for 10 weeks. The subjects consuming fructose exhibited higher fasting and postprandial plasma apoCIII concentrations than the subjects consuming glucose ($p < 0.05$ for both). They also had higher concentrations of postprandial TG in all TRL subfractions ($p < 0.05$, effect of sugar), with the highest increases occurring in the largest TRL particles ($p < 0.0001$ for fructose linear trend). Compared to glucose consumption, fructose consumption increased postprandial TG in low-density lipoprotein (LDL) particles ($p < 0.05$, effect of sugar), especially in the smaller particles ($p < 0.0001$ for fructose linear trend). The increases of both postprandial apoCIII and TG in large TRL subfractions were associated with fructose-induced increases of fasting cholesterol in the smaller LDL particles. In conclusion, 10 weeks of fructose consumption increased the circulating apoCIII and postprandial concentrations of large TRL particles compared with glucose consumption.

Keywords: sugar; atherosclerosis risk factors; lipoprotein fractions; TG-rich lipoproteins; clinical studies; LDL; lipid and lipoprotein metabolism; nutrition/carbohydrates

1. Introduction

The incidence and prevalence of undesirable health outcomes including obesity, type-2 diabetes, cardiovascular disease (CVD), and metabolic syndrome are increasing in developing and developed countries alike, with CVD being the number one cause of death globally [1]. Dietary habits affect cardiometabolic risk [2], but we lack a full understanding of how dietary patterns influence the development of undesirable lipid profiles that lead to metabolic diseases. Understanding the mechanisms that link specific dietary components and patterns to atherogenic dyslipidemia will promote the implementation of dietary policies to reduce CVD risk.

We earlier reported the results from a 10-week intervention trial with women and men (age: 54 ± 8 years; body mass index (BMI): 29.1 ± 2.9 kg/m^2 (mean ± SD)) who consumed 25% of their energy requirement from fructose- or glucose-sweetened beverages [3]. Despite comparable weight gain in both groups, fructose consumption promoted lipid dysregulation, while glucose consumption did not [3]. Compared with glucose, the consumption of fructose increased the circulating concentrations of postprandial triglycerides (TG), remnant-like particle lipoprotein (RLP)-TG, and RLP-cholesterol (chol), as well as those of fasting total chol, low-density lipoprotein (LDL)-chol, apolipoprotein B (apoB), small dense LDL-chol (sdLDL-chol), and oxidized LDL [3]. Subjects consuming fructose also exhibited increased postprandial hepatic de novo lipogenesis (DNL) and decreased insulin sensitivity compared with subjects consuming glucose [3].

We and others have suggested that these results are mediated by the preferential and unregulated metabolism of fructose in the liver [4–7]. Hepatic fructose overload leads to upregulated DNL [3,8–10], reduced fat oxidation [8,9,11], and increased liver fat content [8,9,12], which are associated with increased synthesis and secretion of TG-rich $VLDL_1$ (very low density lipoprotein) [13]. At high concentrations, $VLDL_1$ becomes the favored substrate of cholesteryl ester transfer protein (CETP) [14] that catalyzes lipid transfer between lipoproteins. This leads to TG enrichment of LDL. TG-enriched LDL particles are the preferential substrate for the lipolytic action of hepatic lipase, which leads to smaller, denser particles [15]. However, whether sustained fructose consumption causes an increase in large TRL or TG enrichment of LDL particles has not been determined. Furthermore, apoCIII has been implicated as a major mediator of the metabolic processes that increase CVD risk [16,17] by causing reduced lipoprotein flux through clearance pathways and increased flux through the lipolysis pathways that lead to sdLDL [17]. In support of this, it was recently reported that the increase in LDL particle size caused by a weight loss intervention and the decrease in LDL particle size caused by a high-carbohydrate (32.5% of energy as complex, 32.5% as simple) dietary intervention, were both inversely correlated to the changes in apoCIII concentrations [18]. While it has been shown that consumption of both fructose [8,19] and fructose-containing sugar [20] leads to increased plasma apoCIII concentrations, it is not known if this effect is general for all carbohydrates or specific to fructose. Therefore, our objective was to determine the effects of sustained consumption of fructose-sweetened compared with glucose-sweetened beverages on fasting and postprandial circulating apoCIII and the TG-enrichment of large lipoproteins and LDL. We analyzed apoCIII concentrations and the TG and chol content of 20 lipoprotein fractions separated by size in fasting and postprandial plasma collected before and after intervention from subjects who consumed glucose- or fructose-sweetened beverages for 10 weeks [3].

2. Experimental Section

As previously reported [3], this was a matched, parallel-arm, dietary intervention study that consisted of three phases: (1) a two-week inpatient baseline period during which the subjects consumed an energy-balanced diet; (2) an eight-week outpatient intervention period during which the subjects consumed 25% of daily energy requirement as either glucose- (n = 15) or fructose-sweetened (n = 17) beverages, divided into three servings, along with their usual ad libitum diet; and (3) a two-week inpatient intervention period during which the subjects consumed 25% of their daily energy requirement as the assigned sugar-sweetened beverage along with an energy-balanced diet (Figure 1). Daily energy requirement was calculated by the Mifflin equation ([21]), with an adjustment of 1.3 for the days of the 24 h blood collections and an adjustment of 1.5 for the other days. Subjects resided in the University of California, Davis, (UCD), Clinical and Translational Science Center's Clinical Research

Center (CCRC) during the two-week baseline and two-week intervention inpatient periods of the study (Figure 1). Energy-balanced breakfast accounted for 25% of the subjects' energy requirement, lunch for 35%, and dinner for 40%. The baseline diet consisted of 55% of energy as mainly complex carbohydrate, 30% fat, and 15% protein. Intervention meals mimicked the respective baseline meals in all but the carbohydrate composition, which consisted of 30% complex carbohydrate and 25% glucose- or fructose-sweetened beverages. During the eight-week outpatient intervention period, the subjects were instructed to drink three servings of the assigned beverages, one with each meal, and to refrain from drinking other sugar-containing beverages including fruit juices. We have previously reported that during the eight-week outpatient period, both groups gained comparable amounts of body weight (approximately 1.4 kg) [3].

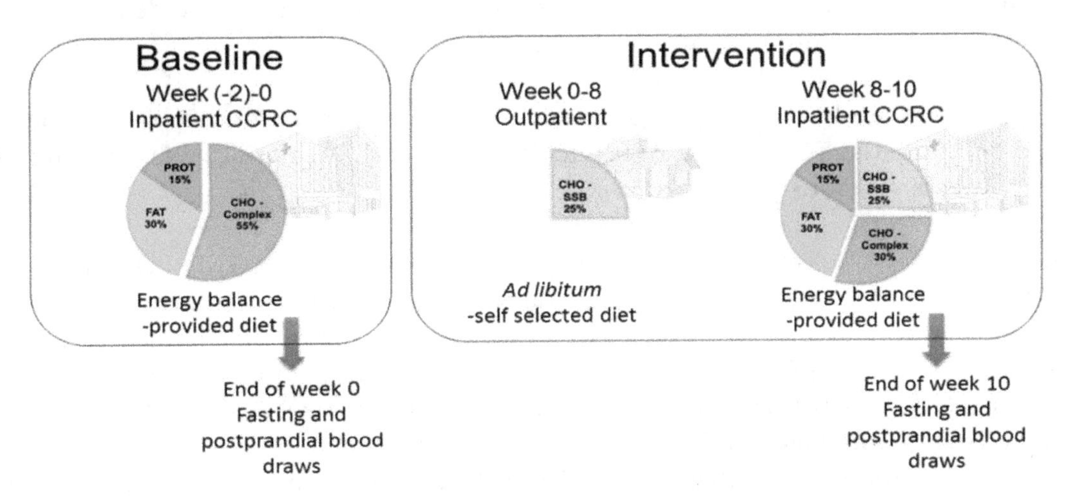

Figure 1. Study design and dietary protocol. CCRC: Clinical and Translational Science Center's Clinical Research Center.

Subjects: Participants were recruited through newspaper advertisements and underwent a telephone and an in-person interview with medical history, a complete blood count, and a serum biochemistry panel to assess eligibility. Inclusion criteria included age 40–72 years and BMI 25–35 kg/m^2, with a self-report of stable body weight during the prior six months. Women were post-menopausal on the basis of a self-report of no menstruation for at least one year. Exclusion criteria included: evidence of diabetes, renal or hepatic disease, fasting serum TG concentrations >400 mg/dL, hypertension (>140/90 mg Hg), and surgery for weight loss. Also excluded were individuals who smoked, reported exercise of more than 3.5 h/week at a level more vigorous than walking, or having used thyroid, lipid-lowering, glucose-lowering, anti-hypertensive, anti-depressant, or weight loss medications. Diet-related exclusion criteria included habitual consumption of more than one sugar-sweetened beverage/day or more than two alcoholic beverages/day. All experimental procedures were in accordance with the Helsinki Declaration and approved by the UCD Institutional Review Board. All subjects provided informed written consent to participate in the study. Thirty-nine subjects enrolled in the study, and experimental groups were matched for gender, BMI, and fasting TG and insulin concentrations. Seven subjects (three in the glucose group, four in the fructose group) failed to complete the study due to inability/unwillingness to comply with the protocol or due to personal or work-related conflicts. The baseline anthropometric and metabolic parameters of the subjects were previously reported [3] and were equal between the experimental groups. The mean age, BMI, and baseline fasting plasma TG concentration of all subjects was 53.7 ± 1.4 years, 30.8 ± 1.0 kg/m^2, and 145.2 ± 12.3 mg/dL, respectively.

After 10 days of energy-balanced feeding, 24 h serial blood collections were conducted during baseline (0 week) and the 10th week of intervention (10 week). Meals were served at 9:00 a.m., 1:00 p.m. and 6:00 p.m. The plasma from the three fasting samples (8:00 a.m., 8:30 a.m., 9:00 a.m.) was pooled, as was the plasma from three postprandial blood samples (10:00 p.m., 11:00 p.m., 11:30 p.m.).

We chose 10:00–11:30 p.m. as the postprandial time-points because it was during this period that fructose had the most marked effects on TG concentrations compared with glucose during our previous study [22]. The 0-week and 10-week fasting and postprandial plasma samples from 31 of the 32 subjects (insufficient plasma obtained from one subject in the fructose group) were classified and quantified for chol and TG concentrations in 20 subfractions by high-performance liquid chromatography at Skylight Biotech (LipoSEARCH; Skylight Bio-tech Inc., Akita, Japan) to examine the lipoprotein profiles by subclass [23–25]. The subfractions were termed TRLp1-7, LDLp1-6, and HDLp1-7, respectively, and were classified by particle diameter (Table 1). The results pertaining to the HDLp1-7 subfractions are not reported in this paper. Apolipoprotein CIII (apoCIII) was measured in the same pooled samples used to determine fasting (8:00, 8:30, 9:00 a.m.) and postprandial (10:00, 11:00, 11:30 p.m.) lipoproteins. The concentrations were assessed with a Polychem Chemistry Analyzer (PolyMedCo Inc., Cortlandt Manor, NY, USA) with reagents from MedTest DX.

The effects of 2-, 8- and 10-week glucose and fructose consumption on the plasma concentrations of fasting and postprandial TG and apoB100, and fasting total, LDL, high-density lipoprotein (HDL), and sdLDL-chol were previously reported [3].

Statistical Analysis: Differences in the percent changes (delta Δ) in the TRL, LDL fractions (Table 2), and apoCIII (Figure 2) were analyzed with a generalized linear two-factor (sugar and gender) method. The percent changes of chol and TG in TRL (chylomicron, VLDL) and LDL subfractions at 10 weeks compared to baseline (Figures 3 and 4) were analyzed by three-factor (sugar, subfraction size, gender), mixed procedures (PROC MIXED) repeated measures (subfraction size) ANOVA (SAS 9.4). Significant within-group changes from baseline for the individual subfractions were identified by least-squares means (LS means) of the percent changes significantly different from zero. Trend contrasts were used to identify linear relationships between particle size and glucose or fructose consumption. The symbols designating a significant effect of ANOVA factors are consistent for Figures 2–4: a = sugar, b = particle size, c = gender, d = sugar × size, f = fructose-induced linear trend, g = glucose-induced linear trend. Pearson's correlation coefficients were calculated for the changes of total postprandial TG, total and subfraction TRL TG, fasting and postprandial apoCIII, and total fasting LDL and LDLp3-6 chol (SAS 9.4). The data are presented as mean ± SEM.

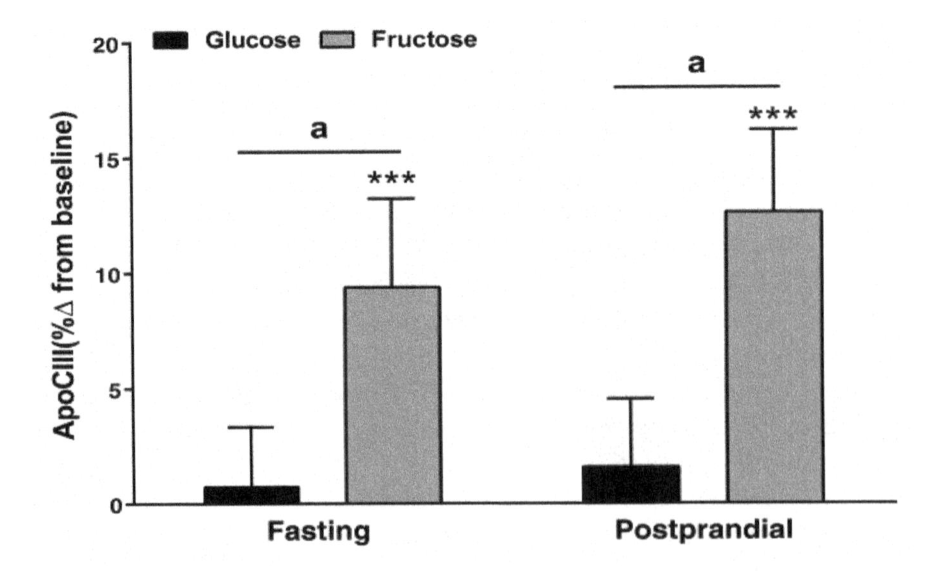

Figure 2. Percent (%) changes (10 weeks vs. 0 weeks) of apoCIII in the serum of subjects consuming glucose- ($n = 15$) or fructose-sweetened beverages ($n = 16$) for 10 weeks. [a] $p < 0.05$ effect of sugar, least squares (LS) means different from zero; *** $p < 0.001$, LS means different from zero—change from baseline. Data shown as mean ± SEM.

Table 1. Baseline values of fasting and postprandial cholesterol (chol) and triglycerides (TG) in TG-rich lipoproteins (TRL) and low-density lipoprotein (LDL) subfractions.

	Diameter	Cholesterol (mg/dL)				TG (mg/dL)			
		Fasting		Postprandial		Fasting		Postprandial	
	(nm)	Glucose	Fructose	Glucose	Fructose	Glucose	Fructose	Glucose	Fructose
TRLp1	>90	2.7 ± 0.6	3.2 ± 0.8	3.4 ± 0.7	3.6 ± 0.9	10.0 ± 2.6	14.1 ± 3.4	19.0 ± 4.1	22.1 ± 5.0
TRLp2	75	1.4 ± 0.2	1.5 ± 0.3	1.6 ± 0.2	1.6 ± 0.3	6.6 ± 1.3	6.9 ± 1.3	10.1 ± 1.7	10.3 ± 2.1
TRLp3	64	3.8 ± 0.5	3.7 ± 0.5	4.1 ± 0.5	3.7 ± 0.6	14.9 ± 2.6	14.1 ± 2.3	18.4 ± 2.7	17.9 ± 2.9
TRLp4	53.6	7.4 ± 0.7	6.8 ± 0.7	7.1 ± 0.7	6.4 ± 0.8	27.1 ± 4.0	23.9 ± 3.4	29.7 ± 4.0	28.0 ± 4.0
TRLp5	44.5	16.5 ± 1.0	14.6 ± 1.0	14.4 ± 1.2	12.6 ± 1.1	33.9 ± 4.4	28.9 ± 3.5	35.0 ± 4.3	32.7 ± 3.9
TRLp6	36.8	12.9 ± 1.1	11.5 ± 1.2	10.6 ± 1.4	9.5 ± 1.3	17.7 ± 2.0	15.1 ± 1.7	18.5 ± 2.0	17.6 ± 1.9
TRLp7	31.3	6.0 ± 0.4	5.5 ± 0.6	6.4 ± 0.5	6.0 ± 0.5	5.0 ± 0.5	4.3 ± 0.5	5.6 ± 0.5	5.5 ± 0.5
LDLp1	28.6	19.4 ± 1.1	18.2 ± 1.2	20.7 ± 1.6	19.1 ± 1.2	7.6 ± 0.6	6.9 ± 0.7	8.7 ± 0.7	8.5 ± 0.7
LDLp2	25.5	39.0 ± 1.3	36.3 ± 2.1	36.6 ± 1.6	35.7 ± 2.1	8.4 ± 0.6	8.0 ± 0.8	9.4 ± 0.7	9.6 ± 1.0
LDLp3	23.0	21.7 ± 1.3	20.2 ± 1.9	19.0 ± 1.6	18.6 ± 1.7	5.5 ± 0.5	5.1 ± 0.6	5.9 ± 0.6	6.0 ± 0.8
LDLp4	20.7	6.3 ± 0.5	5.8 ± 0.6	5.6 ± 0.7	5.2 ± 0.5	2.1 ± 0.2	1.9 ± 0.2	2.2 ± 0.3	2.2 ± 0.3
LDLp5	18.6	2.5 ± 0.2	2.4 ± 0.2	2.3 ± 0.2	2.2 ± 0.2	1.1 ± 0.1	1.1 ± 0.1	1.4 ± 0.2	1.3 ± 0.2
LDLp6	16.7	1.4 ± 0.1	1.3 ± 0.1	1.3 ± 0.1	1.2 ± 0.1	0.7 ± 0.1	0.7 ± 0.1	1.0 ± 0.1	0.9 ± 0.1

Mean ± SEM.

Table 2. Total fasting (FST) and postprandial (PP) TG and cholesterol concentrations in TRL and LDL fractions before and after consumption of glucose- and fructose-sweetened beverages for 10 weeks.

	Glucose			Fructose		
	0 weeks	10 weeks	% change	0 weeks	10 weeks	% change
Lipoprotein TG (mg/dL)						
TRL TG–FST	116.4 ± 17.3	122.8 ± 16.6	14.3 ± 6.0 *	107.3 ± 14.5	111.9 ± 15.4	7.2 ± 6.8
TRL TG–PP	138.3 ± 19.4	149.8 ± 18.9	11.4 ± 6.1	134.2 ± 18.8	180.9 ± 22.4	42.9 ± 8.3 aa,****
LDL TG–FST	24.7 ± 2.3	26.1 ± 2.2	6.3 ± 6.3	23.7 ± 2.5	26.8 ± 2.9	13.9 ± 5.3 ****
LDL TG–PP	27.3 ± 2.7	30.6 ± 2.2	8.8 ± 4.4 *	28.5 ± 2.9	33.2 ± 3.1	18.6 ± 3.1 ****
Lipoprotein Chol (mg/dL)						
TRL Chol–FST	51.3 ± 43.7	46.3 ± 5.3	−4.1 ± 3.0	46.7 ± 4.0	47.9 ± 4.7	2.6 ± 3.8
TRL Chol–PP	48.1 ± 4.3	46.4 ± 6.1	−2.7 ± 3.6	43.4 ± 4.5	49.8 ± 4.7	16.3 ± 5.1 aa,***
LDL Chol–FST	90.4 ± 3.3	96.1 ± 3.9	7.0 ± 3.7	84.3.0 ± 5.3	101 ± 7	19.3 ± 2.9 a,****
LDL Chol–PP	86.0 ± 3.9	90.3 ± 3.4	7.1 ± 2.6 **	82.1 ± 5.0	94.3 ± 6.1	14.7 ± 1.9 a,****

[a] $p < 0.05$, [aa] $p < 0.01$, effect of sugar. * $p < 0.05$, ** $p < 0.01$, *** $p < 0.001$, **** $p < 0.0001$, LS mean of % change different than zero. Mean ± SEM.

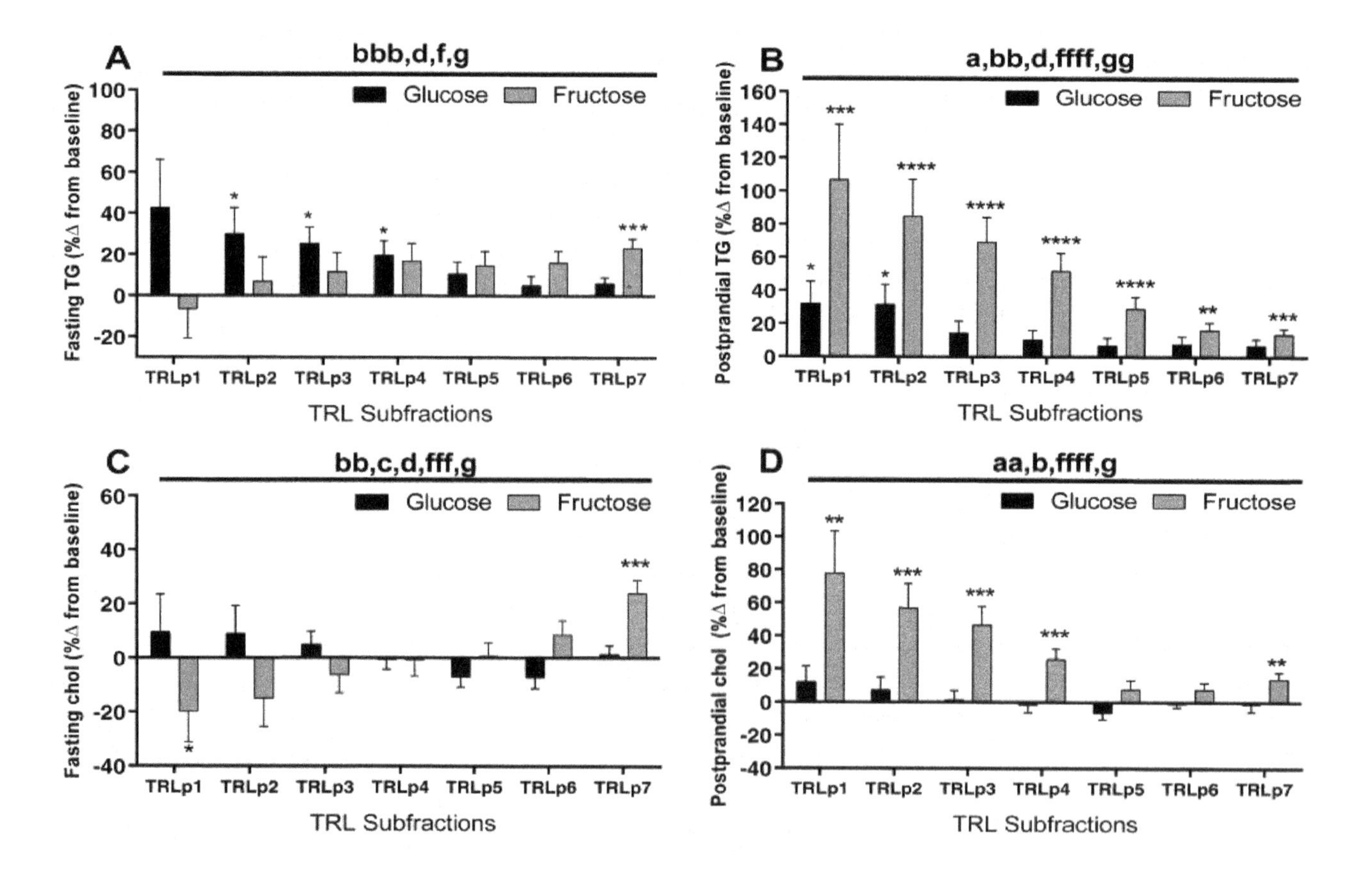

Figure 3. Percent (%) changes (10 weeks vs. 0 weeks) of fasting (**A**) and postprandial (**B**) TG and fasting (**C**) and postprandial (**D**) chol in TRL subfractions (chylomicrons (CM) and very low density lipoprotein (VLDL)) in subjects consuming glucose- ($n = 15$) or fructose-sweetened beverages ($n = 16$) for 10 weeks. [a] $p < 0.05$, [aa] $p < 0.01$, effect of sugar; [b] $p < 0.05$, [bb] $p < 0.01$, [bbb] $p < 0.001$, effect of particle size, [c] $p < 0.05$, effect of gender, [d] $p < 0.05$, effect of sugar x size; [f] $p < 0.05$, [fff] $p < 0.00$, [ffff] $p < 0.0001$ for fructose-induced lineal trend, [g] $p < 0.05$, [gg] $p < 0.01$ for glucose-induced lineal trend. * $p < 0.05$, ** $p < 0.01$, *** $p < 0.001$, **** $p < 0.0001$, LS means different from zero—within-group change from baseline. Data shown as mean ± SEM. Note the differences in scales.

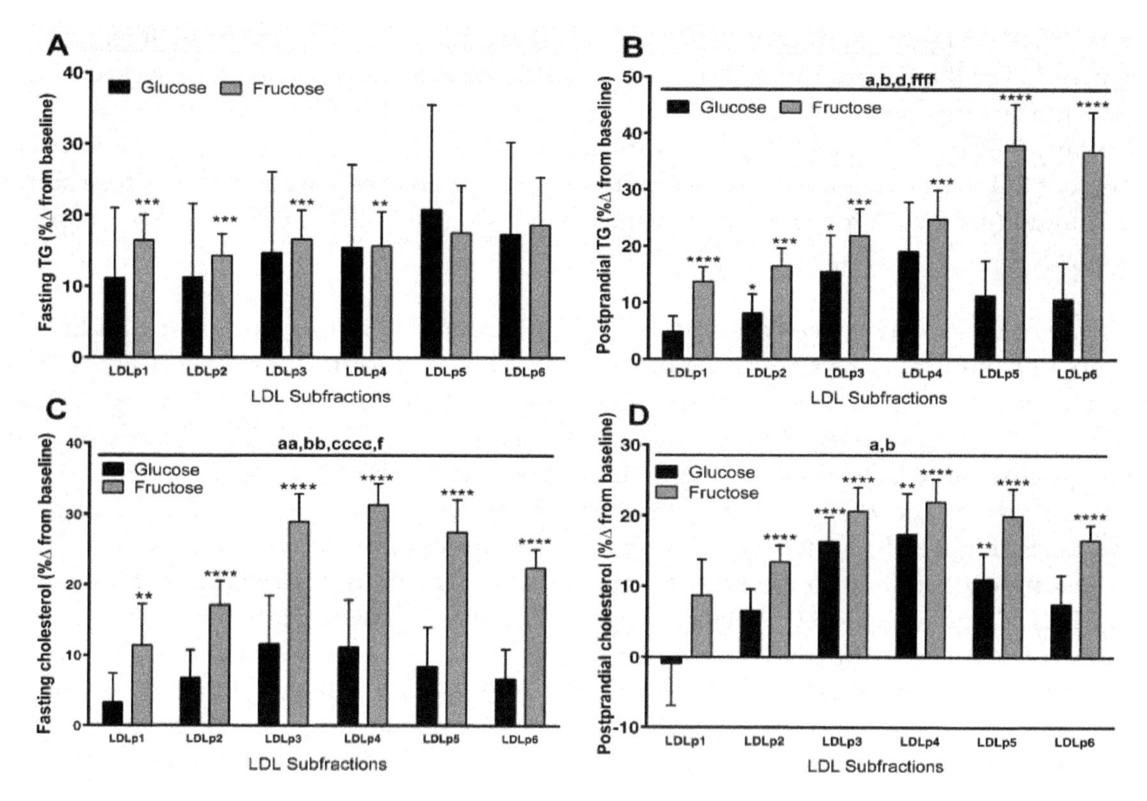

Figure 4. Percent (%) changes (10 weeks vs. 0 weeks) of fasting (**A**) and postprandial (**B**) TG and fasting (**C**) and postprandial (**D**) chol in LDL subfractions in subjects consuming glucose-sweetened beverages (n = 15) or fructose-sweetened beverages (n = 16) for 10 weeks. ^{a} $p < 0.05$, ^{aa} $p < 0.01$, effect of sugar; ^{b} $p < 0.05$, ^{bb} $p < 0.01$, effect of particle size; ^{cccc} $p < 0.0001$, effect of gender, ^{d} $p < 0.05$, effect of sugar × size, ^{f} $p < 0.05$; ^{ffff} $p < 0.0001$ for fructose-induced lineal trend, ^{g} $p < 0.05$ for glucose-induced lineal trend. * $p < 0.05$, ** $p < 0.01$, *** $p < 0.001$, **** $p < 0.0001$, LS means different from zero—within group change from baseline. Data shown as mean ± SEM. Note the differences in scales.

3. Results

Figure 2 shows the percent changes of plasma apoCIII concentrations after glucose or fructose intervention. Fasting and postprandial apoCIII levels increased in subjects consuming fructose compared with subjects consuming glucose ($p < 0.05$ for both fasting and postprandial, effect of sugar).

The baseline fasting and postprandial contents of chol and TG were not significantly different between the groups in any of the TRL or LDL subfractions (Table 1). The baseline and intervention values and percent changes in the overall TRL and LDL fractions are shown in Table 2. The subjects consuming fructose had increased postprandial levels of chol and TG in both overall particle fractions. In addition, chol and TG were increased in fasting LDL fractions after fructose consumption. In the glucose group, fasting TRL TG and postprandial LDL TG and chol levels increased after the intervention compared to baseline. The fructose-induced increases were significantly higher than those induced by glucose for postprandial TG in TRL, postprandial chol in TRL and LDL, and fasting chol in LDL.

The percent changes of TG and chol (week 10 compared to baseline) in the TRL subfractions are shown in Figure 3. The two sugars induced opposite linear trends for the changes of fasting TG within the TRL subfractions (Figure 3A: $p < 0.05$, sugar × size; $p < 0.05$, both fructose and glucose linear trend). The subjects consuming glucose had increased TG content in the larger TRL particles (TRLp2–4), while those consuming fructose had increased TG content only in the smallest particles (TRLp7). The same opposing linear trends occurred for fasting chol in TRL (Figure 3C: $p < 0.001$, fructose linear trend; $p < 0.05$, glucose linear trend). In the postprandial state, the subjects consuming fructose had increased TG content in all TRL subfractions, with the highest changes in the largest TRL subfractions. This increase exhibited a highly significant linear trend (Figure 3B; $p < 0.0001$, fructose linear trend) in the opposite direction of the fasting trend. The effects of glucose consumption on postprandial TG content in the TRL subfractions were significantly lower, ($p < 0.05$, effect of sugar; $p < 0.05$ effect of sugar x size), with only TRLp1 and 2 showing a significant increase. The postprandial changes in TRL chol content (Figure 3D) paralleled the changes in TRL TG. The increases induced by fructose showed the same linear trend ($p < 0.0001$ for linear trend) and were higher than those induced by glucose ($p < 0.01$, effect of sugar).

The percent change at 10 weeks compared with baseline of fasting and postprandial chol and TG in the six LDL subfractions are shown in Figure 4. The fructose-induced increases of fasting TG content in LDL were comparable among the subfractions and were not significantly higher than those induced by glucose (Figure 4A). In contrast to the fasting state (Figure 4A), the fructose-induced increases in postprandial LDL TG were higher than those induced by glucose ($p < 0.05$, effect of sugar, effect of sugar x size) and displayed a highly significant linear trend with higher increases in the smaller particles (Figure 4B; $p < 0.0001$). Compared with glucose, fructose consumption significantly increased fasting chol content in the LDL subfractions, especially in the smaller subfractions (small dense (sd)LDL) (Figure 4C; $p < 0.01$, effect of sugar). The changes were higher in men than in women (Figure 4C; $p < 0.0001$, effect of gender). In the postprandial state, both sugars increased LDL TG and chol content, but the increases were higher and more significant in subjects consuming fructose than in subjects consuming glucose (Figure 4B-TG: $p < 0.05$, effect of sugar; $p < 0.05$, effect of sugar × size; Figure 4D-chol: $p < 0.05$, effect of sugar).

In order to compare the relationships of postprandial TG-rich particles and apoCIII to fasting sdLDL-chol, we performed regression analysis. Table 3 lists the regression coefficients and *p*-values for the relationships between the changes of fasting and postprandial apoCIII, total TG, total TLR TG, and TG in each TRL subfraction and the changes of total fasting LDL chol and fasting chol in the small LDL particles (LDLp3–6). In subjects consuming fructose, postprandial apoCIII correlated with total fasting LDL-chol ($p < 0.03$), while the individual TRL subfractions and total TG did not. There were significant associations (all $p < 0.05$) between the increase in fasting LDLp3–6 chol (sdLDL-chol) and the increase in postprandial apoCIII and postprandial TG in TRLp2 and TRLp3 in subjects consuming fructose, but not in subjects consuming glucose. In multivariate regression that included both postprandial apoCIII and TRLp2 or TRLp3, the significance of both were attenuated (apoCIII and TRLp2 $p = 0.16$ and $p = 0.13$; apoCIII and TRLp3 $p = 0.20$ and $p = 0.20$). There were significant positive correlations between postprandial apoCIII and total TRL TG ($p < 0.0001$) and between postprandial apoCIII and TRLp2 or TRLp3 TG ($p < 0.05$ for both).

Table 3. The relationship of percent change of postprandial total, TRL subfraction TG, and fasting and postprandial apoCIII to the absolute increase of total fasting LDL and LDLp3–6 cholesterol.

	Total FST LDL Cholesterol				FST LDLp3-6 Cholesterol			
	Glucose *r*	*P* Value	Fructose *r*	*P* Value	Glucose *r*	*P* Value	Fructose *r*	*P* Value
Total TG–PP	0.03	0.91	0.21	0.44	−0.13	0.65	0.21	0.43
Total TRL TG–PP	0.04	0.88	0.01	0.97	−0.14	0.64	0.28	0.29
TRLp1 TG–PP	−0.07	0.82	−0.08	0.77	−0.21	0.47	0.40	0.12
TRLp2 TG–PP	0.02	0.94	−0.04	0.88	−0.23	0.42	0.53	**0.04**
TRLp3 TG–PP	0.10	0.72	0.01	0.96	0.03	0.91	0.51	**0.05**
TRLp4 TG–PP	0.06	0.83	0.07	0.78	−0.04	0.88	0.39	0.14
TRLp5 TG–PP	0.08	0.78	0.06	0.84	−0.09	0.75	0.33	0.21
TRLp6TG–PP	0.04	0.88	−0.17	0.53	−0.14	0.63	0.16	0.54
TRLp7 TG–PP	−0.07	0.82	−0.27	0.30	−0.22	0.44	−0.06	0.82
ApoCIII FST	−0.27	0.36	0.44	0.09	−0.37	0.20	0.44	0.09
ApoCIII PP	−0.32	0.26	0.53	**0.03**	−0.48	0.08	0.51	**0.04**

r: Pearson's correlation coefficient; FST: fasting state; PP: postprandial state. Bold: indicates significance ($p < 0.05$).

4. Discussion

In the present study, we explored differences between circulating apoCIII and the TG and chol composition of lipoprotein fractions in subjects consuming glucose- or fructose-sweetened beverages for 10 weeks. The changes in apoCIII and in the patterns of TG and chol within the different lipoprotein fractions varied markedly between the two groups, despite their consuming standardized inpatient diets for 10 days prior to both baseline and 10-week intervention blood collections. The intervention diets differed solely in the composition of the beverages, specifically, in the type of added sugar, i.e., glucose or fructose.

ApoCIII is associated with increased CVD risk through various mechanisms, and several studies suggest it to be a robust and reliable predictor of CVD risk [26,27]. Our data show fasting and postprandial apoCIII levels increased after fructose consumption compared with the levels after glucose consumption. To the best of our knowledge, this is the first study to report increased responses of circulating apoCIII to fructose consumption compared with glucose consumption. The results suggest that the previously reported increases of plasma apoCIII concentrations in human subjects consuming fructose [8] or fructose-containing sugar [20] are specific to fructose rather than to carbohydrate in general. A possible explanation for these results may involve insulin, which is a negative transcriptional regulator of apoCIII expression [28]. We have previously reported that the two sugars had highly significant and opposite effects on circulating insulin, with glucose consumption increasing, and fructose consumption decreasing 24 h area under the curve (AUC) and post-meal insulin responses [29]. Cell culture experiments showed apoCIII expression is induced by glucose via hepatocyte nuclear factor 4 alpha (HNF-4α) and carbohydrate-responsive element-binding protein (ChREBP) [30] and is reduced by insulin via Forkhead Box O1 (FOXO1) [28]. This regulation takes place in the liver but not in the intestine, which are the two main sites of apoCIII expression [31]. Thus, it is possible that the failure of glucose consumption to increase circulating apoCIII is due to insulin's negative feedback on hepatic apoCIII transcription. Fructose also activates ChREBP [32,33]. This activation, in the absence of negative feedback by insulin on apoCIII transcription [34], may explain the increased levels of circulating apoCIII after fructose consumption compared with glucose consumption.

It has been recently reported that apoCIII is the strongest predictor of hypertriglyceridemia in a large cohort of rhesus primates and that inhibition of apoCIII by RNA interference lowered fructose-induced hypertriglyceridemia [35]. ApoCIII may affect the lipid metabolism by promoting hepatic DNL and $VLDL_1$ production [27,34,36–40] and by interfering with hepatic clearance of TRL through masking apoB/apoE receptors [16,17,41,42]. Both processes lead to increased and sustained TRL levels in the circulation, which are associated with CVD development and progression [43,44]. Therefore, to investigate the effects of fructose on the fasting and postprandial levels of TRL and other indicators of CVD risk, we measured TG and chol in lipoprotein particles separated by size. The subjects consuming glucose had increased fasting TG in large TRL particles, while those consuming fructose had increased fasting TG in small TRL particles. Thus, if our study only investigated the changes that occurred in the fasting state, these results could lead to the suggestion that consumption of glucose is associated with CVD risk to a larger extent than consumption of fructose. However, the postprandial changes induced by the two sugars in the TG content of the TRL subfractions differed dramatically from the changes in the fasting state with regard to the direction of the linear trend, the magnitude of the increases, and the differential effects of the beverages. Overall, they clearly demonstrate that, compared with glucose consumption, the consumption of fructose increased postprandial TG content in all TRL subfractions, with the increases being most marked in the largest particles. Given that people spend up to 18 h per day in a nonfasted state [45], these results from samples collected postprandially are likely to be more relevant to CVD risk than the fasting results. Furthermore, epidemiology studies provide evidence that non-fasting TG is a more reliable index of CVD risk than fasting TG [46,47]. Compared with glucose, fructose also increased postprandial chol content in the TRL subfractions, with the increases being most marked in the largest particles. This too may promote CVD risk. A prospective study on 90,000 individuals showed a dose-dependent effect of non-fasted remnant cholesterol on later ischemic heart disease and myocardial infarction [48].

The prominently increased postprandial TRL TG and chol in the subjects consuming fructose may result from impaired TRL clearance or increased TRL synthesis—or a combination of both. As stated above, apoCIII could be involved in TRL clearance and/or increased TRL synthesis. Other possible mechanisms not involving apoCIII include a direct effect of fructose overload on the upregulation of hepatic DNL. We have previously reported that postprandial hepatic DNL was significantly increased in the subjects consuming fructose compared to those consuming glucose [3]. Also, it has been suggested, although the available evidence to date is limited, that disruption of enterocyte lipid metabolism may make a meaningful contribution to the hypertriglyceridemia often associated with fructose consumption [49,50]. Fructose feeding has been shown to increase chylomicron synthesis in enterocytes via upregulated DNL and reduced apoB48 degradation in a hamster model of insulin resistance [49]. Impaired TRL clearance could be mediated by decreased lipoprotein lipase (LPL) activity [3], which catalyzes the lipolysis of TG from TRL in the circulation. ApoCII is an important cofactor for LPL activation [51,52] and could be involved in the in differential effects of the two beverages on TRL clearance; however, the effects of fructose compared with those of glucose on apoCII have yet to be investigated.

We previously reported that sdLDL cholesterol was increased in the subjects consuming fructose compared with those consuming glucose [3], and the current data confirm this. The high levels of apoCIII may be involved in generating sdLDL by inhibiting lipoprotein clearance pathways and promoting the lipolytic conversion of TRL, IDL, and LDL to smaller, denser LDL particles [17]. However, the traditional view on the generation of sdLDL involves cholesteryl ester transfer protein (CETP) -mediated TG transfer from TRL to LDL [15,53,54]. Supportive of this, our results showed an increase in the TG content of all LDL subfractions during the postprandial period after fructose consumption compared to glucose consumption. TG-enriched LDL has reduced affinity for the LDL receptor and a longer residence time in the circulation compared to LDL with normal TG content [55]. It is therefore exposed to hepatic lipase, which lyses TG. Accordingly, the LDL particles from subjects consuming fructose were less enriched with TG in the fasting state than in the postprandial state ($p < 0.001$ for all individual LDL subfractions, paired t tests). At the same time, these fasting particles had increased cholesterol content compared to the LDL particles from subjects consuming glucose, especially in the smaller particles (LDLp3-6).

Regression analyses showed associations between the changes in fasting sdLDL-chol and postprandial apoCIII and large particle TRLs (TRLp2 and TRLp3) only in subjects consuming fructose. The results are in agreement with the hypothesis that increased and sustained concentrations of large TRL particles lead to lipoprotein changes that result in the formation of sdLDL-chol [15,56,57] and the possibility that apoCIII has a major role in mediating these metabolic processes [17]. A recent intervention trial showed apoCIII was positively associated with sdLDL formation after a high-carbohydrate diet that contained equal amounts of complex and simple carbohydrate [18]. Here, we expand on these results showing that the elevation of apoCIII and its association with sdLDL formation occurred after fructose, but not glucose, consumption. The results showing that apoCIII also correlated with the changes in total LDL-chol may suggest that apoCIII impairs clearance of all LDL particles. In contrast, neither TRLp2 nor TRLp3 correlated with total LDL-chol. Possibly, the effects of TRLp2 and TRLp3 were more specific to LDLp3–6 because they mediated higher TG-enrichment in LDLp3-6 than in LDLp1 (p = 0.003–0.04) or p2 (p = 0.003–0.06, all comparisons, paired t tests)). However, the attenuated effects of both apoCIII and TRLp2 or TRLp3, when included in the same multi-regression analysis, suggests that their effects on the increase in fasting chol in LDLp3–6 are mediated by dependent pathways.

Elevated levels of sdLDL have been described as independent predictors of cardiovascular events in patients with non-coronary atherosclerosis [58–60] and also of cardio- and cerebro-vascular events in patients with metabolic syndrome [59]. Increased sdLDL, along with elevated levels of TRL, LDL cholesterol, oxidized LDL, and apoB and low levels of HDL-chol constitute the 'atherogenic dyslipidemia complex', a feature of type 2 diabetes and the metabolic syndrome [61]. The subjects consuming fructose-sweetened beverages for 10 weeks exhibited adverse changes in all components of the 'atherogenic dyslipidemia complex', excepting lowered HDL-chol concentrations. As previously reported, plasma HDL concentrations were unchanged at 10 weeks in the subjects consuming fructose- or glucose-sweetened beverages [3].

A limitation to our study is the selective inclusion of older and overweight subjects, which may limit our findings to this group. However, as this demographic is increasing and already at a high risk for CVD, our reported findings are valuable even if younger and healthier subjects react differently to sugar consumption. The modest sample size limited the exploration of gender effects, which should be studied further with increased subject numbers. Finally, this study does not investigate the effects of sugar-sweetened beverage consumption as they are commonly consumed in this country, with regard to both the amount of sugar consumed and the types of sugars consumed. Self-reported intake data suggest that only 13% of the US population consumes >25% of energy from added sugars (41), and the majority of the added sugar is not pure fructose or glucose, but rather high fructose corn syrup (HFCS) (55% fructose, 45% glucose) and sucrose (50% fructose, 50% glucose). However, the study of fructose and glucose separately allowed us to demonstrate that fructose increases circulating apoCIII compared to glucose, thus, it is the likely mediator of the increases in apoCIII induced by a high-carbohydrate diet [18] or HFCS-sweetened beverages [20].

Furthermore, mechanistic insights gleaned from investigations of fructose compared to glucose are relevant to explaining the observed increases in postprandial TG, fasting and/or postprandial apoCIII, LDL-chol, sdLDL, and apoB observed in subjects consuming HFCS or sucrose-sweetened beverages [12,20,62,63].

5. Conclusions

The results from this study demonstrate that consumption of fructose increases fasting and postprandial plasma concentrations of apoCIII compared with the consumption of glucose and support the involvement of apoCIII in the development of sdLDL and CVD risk [17]. The results also show that fructose markedly increases large TRL particles and the TG-enrichment of LDL in the late postprandial period, which may also affect the development of sdLDL and CVD risk [3,15,56,57]. As the adverse effects of fructose compared with glucose occurred after 10 days of controlled dietary conditions, the results do not support the often-repeated belief that "a calorie is a calorie" independent of its source. While more research is required to determine the levels of fructose-containing sugar that can be consumed without increased risk, it is prudent to advise patients at risk for CVD to refrain from drinking beverages sweetened with fructose-containing sugars.

Author Contributions: Conceptualization, P.J.H. and K.L.S.; Data curation, B.H.; Formal analysis, K.L.S.; Funding acquisition, N.L.K., L.B., P.J.H., and K.L.S.; Investigation, S.C.G., N.L.K., A.A.B., L.B., K.N., and K.L.S.; Methodology, S.C.G., A.A.B., K.A., P.J.H., and K.L.S.; Project administration, K.L.S.; Supervision, K.L.S.; Visualization, B.H.; Writing, original draft, B.H. and K.L.S.; Writing, review & editing, B.H., S.C.G., N.L.K., A.A.B., L.B., K.A., P.J.H., and K.L.S.

References

1. World Heal Organ (WHO). *Global Status Report on Noncommunicable Diseases 2014*; World Heal Organ: Geneva, Switzerland, 2014; p. 176.
2. Mozaffarian, D.; Benjamin, E.J.; Go, A.S.; Arnett, D.K.; Blaha, M.J.; Cushman, M.; Das, S.R.; De Ferranti, S.; Després, J.P.; Fullerton, H.J.; et al. Executive summary: Heart disease and stroke statistics-2016 update: A Report from the American Heart Association. *Circulation* **2016**, *133*, 447–454. [CrossRef] [PubMed]
3. Stanhope, K.L.; Schwarz, J.M.; Keim, N.L.; Griffen, S.C.; Bremer, A.A.; Graham, J.L.; Hatcher, B.; Cox, C.L.; Dyachenko, A.; Zhang, W.; et al. Consuming fructose-sweetened, not glucose-sweetened, beverages increases visceral adiposity and lipids and decreases insulin sensitivity in overweight/obese humans. *J. Clin. Investig.* **2009**, *119*, 1322–1334. [CrossRef] [PubMed]
4. Stanhope, K.L.; Havel, P.J. Fructose consumption: Potential mechanisms for its effects to increase visceral adiposity and induce dyslipidemia and insulin resistance. *Curr. Opin. Lipidol.* **2008**, *19*, 16–24. [CrossRef] [PubMed]
5. Stanhope, K.L. Sugar consumption, metabolic disease and obesity: The state of the controversy. *Crit. Rev. Clin. Lab. Sci.* **2016**, *53*, 52–67. [CrossRef] [PubMed]
6. Softic, S.; Cohen, D.E.; Kahn, C.R. Role of Dietary Fructose and Hepatic De Novo Lipogenesis in Fatty Liver Disease. *Dig. Dis. Sci.* **2016**, *61*, 1282–1293. [CrossRef] [PubMed]
7. Mirtschink, P.; Jang, C.; Arany, Z.; Krek, W. Fructose metabolism, cardiometabolic risk, and the epidemic of coronary artery disease. *Eur. Heart J.* **2018**, *39*, 2497–2505. [CrossRef] [PubMed]
8. Taskinen, M.-R.; Söderlund, S.; Bogl, L.H.; Hakkarainen, A.; Matikainen, N.; Pietiläinen, K.H.; Räsänen, S.; Lundbom, N.; Björnson, E.; Eliasson, B.; et al. Adverse effects of fructose on cardiometabolic risk factors and hepatic lipid metabolism in subjects with abdominal obesity. *J. Intern. Med.* **2017**, *140*, 874–888. [CrossRef] [PubMed]
9. Schwarz, J.M.; Noworolski, S.M.; Wen, M.J.; Dyachenko, A.; Prior, J.L.; Weinberg, M.E.; Herraiz, L.A.; Tai, V.W.; Bergeron, N.; Bersot, T.P.; et al. Effect of a high-fructose weight-maintaining diet on lipogenesis and liver fat. *J. Clin. Endocrinol. Metab.* **2015**, *100*, 2434–2442. [CrossRef] [PubMed]
10. Faeh, D.; Minehira, K.; Schwarz, J.M.; Periasami, R.; Seongsu, P.; Tappy, L. Effect of fructose overfeeding and fish oil administration on hepatic de novo lipogenesis and insulin sensitivity in healthy men. *Diabetes* **2005**, *54*, 1907–1913. [CrossRef] [PubMed]
11. Cox, C.L.; Stanhope, K.L.; Schwarz, J.M.; Graham, J.L.; Hatcher, B.; Griffen, S.C.; Bremer, A.A.; Berglund, L.; McGahan, J.P.; Havel, P.J.; et al. Consumption of fructose-sweetened beverages for 10 weeks reduces net fat oxidation and energy expenditure in overweight/obese men and women. *Eur. J. Clin. Nutr.* **2012**, *66*, 201–208. [CrossRef]
12. Maersk, M.; Belza, A.; Stodkilde-Jorgensen, H.; Ringgaard, S.; Chabanova, E.; Thomsen, H.; Pedersen, S.B.; Astrup, A.; Richelsen, B. Sucrose-sweetened beverages increase fat storage in the liver, muscle, and visceral fat depot: A 6-mo randomized intervention study. *Am. J. Clin. Nutr.* **2012**, *95*, 283–289. [CrossRef] [PubMed]
13. Adiels, M.; Taskinen, M.-R.; Packard, C.; Caslake, M.J.; Soro-Paavonen, A.; Westerbacka, J.; Vehkavaara, S.; Hakkinen, A.; Olofsson, S.-O.; Yki-Jarvinen, H.; et al. Overproduction of large VLDL particles is driven by increased liver fat content in man. *Diabetologia* **2006**, *49*, 755–765. [CrossRef] [PubMed]
14. Chapman, M.J.; Le Goff, W.; Guerin, M.; Kontush, A. Cholesteryl ester transfer protein: At the heart of the action of lipid-modulating therapy with statins, fibrates, niacin, and cholesteryl ester transfer protein inhibitors. *Eur. Heart J.* **2010**, *31*, 149–164. [CrossRef] [PubMed]
15. Packard, C.J. Triacylglycerol-rich lipoproteins and the generation of small, dense low-density lipoprotein. *Biochem. Soc. Trans.* **2003**, *31*, 1066–1069. [CrossRef] [PubMed]
16. Zheng, C.; Khoo, C.; Furtado, J.; Sacks, F.M. Apolipoprotein C-III and the metabolic basis for hypertriglyceridemia and the dense low-density lipoprotein phenotype. *Circulation* **2010**, *121*, 1722–1734. [CrossRef] [PubMed]
17. Sacks, F.M. The crucial roles of apolipoproteins E and C-III in apoB lipoprotein metabolism in normolipidemia and hypertriglyceridemia. *Curr. Opin. Lipidol.* **2015**, *26*, 56–63. [CrossRef] [PubMed]
18. Mendoza, S.; Trenchevska, O.; King, S.M.; Nelson, R.W.; Nedelkov, D.; Krauss, R.M.; Yassine, H.N. Changes in low-density lipoprotein size phenotypes associate with changes in apolipoprotein C-III glycoforms after dietary interventions. *J. Clin. Lipidol.* **2017**, *11*, 224–233.e2. [CrossRef]

19. Bremer, A.A.; Stanhope, K.L.; Graham, J.L.; Cummings, B.P.; Wang, W.; Saville, B.R.; Havel, P.J. Fructose-fed rhesus monkeys: A nonhuman primate model of insulin resistance, metabolic syndrome, and type 2 diabetes. *Clin. Transl. Sci.* **2011**, *4*, 243–252. [CrossRef] [PubMed]
20. Stanhope, K.L.; Medici, V.; Bremer, A.A.; Lee, V.; Lam, H.D.; Nunez, M.V.; Chen, G.X.; Keim, N.L.; Havel, P.J. A dose-response study of consuming high-fructose corn syrup-sweetened beverages on lipid/lipoprotein risk factors for cardiovascular disease in young adults. *Am. J. Clin. Nutr.* **2015**, *101*, 1144–1154. [CrossRef]
21. Gonzalez-granda, A.; Damms-machado, A.; Basrai, M.; Bischoff, S.C. Changes in Plasma Acylcarnitine and Lysophosphatidylcholine Levels Following a High-Fructose Diet: A Targeted Metabolomics Study in Healthy Women. *Nutrients* **2018**, *10*, 1254. [CrossRef]
22. Teff, K.L.; Elliott, S.S.; Tschöp, M.; Kieffer, T.J.; Rader, D.; Heiman, M.; Townsend, R.R.; Keim, N.L.; D'Alessio, D.; Havel, P.J. Dietary fructose reduces circulating insulin and leptin, attenuates postprandial suppression of ghrelin, and increases triglycerides in women. *J. Clin. Endocrinol. Metab.* **2004**, *89*, 2963–2972. [CrossRef] [PubMed]
23. Okazaki, M.; Usui, S.; Ishigami, M.; Sakai, N.; Nakamura, T.; Matsuzawa, Y.; Yamashita, S. Identification of unique lipoprotein subclasses for visceral obesity by component analysis of cholesterol profile in high-performance liquid chromatography. *Arterioscler. Thromb. Vasc. Biol.* **2005**, *25*, 578–584. [CrossRef] [PubMed]
24. Toshima, G.; Iwama, Y.; Kimura, F.; Matsumoto, Y.; Miura, M. LipoSEARCH®; Analytical GP-HPLC method for lipoprotein profiling and its applications. *J. Biol. Macromol.* **2013**, *13*, 21–32.
25. Araki, E.; Yamashita, S.; Arai, H.; Yokote, K.; Satoh, J.; Inoguchi, T.; Nakamura, J.; Maegawa, H.; Yoshioka, N.; Yukio, T.; et al. Effects of Pemafibrate, a Novel Selective PPARα Modulator, on Lipid and Glucose Metabolism in Patients With Type 2 Diabetes and Hypertriglyceridemia: A Randomized, Double-Blind, Placebo-Controlled, Phase 3 Trial. *Diabetes Care* **2018**, *41*, 538–546. [CrossRef] [PubMed]
26. Lee, S.J.; Campos, H.; Moye, L.A.; Sacks, F.M. LDL containing apolipoprotein CIII is an independent risk factor for coronary events in diabetic patients. *Arterioscler. Thromb. Vasc. Biol.* **2003**, *23*, 853–858. [CrossRef] [PubMed]
27. Ooi, E.M.M.; Barrett, P.H.R.; Chan, D.C.; Watts, G.F. Apolipoprotein C-III: Understanding an emerging cardiovascular risk factor. *Clin. Sci.* **2008**, *114*, 611–624. [CrossRef] [PubMed]
28. Altomonte, J.; Cong, L.; Harbaran, S.; Richter, A.; Xu, J.; Meseck, M.; Dong, H.H. Foxo1 mediates insulin action on apoC-III and triglyceride metabolism. *J. Clin. Investig.* **2004**, *114*, 1493–1503. [CrossRef] [PubMed]
29. Stanhope, K.L.; Griffen, S.C.; Bremer, A.A.; Vink, R.G.; Schaefer, E.J.; Nakajima, K.; Schwarz, J.M.; Beysen, C.; Berglund, L.; Keim, N.L.; et al. Metabolic responses to prolonged consumption of glucose- and fructose-sweetened beverages are not associated with postprandial or 24-h glucose and insulin excursions. *Am. J. Clin. Nutr.* **2011**, *94*, 112–119. [CrossRef]
30. Caron, S.; Verrijken, A.; Mertens, I.; Samanez, C.H.; Mautino, G.; Haas, J.T.; Duran-Sandoval, D.; Prawitt, J.; Francque, S.; Vallez, E.; et al. Transcriptional activation of apolipoprotein CIII expression by glucose may contribute to diabetic dyslipidemia. *Arterioscler. Thromb. Vasc. Biol.* **2011**, *31*, 513–519. [CrossRef]
31. West, G.; Rodia, C.; Li, D.; Johnson, Z.; Dong, H.; Kohan, A.B. Key differences between apoC-III regulation and expression in intestine and liver. *Biochem. Biophys. Res. Commun.* **2017**, *491*, 747–753. [CrossRef]
32. Kim, M.; Lai, M.; Herman, M.A.; Kim, M.; Krawczyk, S.A.; Doridot, L.; Fowler, A.J.; Wang, J.X.; Trauger, S.A.; Noh, H.; et al. ChREBP regulates fructose-induced glucose production independently of insulin signaling. *J. Clin. Investig.* **2016**, *126*, 4372–4386. [CrossRef] [PubMed]
33. Koo, H.Y.; Wallig, M.A.; Chung, B.H.; Nara, T.Y.; Cho, B.H.S.; Nakamura, M.T. Dietary fructose induces a wide range of genes with distinct shift in carbohydrate and lipid metabolism in fed and fasted rat liver. *Biochim. Biophys. Acta Mol. Basis Dis.* **2008**, *1782*, 341–348. [CrossRef] [PubMed]
34. Ramms, B.; Gordts, P.L.S.M. Apolipoprotein C-III in triglyceride-rich lipoprotein metabolism. *Curr. Opin. Lipidol.* **2018**, *29*, 171–179. [CrossRef] [PubMed]
35. Butler, A.A.; Price, C.A.; Graham, J.L.; Stanhope, K.L.; King, S.; Hung, Y.-H.; Sethupathy, P.; Wong, S.; Hamilton, J.; Krauss, R.M.; et al. Fructose-induced hypertriglyceridemia in rhesus macaques is attenuated with fish oil or apoC3 RNA interference. *J. Lipid Res.* **2019**, *60*, jlr.M089508. [CrossRef] [PubMed]
36. Batal, R.; Tremblay, M.; Barrett, P.H.R.; Jacques, H.; Fredenrich, A.; Mamer, O.; Davignon, J.; Cohn, J.S. Plasma kinetics of apoC-III and apoE in normolipidemic and hypertriglyceridemic subjects. *J. Lipid Res.* **2000**, *41*, 706–718. [PubMed]

37. Yao, Z. Human apolipoprotein C-III—A new intrahepatic protein factor promoting assembly and secretion of very low density lipoproteins. *Cardiovasc. Hematol. Disord. Drug Targets* **2012**, *12*, 133–140. [CrossRef] [PubMed]
38. Sundaram, M.; Yao, Z. Recent progress in understanding protein and lipid factors affecting hepatic VLDL assembly and secretion. *Nutr. Metab.* **2010**, *7*, 1–17. [CrossRef]
39. Sundaram, M.; Curtis, K.R.; Amir Alipour, M.; LeBlond, N.D.; Margison, K.D.; Yaworski, R.A.; Parks, R.J.; McIntyre, A.D.; Hegele, R.A.; Fullerton, M.D.; et al. The apolipoprotein C-III (Gln38Lys) variant associated with human hypertriglyceridemia is a gain-of-function mutation. *J. Lipid Res.* **2017**, *58*, 2188–2196. [CrossRef]
40. Matikainen, N.; Adiels, M.; Söderlund, S.; Stennabb, S.; Ahola, T.; Hakkarainen, A.; Borén, J.; Taskinen, M.R. Hepatic lipogenesis and a marker of hepatic lipid oxidation, predict postprandial responses of triglyceride-rich lipoproteins. *Obesity* **2014**, *22*, 1854–1859. [CrossRef]
41. Gordts, P.L.S.M.; Nock, R.; Son, N.-H.; Ramms, B.; Lew, I.; Gonzales, J.C.; Thacker, B.E.; Basu, D.; Lee, R.G.; Mullick, A.E.; et al. ApoC-III Modulates Clearance of Triglyceride-Rich Lipoproteins in Mice Through Low Density Lipoprotein Family Receptors. *J. Clin. Investig.* **2016**, *126*, 2855–2866. [CrossRef]
42. Talayero, B.; Wang, L.; Furtado, J.; Carey, V.J.; Bray, G.A.; Sacks, F.M. Obesity favors apolipoprotein E- and C-III-containing high density lipoprotein subfractions associated with risk of heart disease. *J. Lipid Res.* **2014**, *55*, 2167–2177. [CrossRef] [PubMed]
43. Hodis, H.N. Triglyceride-rich lipoprotein remnant particles and risk of atherosclerosis. *Circulation* **1999**, *99*, 2852–2854. [CrossRef] [PubMed]
44. Sacks, F.M.; Alaupovic, P.; Moye, L.A.; Cole, T.G.; Sussex, B.; Stampfer, M.J.; Pfeffer, M.A.; Braunwald, E. VLDL, apolipoproteins B, CIII, and E, and risk of recurrent coronary events in the Cholesterol and Recurrent Events (CARE) trial. *Circulation* **2000**, *102*, 1886–1892. [CrossRef] [PubMed]
45. Sharrett, A.R.; Heiss, G.; Chambless, L.E.; Boerwinkle, E.; Coady, S.A.; Folsom, A.R.; Patsch, W. Metabolic and lifestyle determinants of postprandial lipemia differ from those of fasting triglycerides the Atherosclerosis Risk in Communities (ARIC) study. *Arterioscler. Thromb. Vasc. Biol.* **2001**, *21*, 275–281. [CrossRef] [PubMed]
46. Bansal, S.; Buring, J.E.; Rifai, N.; Mora, S.; Sacks, F.M.; Ridker, P.M. Fasting compared with nonfasting triglyceride and risk of cardiovascular events in women. *JAMA* **2007**, *298*, 309–316. [CrossRef] [PubMed]
47. Nordestgaard, B.G.; Benn, M.; Schnohr, P.; Tybjærg-hansen, A. Nonfasting Triglycerides and Risk of Myocardial Infarction, Ischemic Heart. *JAMA* **2007**, *298*, 299–308. [CrossRef] [PubMed]
48. Varbo, A.; Freiberg, J.J.; Nordestgaard, B.G. Extreme nonfasting remnant cholesterol vs extreme LDL cholesterol as contributors to cardiovascular disease and all-cause mortality in 90000 individuals from the general population. *Clin. Chem.* **2015**, *61*, 533–543. [CrossRef]
49. Haidari, M.; Leung, N.; Mahbub, F.; Uffelman, K.D.; Kohen-Avramoglu, R.; Lewis, G.F.; Adeli, K. Fasting and postprandial overproduction of intestinally derived lipoproteins in an animal model of insulin resistance: Evidence that chronic fructose feeding in the hamster is accompanied by enhanced intestinal de novo lipogenesis and ApoB48-containing li. *J. Biol. Chem.* **2002**, *277*, 31646–31655. [CrossRef]
50. Steenson, S.; Umpleby, A.M.; Lovegrove, J.A.; Jackson, K.G.; Fielding, B.A. Role of the enterocyte in fructose-induced hypertriglyceridaemia. *Nutrients* **2017**, *9*, 349. [CrossRef]
51. Nestel, P.J.; Fidge, N.H. Apoprotein C Metabolism in Man. *Adv. Lipid Res.* **1982**, *19*, 55–83.
52. Wolska, A.; Dunbar, R.L.; Freeman, L.A.; Ueda, M.; Amar, M.J.; Sviridov, D.O.; Remaley, A.T. Apolipoprotein C-II: New findings related to genetics, biochemistry, and role in triglyceride metabolism. *Atherosclerosis* **2017**, *267*, 49–60. [CrossRef] [PubMed]
53. Taskinen, M.R. Diabetic dyslipidaemia: From basic research to clinical practice. *Diabetologia* **2003**, *46*, 733–749. [CrossRef] [PubMed]
54. Eisenberg, S. Preferential enrichment of large-sized very low density lipoprotein populations with transferred cholesteryl esters. *J. Lipid Res.* **1985**, *26*, 487–494. [PubMed]
55. Krauss, R.M. Dietary and genetic probes of atherogenic dyslipidemia. *Arterioscler. Thromb. Vasc. Biol.* **2005**, *25*, 2265–2272. [CrossRef] [PubMed]
56. Adiels, M.; Olofsson, S.O.; Taskinen, M.R.; Borén, J. Overproduction of very low-density lipoproteins is the hallmark of the dyslipidemia in the metabolic syndrome. *Arterioscler. Thromb. Vasc. Biol.* **2008**, *28*, 1225–1236. [CrossRef] [PubMed]
57. Berneis, K.K.; Krauss, R.M. Metabolic origins and clinical significance of LDL heterogeneity. *J. Lipid Res.* **2002**, *43*, 1363–1379. [CrossRef] [PubMed]

58. Berneis, K.; Rizzo, M.; Spinas, G.A.; Di Lorenzo, G.; Di Fede, G.; Pepe, I.; Pernice, V.; Rini, G.B. The predictive role of atherogenic dyslipidemia in subjects with non-coronary atherosclerosis. *Clin. Chim. Acta* **2009**, *406*, 36–40. [CrossRef]
59. Rizzo, M.; Pernice, V.; Frasheri, A.; Di Lorenzo, G.; Rini, G.B.; Spinas, G.A.; Berneis, K. Small, dense low-density lipoproteins (LDL) are predictors of cardio- and cerebro-vascular events in subjects with the metabolic syndrome. *Clin. Endocrinol.* **2009**, *70*, 870–875. [CrossRef]
60. Ivanova, E.A.; Myasoedova, V.A.; Melnichenko, A.A.; Grechko, A.V.; Orekhov, A.N. Small Dense Low-Density Lipoprotein as Biomarker for Atherosclerotic Diseases. *Oxid. Med. Cell. Longev.* **2017**, *2017*, 1273042. [CrossRef]
61. Xiao, C.; Dash, S.; Morgantini, C.; Hegele, R.A.; Lewis, G.F. Pharmacological targeting of the atherogenic dyslipidemia complex: The next frontier in CVD prevention beyond lowering LDL cholesterol. *Diabetes* **2016**, *65*, 1767–1778. [CrossRef]
62. Aeberli, I.; Hochuli, M.; Gerber, P. Moderate Amounts of Fructose Consumption Impair Insulin Sensitivity in Healthy Young Men A randomized controlled trial. *Diabetes Care* **2013**, *36*, 150–156. [CrossRef] [PubMed]
63. Aeberli, I.; Gerber, P.A.; Hochuli, M.; Kohler, S.; Haile, S.R.; Gouni-Berthold, I.; Berthold, H.K.; Spinas, G.A.; Berneis, K. Low to moderate sugar-sweetened beverage consumption impairs glucose and lipid metabolism and promotes inflammation in healthy young men: A randomized controlled trial. *Am. J. Clin. Nutr.* **2011**, *94*, 479–485. [CrossRef] [PubMed]

9

We are What We Eat: Impact of Food from Short Supply Chain on Metabolic Syndrome

Gaetano Santulli [1,2,3,*], Valeria Pascale [4], Rosa Finelli [4], Valeria Visco [4], Rocco Giannotti [4], Angelo Massari [5], Carmine Morisco [2], Michele Ciccarelli [4], Maddalena Illario [6,7], Guido Iaccarino [2,3,*] and Enrico Coscioni [5]

[1] Dept. of Medicine, Division of Cardiology, and Dept. of Molecular Pharmacology, Montefiore University Hospital, Fleischer Institute for Diabetes and Metabolism (FIDAM), Albert Einstein College of Medicine (AECOM), New York, NY 10461, USA
[2] Dept. of Advanced Biomedical Science, Federico II University, 80131 Naples, Italy; carmine.morisco@unina.it
[3] International Translational Research and Medical Education Consortium (ITME), 80131 Naples, Italy
[4] Dept. of Medicine, Surgery and Dentistry, University of Salerno, 8408 Baronissi, Italy; pascalevaleria@gmail.com (V.P.); rosafinelli1@gmail.com (R.F.); valeriavisco1991@libero.it (V.V.); tintorangocico@live.it (R.G.); mciccarelli@unisa.it (M.C.)
[5] "San Giovanni di Dio e Ruggi d'Aragona" University Hospital, 84131 Salerno, Italy; angelo.massari@sangiovannieruggi.it (A.M.); enrico.coscioni@regione.campania.it (E.C.)
[6] Health's Innovation, Campania Regional Government, 80132 Naples, Italy; illario@unina.it
[7] Dept. of Public Health, Federico II University, 80131 Naples, Italy
* Correspondence: gaetano.santulli@einsteinmed.org or gsantulli001@gmail.com (G.S.); guiaccar@unina.it (G.I.)

Abstract: Food supply in the Mediterranean area has been recently modified by big retail distribution; for instance, industrial retail has favored shipments of groceries from regions that are intensive producers of mass food, generating a long supply chain (LSC) of food that opposes short supply chains (SSCs) that promote local food markets. However, the actual functional role of food retail and distribution in the determination of the risk of developing metabolic syndrome (MetS) has not been studied hitherto. The main aim of this study was to test the effects of food chain length on the prevalence of MetS in a population accustomed to the Mediterranean diet. We conducted an observational study in Southern Italy on individuals adhering to the Mediterranean diet. We examined a total of 407 subjects (41% females) with an average age of 56 ± 14.5 years (as standard deviation) and found that being on the Mediterranean diet with a SSC significantly reduces the prevalence of MetS compared with the LSC (SSC: 19.65%, LSC: 31.46%; *p*: 0.007). Our data indicate for the first time that the length of food supply chain plays a key role in determining the risk of MetS in a population adhering to the Mediterranean diet.

Keywords: mediterranean diet; supply chain of food; metabolic syndrome; food retail; cardiovascular risk

1. Introduction

Several studies have demonstrated that the Mediterranean diet significantly reduces the risk of developing metabolic syndrome (MetS) [1–4], a cluster of clinical conditions that occur together and increase the risk of heart disease, stroke, and type 2 diabetes [5–7]. However, the exact role of food retail and distribution in the risk of developing MetS has not yet been fully determined.

Recently, the development of big retail food distribution has deeply modified food supply in the Mediterranean area [8,9]. Indeed, industrial retail has favored shipments of groceries from regions that are intensive producers of mass foods, generating the long supply chain (LSC) of food [10]; on the other hand, short supply chains (SSCs) involve local self-producers that promote local food markets [8]. The origin of food, the long period of time elapsing from production to consumption, the need to add preservatives, as well as the loss of perishable nutrients such as vitamins, can all contribute to reducing the quality of food. Nevertheless, whether food quality loss has an impact on the health of the population remains to be determined.

The increasing availability of foods from big retail is a revolutionary event that has impacted health on a population-size level. In particular, the adherence to the Mediterranean diet is decreasing even within those regions where it was first discovered [11,12], and such a change in the alimentary habit is generally seen as one of the potential causes of the obesity epidemic [13], especially among adolescents [14].

The overarching aim of our study was to test the effects of food chain length on metabolic alterations in a population accustomed to the Mediterranean diet. Specifically, we compared SSCs of food—in which aliments are produced *in loco*, usually with traditional and low-technology methodologies—to the LSC of food.

2. Methods

2.1. Subjects

We conducted an observational, cross-sectional study on the general population of Salerno (population: 138,000 inhabitants) and of five nearby villages (population <6000 inhabitants): Castelnuovo Cilento, Polla, Sapri, San Gregorio Magno, and Satriano di Lucania. In order to be considered eligible, subjects had to be currently and stably (for at least 10 years) living in the cities indicated, and to have signed the informed consent.

2.2. Study Approval

The study was approved by the Institutional Ethical Committee of Salerno University Hospital. Written informed consent was obtained from all participants. The study is registered in the ClincalTrial.gov database (Trial number: NCT03305276).

2.3. Data Acquisition

On the occasion of 2015–2017 World Hypertension Day (May 17th), booths were organized in the major squares of the mentioned villages, harnessing a collaborative effort of the Medical School of Salerno and local authorities [15]. The event was successfully publicized with a 15-day notice via local media advertisements, and we had the partnership of local authorities and patient associations, as well as parishes. The population was instructed to show up on the day of the event at the booths, where subjects were asked to sign the informed consent to participate in the survey and to donate blood samples for analysis. Anamnesis and anthropometric parameters were obtained including weight, height, waist and hip circumferences, and BMI. Blood pressure was detected according to the Guidelines of the European Society of Cardiology and European Society of Hypertension (ESC/ESH) [16]. Current smokers were defined as those reporting having smoked at least 100 cigarettes during their lifetime and currently smoking every day or some days [17]. Dietary habits were collected by means of a questionnaire previously described by Trichopoulou et al. [18]. This nine-question questionnaire allows a score (Trichopoulou score) to be attributed to each subject. To determine the use of SSCs or the LSC, we formulated a questionnaire that included the following eight questions: (1) "Do the vegetables you consume come mainly from your vegetable garden?" (Yes = 1); (2) "Do you buy fruit grown in your area?" (Yes = 1); (3) "Do you eat seasonal fruit?" (Yes = 1); (4) "Does the meat you consume come mainly from local farms or from butchers in your area?" (Yes = 1); (5) "Do you eat mostly fresh, unpackaged food?" (Yes = 1); (6) "Do you eat cookies, snacks, and/or sweets more than once a week?" (No = 1); (7) "Do you use canned or frozen food?" (No = 1); and (8) "Do you drink carbonated or sweetened drinks?" (No = 1). These questions were derived from preliminary interviews performed by experienced personnel to relatives and families of volunteers in order to verify the kinds of food that are more frequently acquired from small business stores, as well as the ones mostly purchased from big food retail shops. According to this survey, fruits, vegetables, and meats were purchased more often from small business shops, whereas preserved and canned foods, as well as frozen food, sodas, cookies, and snacks, were mainly obtained from big resellers. In a second phase, we asked one big food retailer from the city of Salerno and two small business of the city of San Gregorio Magno to provide us with the suppliers of the listed products, so as to substantiate the actual length of the supply chain of food. The optimal cut-off of the score (5) was determined by receiver operating characteristic (ROC) curves (see Supplementary Figure S1), applying Youden's index [19,20]; with a score ≥5, the subject was included in the SSC group, whereas with a score <5 the subject was included in the LSC group. MetS was diagnosed according to the 2009 Harmonized Criteria, implementing the criteria of the International Diabetes Federation (IDF) to evaluate abdominal obesity [7,21].

2.4. *Blood Sample Laboratory Analysis*

A venous blood sample was collected from the antecubital vein in a dedicate booth from experienced volunteer nurses in two tubes of 5.0 mL and centrifuged the same day. The time of the last meal was recorded during data collection. We measured blood glucose, insulin, total cholesterol, HDL cholesterol, LDL cholesterol, and triglycerides. The homeostatic model assessment (HOMA) index was calculated as previously described, based on an adequate fasting time (6 h) [22].

2.5. *Statistical Analysis*

Continuous data are presented as mean ± SE. Categorical data are presented as absolute values and/or frequencies. To observe a change of one quartile in frequency with an α cut-off of 5% and a β cut-off of 20%, and given an estimated incidence of MetS of 26% in our population [23], we calculated that a $n = 398$ would have been necessary to reach statistical significance. A Kolmogorov–Smirnov test was used to verify the normality of distributions of continuous variables. A chi-square (χ^2) test was used to compare frequencies. Independent sample t-tests were used for between-group comparisons. In all the above-mentioned tests, $p < 0.05$ was considered statistically significant. Statistical analysis was performed with SPSS (Statistical Package for the Social Sciences) 24.0 (IBM, Armonk, NY, USA) and Prism 7 (GraphPad Software, San Diego, CA, USA).

3. Results

3.1. *Clinical Features of Study Population*

A total of 808 subjects (45% male and 55% female, 14–85 years) were recruited during the XI, XII, and XIII editions of World Hypertension Day, which is celebrated every year on 17 May. We excluded from the analysis patients younger than 30 ($n = 70$) and older than 80 years ($n = 30$) because of the previously reported relatively low adherence to the Mediterranean diet by populations at those ages [12,24–26]. We also excluded those with an incomplete database, thereby precluding the calculation of adherence to the Mediterranean diet, SSCs or the LSC, or the HOMA index ($n = 269$), as well as 28 outliers (3 SD over/below mean) in MetS determinants.

The main characteristics of our population (407 subjects, 41% females, with an average age of ~56 years) are depicted in Table 1.

3.2. *Effects of SSCs on Clinical Features*

We divided the population according to the eight-point questionnaire indicated above, using the score of 5 as a cutoff to indicate adherence to SSCs (≥5) or the LSC (<5). Data are indicated in Table 1.

Table 1. Impact of SSCs and the LSC on anthropometric and clinical characteristics.

	Total	LSC	SSC	*p*
N	407	178	229	-
Age (years)	55.9 ± 0.58	56.4 ± 0.8	55.52 ± 0.8	0.422
Sex (M, %)	59	60	58	0.765
Weight (Kg)	73.8 ± 0.82	72.2 ± 1.2	75.1 ± 1.08	0.085
Height (cm)	163.7 ± 0.6	164.2 ± 0.6	163.3 ± 0.91	0.399
Waist (cm)	96.3 ± 0.74	96.4 ± 0.84	96,0 ± 1.49	0.803
BMI (Kg/m^2)	27.6 ± 0.25	27.1 ± 0.39	27.9 ± 0.34	0.098
SBP (mmHg)	130.6 ± 0.9	131.2 ± 1.3	130.1 ± 1.2	0.523
DBP (mmHg)	79.8 ± 0.5	80.5 ± 0.8	79.2 ± 0.69	0.220
HR (bpm)	72.2 ± 0.6	72.1 ± 0.8	72.28 ± 0.82	0.877
Fasting Glucose (mg/dl)	84.4 ± 1.2	91.28 ± 1.7	79.41 ± 1.5	0.001
Serum Insulin (μU/dl)	17.7 ± 0.97	21.4 ± 1.7	14.9 ± 1.1	0.001
Creatinine (mg/dl)	0.85 ± 0.02	0.88 ± 0.05	0.82 ± 0.01	0.19
Current Smokers (%)	32.0	30.0	34.0	0.427
Cholesterol (Total, mg/dl)	201.4 ± 1.9	201.36 ± 3.2	201.48 ± 2.5	0.977
Cholesterol (HDL, mg/dl)	59.3 ± 0.7	59.03 ± 1.2	59.56 ± 1.0	0.737
Cholesterol (LDL, mg/dl)	124.6 ± 2.1	127.02 ± 3.9	123.43 ± 2.4	0.418
TG (mg/dl)	121.7 ± 3.6	136.14 ± 5.9	110.95 ± 4.3	0.001
Metabolic Syndrome (%)	24.81	31.46	19.65	0.007
Trichopoulous Score	4.98 ± 0.08	4.86 ± 0.13	5.08 ± 0.10	0.180

Frequencies are reported as %, continuous variables as mean ± SE; DBP: Diastolic/systolic blood pressure; HR: Heart rate; HDL/LDL: High-density/low-density lipoproteins; LSC/SSC: Long/short supply chain; TG: Triglycerides; Trichopoulous Score: Score of the adherence to a Mediterranean-style diet (9 = max, 0 = min; *p* value was calculated applying the *t* test or χ^2, as appropriate).

Our data indicate that SSCs are associated with lower levels of triglycerides and glucose, and therefore have a marked impact on the occurrence of MetS: indeed, MetS is less frequent among populations that consume SSC food. Interestingly, adherence to the Mediterranean diet, assessed using a validated questionnaire, was similar between the two populations, indicating a homogenous high adherence between the consumers of SSC and LSC foods.

3.3. *Effects of SSCs on Insulin Sensitivity*

Given the notion that MetS is a hallmark of insulin resistance, we assayed insulin resistance by means of the HOMA index. As shown in Figure 1, the HOMA index was lower in the SSC than in the LSC group (2.67 ± 0.20 vs. 4.66 ± 0.44, respectively; $p = 0.0002$).

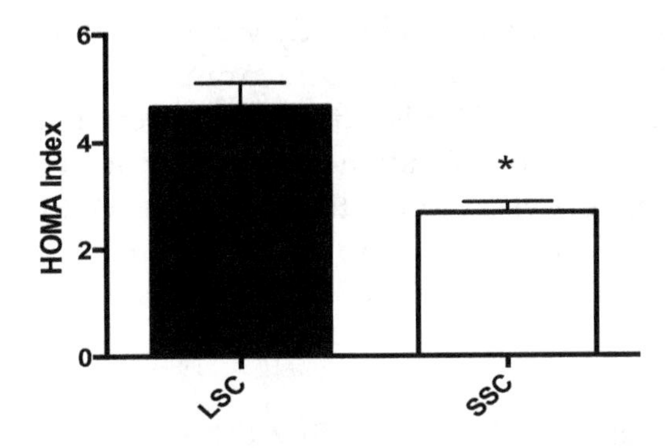

Figure 1. Impact of SSCs and the LSC on insulin resistance. LSC: Long supply chain; SSC: Short supply chain; * $p = 0.0002$.

4. Discussion

Our results indicate that the Mediterranean diet with food from a SSC significantly reduces the prevalence of MetS. These results are consistent with recent observations suggesting that local food environments might affect health outcomes [27]. Our data are corroborated by the evidence that insulin resistance is significantly more common among LSC subjects compared with SSC individuals. With our data, we are among the first investigators to introduce the concept that freshness of food is a key determinant of health outcomes.

Prevalence of MetS in Southern Italy is reported to be ~25% in young adults [23] and ~65% in older women after menopause [28]; of note, the area of assessment might slightly impact the occurrence of MetS [29]. Our population showed overall a prevalence of 35%, and we consider this number to be fairly representative, given the large age range (from 30 to 80 years) of our population.

Substantial evidence indicates that local food environments might affect health outcomes [27,30–36]. It is therefore possible to speculate that length of a food supply chain might affect cardiovascular risk. To verify this hypothesis, it is crucial to compare populations that present similar dietary patterns that derive from different sources (i.e., retail market vs. locally grown food). In this sense, Southern Italy features examples of urbanization, where retail food is the most important source of food, which is the opposite to rural areas, where consuming locally grown, seasonal vegetables, as well as meat of courtyard animals is a fairly regular habit [28,29,37]. These contrasting local food environments, somehow superimposed on the Mediterranean diet, represent a unique setting to test the impact on health phenotypes, such as intermediate metabolism and cardiovascular risk [4,38,39].

Our findings are particularly relevant because they provide for the first time an actual evaluation of how critical the food supply chain is in the context of the Mediterranean diet. Indeed, it is well established that the Mediterranean diet can ameliorate cardiovascular risk [40]. Therefore, to verify the existence of a further improvement in health outcomes from SSCs versus the LSC, it is imperative to compare groups that consume the same diet, with no difference in macro- and micronutrients. Based on our data on insulin resistance, we can speculate that insulin sensitivity is better preserved among subjects adhering to the Mediterranean diet who eat SSC foods. Using a previously published questionnaire [18], we were indeed able to verify the high adherence of Southern Italians to the Mediterranean diet, and no differences were observed when we divided our population according to LSC and SSC groups. Therefore, we can conclude that the difference observed in terms of MetS prevalence cannot be attributable to a different attitude towards the Mediterranean diet.

Our findings should be interpreted in light of several limitations. First and foremost, the cross-sectional design of the study prevents a determination of causality. Another major issue that was not addressed by our questionnaires is the lifestyle that accompanies the provision of SSC food, nor did our questionnaire did not measure the time spent in the production of such food, such as the time spent looking after crops and/or courtyard animals, which would imply a more active lifestyle. Likewise, the use of food from the LSC is more distinctive of urban centers, where alternative healthy lifestyles are also more common (practicing sports, attending the gym). This aspect was also testified by our observation of no significant differences in body weight or waist between the two populations, with a tendency of heavier weights detected in the SSC group. Therefore, while we cannot completely rule out an effect of physical activity on MetS in our study, the evidence that SSC is associated with a lower prevalence of MetS is suggestive of a fundamental impact of fresh food on metabolic parameters.

If confirmed in larger prospective studies, these results could promote public interventions to improve lifestyle, preferring, whenever possible, SSCs to the LSC. Therefore, an assessment of cardiovascular risk should include dietary habits of the studied population.

5. Conclusions

Taken together, our findings indicate for the first time that the length of food supply chain is crucial in determining the risk of developing MetS as well as in the assessment of cardiovascular risk in a population adhering to the Mediterranean diet.

Author Contributions: Methodology, G.S., M.C., and G.I.; validation, G.S., C.M., M.I., G.I., and E.C.; formal analysis, G.S. and G.I.; investigation, V.P., R.F., V.V., R.G., A.M., and M.C.; data curation, G.S., G.I., and E.C.; writing, G.S. and G.I.

References

1. Salas-Salvado, J.; Guasch-Ferre, M.; Lee, C.H.; Estruch, R.; Clish, C.B.; Ros, E. Protective effects of the Mediterranean diet on Type 2 Diabetes and metabolic syndrome. *J. Nutr.* **2016**, *146*, 920S–927S. [CrossRef]
2. Grosso, G.; Mistretta, A.; Marventano, S.; Purrello, A.; Vitaglione, P.; Calabrese, G.; Drago, F.; Galvano, F. Beneficial effects of the Mediterranean diet on metabolic syndrome. *Curr. Pharm. Des.* **2014**, *20*, 5039–5044. [CrossRef] [PubMed]
3. Estruch, R.; Ros, E.; Salas-Salvadó, J.; Covas, M.I.; Corella, D.; Arós, F.; Gómez-Gracia, E.; Ruiz-Gutiérrez, V.; Fiol, M.; Lapetra, J.; et al. Primary prevention of cardiovascular disease with a Mediterranean diet. *N. Engl. J. Med.* **2013**, *368*, 12. [CrossRef] [PubMed]
4. Franquesa, M.; Pujol-Busquets, G.; Garcia-Fernandez, E.; Rico, L.; Shamirian-Pulido, L.; Aguilar-Martinez, A.; Medina, F.X.; Serra-Majem, L.; Bach-Faig, A. Mediterranean diet and cardiodiabesity: A systematic review through evidence-based answers to key clinical questions. *Nutrients* **2019**, *11*, 655. [CrossRef] [PubMed]
5. Santulli, G. Dietary components and metabolic dysfunction: Translating preclinical studies into clinical practice. *Nutrients.* **2016**, *8*, 632. [CrossRef] [PubMed]
6. Smith, G.I.; Mittendorfer, B.; Klein, S. Metabolically healthy obesity: Facts and fantasies. *J. Clin. Investig.* **2019**, *129*, 3978–3989. [CrossRef] [PubMed]
7. Alberti, K.G.; Eckel, R.H.; Grundy, S.M.; Zimmet, P.Z.; Cleeman, J.I.; Donato, K.A.; Fruchart, J.C.; James, W.P.; Loria, C.M.; Smith, S.C., Jr.; et al. Harmonizing the metabolic syndrome: A joint interim statement of the International Diabetes Federation Task Force on Epidemiology and Prevention; National Heart, Lung, and Blood Institute; American Heart Association; World Heart Federation; International Atherosclerosis Society; and International Association for the Study of Obesity. *Circulation* **2009**, *120*, 1640–1645. [PubMed]
8. Hernandez-Rubio, J.; Perez-Mesa, J.C.; Piedra-Munoz, L.; Galdeano-Gomez, E. Determinants of Food Safety Level in Fruit and Vegetable Wholesalers' Supply Chain: Evidence from Spain and France. *Int. J. Environ. Res. Public Health* **2018**, *15*, 2246. [CrossRef]
9. Pettinger, C.; Holdsworth, M.; Gerber, M. 'All under one roof?' differences in food availability and shopping patterns in Southern France and Central England. *Eur. J. Public Health* **2008**, *18*, 109–114. [CrossRef]
10. Wible, B.; Mervis, J.; Wigginton, N.S. The global supply chain. Rethinking the global supply chain. Introduction. *Science* **2014**, *344*, 1100–1103. [CrossRef]
11. Gregorio, M.J.; Rodrigues, A.M.; Graca, P.; de Sousa, R.D.; Dias, S.S.; Branco, J.C.; Canhao, H. Food insecurity is associated with low adherence to the Mediterranean diet and adverse health conditions in Portuguese adults. *Front. Public Health* **2018**, *6*, 38. [CrossRef] [PubMed]
12. Bonaccio, M.; Di Castelnuovo, A.; Bonanni, A.; Costanzo, S.; De Lucia, F.; Persichillo, M.; Zito, F.; Donati, M.B.; de Gaetano, G.; Iacoviello, L. Decline of the Mediterranean diet at a time of economic crisis. Results from the Moli-sani study. *Nutr. Metab. Cardiovasc. Dis.* **2014**, *24*, 853–860. [CrossRef] [PubMed]
13. Agnoli, C.; Sieri, S.; Ricceri, F.; Giraudo, M.T.; Masala, G.; Assedi, M.; Panico, S.; Mattiello, A.; Tumino, R.; Giurdanella, M.C.; et al. Adherence to a Mediterranean diet and long-term changes in weight and waist circumference in the EPIC-Italy cohort. *Nutr. Diabetes* **2018**, *8*, 22. [CrossRef] [PubMed]
14. Theodoridis, X.; Grammatikopoulou, M.G.; Gkiouras, K.; Papadopoulou, S.E.; Agorastou, T.; Gkika, I.; Maraki, M.I.; Dardavessis, T.; Chourdakis, M. Food insecurity and Mediterranean diet adherence among Greek university students. *Nutr. Metab. Cardiovasc. Dis.* **2018**, *28*, 477–485. [CrossRef] [PubMed]
15. Pascale, A.V.; Finelli, R.; Giannotti, R.; Visco, V.; Fabbricatore, D.; Matula, I.; Mazzeo, P.; Ragosa, N.; Massari, A.; Izzo, R.; et al. Vitamin D, parathyroid hormone and cardiovascular risk: The good, the bad and the ugly. *J. Cardiovasc. Med. (Hagerstown)* **2018**, *19*, 62–66. [CrossRef] [PubMed]
16. Williams, B.; Mancia, G.; Spiering, W.; Agabiti Rosei, E.; Azizi, M.; Burnier, M.; Clement, D.L.; Coca, A.; de Simone, G.; Dominiczak, A.; et al. 2018 ESC/ESH Guidelines for the management of arterial hypertension. *Eur. Heart J.* **2018**, *39*, 3021–3104. [CrossRef]

17. Gambardella, J.; Sardu, C.; Sacra, C.; Del Giudice, C.; Santulli, G. Quit smoking to outsmart atherogenesis: Molecular mechanisms underlying clinical evidence. *Atherosclerosis* **2017**, *257*, 242–245. [CrossRef]
18. Trichopoulou, A.; Costacou, T.; Bamia, C.; Trichopoulos, D. Adherence to a Mediterranean diet and survival in a Greek population. *N. Engl. J. Med.* **2003**, *348*, 2599–2608. [CrossRef]
19. Hajian-Tilaki, K. The choice of methods in determining the optimal cut-off value for quantitative diagnostic test evaluation. *Stat. Methods Med. Res.* **2018**, *27*, 2374–2383. [CrossRef]
20. Youden, W.J. Index for rating diagnostic tests. *Cancer* **1950**, *3*, 32–35. [CrossRef]
21. Alberti, K.G.; Zimmet, P.; Shaw, J. Metabolic syndrome—A new world-wide definition. A Consensus Statement from the International Diabetes Federation. *Diabet. Med.* **2006**, *23*, 469–480. [CrossRef] [PubMed]
22. Haffner, S.M.; Kennedy, E.; Gonzalez, C.; Stern, M.P.; Miettinen, H. A prospective analysis of the HOMA model. The Mexico City Diabetes Study. *Diabetes Care* **1996**, *19*, 1138–1141. [CrossRef] [PubMed]
23. Caserta, C.A.; Mele, A.; Surace, P.; Ferrigno, L.; Amante, A.; Messineo, A.; Vacalebre, C.; Amato, F.; Baldassarre, D.; Amato, M.; et al. Association of non-alcoholic fatty liver disease and cardiometabolic risk factors with early atherosclerosis in an adult population in Southern Italy. *Ann. Ist. Super Sanita* **2017**, *53*, 77–81. [PubMed]
24. Ruggiero, E.; Di Castelnuovo, A.; Costanzo, S.; Persichillo, M.; Bracone, F.; Cerletti, C.; Donati, M.B.; de Gaetano, G.; Iacoviello, L.; Bonaccio, M.; et al. Socioeconomic and psychosocial determinants of adherence to the Mediterranean diet in a general adult Italian population. *Eur. J. Public Health* **2019**, *29*, 328–335. [CrossRef] [PubMed]
25. Knoops, K.T.; de Groot, L.C.; Kromhout, D.; Perrin, A.E.; Moreiras-Varela, O.; Menotti, A.; van Staveren, W.A. Mediterranean diet, lifestyle factors, and 10-year mortality in elderly European men and women: The HALE project. *JAMA* **2004**, *292*, 1433–1439. [CrossRef]
26. Cruz, J.A. Dietary habits and nutritional status in adolescents over Europe—Southern Europe. *Eur. J. Clin. Nutr.* **2000**, *54* (Suppl. 1), S29–S35. [CrossRef]
27. Story, M.; Kaphingst, K.M.; Robinson-O'Brien, R.; Glanz, K. Creating Healthy Food and Eating Environments: Policy and Environmental Approaches. *Annu. Rev. Public Health* **2008**, *29*, 253–272. [CrossRef]
28. Maiello, M.; Zito, A.; Ciccone, M.M.; Palmiero, P. Metabolic syndrome and its components in postmenopausal women living in Southern Italy, Apulia region. *Diabetes Metab. Syndr.* **2017**, *11*, 43–46. [CrossRef]
29. Martino, F.; Puddu, P.E.; Pannarale, G.; Colantoni, C.; Zanoni, C.; Martino, E.; Barilla, F. Metabolic syndrome among children and adolescents from Southern Italy: Contribution from the Calabrian Sierras Community Study (CSCS). *Int. J. Cardiol.* **2014**, *177*, 455–460. [CrossRef]
30. Morland, K.B.; Evenson, K.R. Obesity prevalence and the local food environment. *Health Place* **2009**, *15*, 491–495. [CrossRef]
31. Cobb, L.K.; Appel, L.J.; Franco, M.; Jones-Smith, J.C.; Nur, A.; Anderson, C.A. The relationship of the local food environment with obesity: A systematic review of methods, study quality, and results. *Obesity* **2015**, *23*, 1331–1344. [CrossRef] [PubMed]
32. Lamb, K.E.; Thornton, L.E.; Olstad, D.L.; Cerin, E.; Ball, K. Associations between major chain fast-food outlet availability and change in body mass index: A longitudinal observational study of women from Victoria, Australia. *BMJ Open* **2017**, *7*, e016594. [CrossRef] [PubMed]
33. Stark, J.H.; Neckerman, K.; Lovasi, G.S.; Konty, K.; Quinn, J.; Arno, P.; Viola, D.; Harris, T.G.; Weiss, C.C.; Bader, M.D.; et al. Neighbourhood food environments and body mass index among New York City adults. *J. Epidemiol. Community Health* **2013**, *67*, 736–742. [CrossRef] [PubMed]
34. Pitt, E.; Gallegos, D.; Comans, T.; Cameron, C.; Thornton, L. Exploring the influence of local food environments on food behaviours: A systematic review of qualitative literature. *Public Health Nutr.* **2017**, *20*, 2393–2405. [CrossRef] [PubMed]
35. Bibiloni, M.D.M.; Bouzas, C.; Abbate, M.; Martinez-Gonzalez, M.A.; Corella, D.; Salas-Salvado, J.; Zomeno, M.D.; Vioque, J.; Romaguera, D.; Martinez, J.A.; et al. Nutrient adequacy and diet quality in a Mediterranean population with metabolic syndrome: A cross-sectional study. *Clin. Nutr.* **2019**. [CrossRef] [PubMed]
36. Julibert, A.; Bibiloni, M.D.M.; Bouzas, C.; Martinez-Gonzalez, M.A.; Salas-Salvado, J.; Corella, D.; Zomeno, M.D.; Romaguera, D.; Vioque, J.; Alonso-Gomez, A.M.; et al. Total and Subtypes of Dietary Fat Intake and Its Association with Components of the Metabolic Syndrome in a Mediterranean Population at High Cardiovascular Risk. *Nutrients* **2019**, *11*, 1493. [CrossRef] [PubMed]

37. Scuteri, A.; Laurent, S.; Cucca, F.; Cockcroft, J.; Cunha, P.G.; Manas, L.R.; Mattace Raso, F.U.; Muiesan, M.L.; Ryliskyte, L.; Rietzschel, E.; et al. Metabolic syndrome across Europe: Different clusters of risk factors. *Eur. J. Prev. Cardiol.* **2015**, *22*, 486–491. [CrossRef]
38. Lacatusu, C.M.; Grigorescu, E.D.; Floria, M.; Onofriescu, A.; Mihai, B.M. The Mediterranean Diet: From an Environment-Driven Food Culture to an Emerging Medical Prescription. *Int. J. Environ. Res. Public Health* **2019**, *16*, 942. [CrossRef]
39. Salas-Salvado, J.; Diaz-Lopez, A.; Ruiz-Canela, M.; Basora, J.; Fito, M.; Corella, D.; Serra-Majem, L.; Warnberg, J.; Romaguera, D.; Estruch, R.; et al. Effect of a Lifestyle Intervention Program With Energy-Restricted Mediterranean Diet and Exercise on Weight Loss and Cardiovascular Risk Factors: One-Year Results of the PREDIMED-Plus Trial. *Diabetes Care* **2019**, *42*, 777–788. [CrossRef]
40. Kastorini, C.M.; Milionis, H.J.; Esposito, K.; Giugliano, D.; Goudevenos, J.A.; Panagiotakos, D.B. The effect of Mediterranean diet on metabolic syndrome and its components: A meta-analysis of 50 studies and 534,906 individuals. *J. Am. Coll. Cardiol.* **2011**, *57*, 1299–1313. [CrossRef]

10

Resistin and Cardiac Arrest

Raluca M. Tat [1,†], Adela Golea [2,†], Rodica Rahaian [3], Ştefan C. Vesa [4,*] and Daniela Ionescu [1,5]

1 Department of Anesthesia and Intensive Care I, "Iuliu Haţieganu" University of Medicine and Pharmacy, 400012 Cluj-Napoca, Romania; tatralu@yahoo.com
2 Surgical Department of "Iuliu Haţieganu" University of Medicine and Pharmacy, 400012 Cluj-Napoca, Romania; adeg2810@gmail.com
3 Department of Immunology Laboratory, County Emergency Hospital, 400006 Cluj-Napoca, Romania; rodirahaian@yahoo.com
4 Department of Pharmacology, Toxicology and Clinical Pharmacology, "Iuliu Haţieganu" University of Medicine and Pharmacy, 400012 Cluj-Napoca, Romania
5 Outcome Research Consortium, Cleveland, OH 44195, USA; dionescuati@yahoo.com
* Correspondence: stefanvesa@gmail.com
† Authors with equal contributions.

Abstract: The systemic response to ischemia-reperfusion that occurs after a cardiac arrest (CA) followed by the return of spontaneous circulation leads to endothelial toxicity and cytokine production, both responsible for the subsequent occurrence of severe cardiocirculatory dysfunction and early death. Resistin is emerging as a biomarker of proinflammatory status and myocardial ischemic injury and as a mediator of endothelial dysfunction. The study aimed to analyze the possible associations between several clinical and biological variables and the serum levels of resistin in CA survivors. Forty patients with out-of-hospital resuscitated CA, were enrolled in the study. Demographic, clinical and laboratory data (including serum resistin measurements at admission and at 6, 12, 24, 48 and 72 h) were recorded. For resistin, we calculated the area under the curve (AUC) using the trapezoidal method with measurements from 0 to 12 h, 0 to 24 h, 0 to 48 h and 0 to 72 h. Fifteen (37.5%) patients died in the first 72 h after CA. Cardiovascular comorbidities were present in 65% of patients. The majority of patients had post-CA shock (29 (72.5%)). Resistin serum levels rose in the first 12–24 h and decreased in the next 48–72 h. In univariate analysis, advanced age, longer duration of resuscitation, high sequential organ failure assessment score, high lactate levels, presence of cardiovascular comorbidities and the post-CA shock were associated with higher resistin levels. In multivariate analysis, post-CA shock or cardiovascular comorbidities were independently associated with higher AUCs for resistin for 0–12 h and 0–24 h. The only identified variable to independently predict higher AUCs for resistin for 0–48 h and 0–72 h was the presence of post-CA shock. Our data demonstrate strong independent correlation between high serum resistin levels, cardiac comorbidities and post-CA shock. The impact of the post-CA shock on serum concentration of resistin was greater than that of cardiac comorbidities.

Keywords: cardiac arrest; resistin; post-cardiac-arrest shock

---

1. Introduction

One of the relatively common presentations in the emergency department (ED) is that of a patient who suffered an out-of-hospital cardiac arrest (OHCA). Regardless of the etiology of cardiac arrest (CA), the physicians' efforts are centered on the early control of all consequences secondary to the interruption of blood flow to organs and return of spontaneous circulation (ROSC). They are known under the term of post-cardiac-arrest syndrome (PCAS)—which is responsible for the high mortality of post-resuscitation patients [1,2]. In PCAS, four components have been described: post-cardiac-arrest brain injury, post-cardiac-arrest myocardial dysfunction, systemic response to ischemia/reperfusion and persistent precipitating pathology [2]. Although post-cardiac-arrest brain injury remains an important cause of mortality and morbidity among CA patients, the other elements of PCAS (like systemic response to ischemia/reperfusion) also lead to multiple organ failure and early death [2,3].

The pathophysiology of PCAS is very complex and involves ischemia-reperfusion injury and activation of nonspecific mechanisms of systemic inflammatory response. Summarizing the process, the oxygen supply during ischemia is reduced and the cellular metabolism is affected, ultimately resulting in an increase in the intracytoplasmic calcium concentration responsible for the first cellular and tissue lesions. During the reperfusion phase, following restoration of the blood flow, reactive oxygen species formed during the ischemic phase induce cell death through their cytotoxic effect (inactivation of cytochromes, alteration of membrane transport proteins, inducing lipid peroxidation of the membrane). The pro-oxidant state that occurs inside the cells marks the transition to the next stage, characterized by aggressive endothelial toxicity. The onset of vascular endothelial lesions paves the way to systemic inflammation via the ischemia-reperfusion mechanisms: cytokine production, complement activation, arachidonic acid synthesis, leukocyte adhesion to endothelial cells and triggering of activation and chemotaxis of polymorphonuclear neutrophils at the origin of the inflammatory response. All of these are responsible for the subsequent development of multiple organ failure. Of note, the activation of the systemic inflammatory response is also associated with changes in coagulation (intravascular coagulation dissemination), which generate additional endothelial lesions. This creates a vicious circle where inflammatory lesions and coagulation abnormalities induce further organ damage by accentuating pre-existing lesions and enhancing the persistence of the precipitating pathology of CA, more likely in close dependence with the duration of resuscitation and the rhythm of CA [4–7].

In the past few years, the research community has been focused on identifying biomarkers able to adequately predict the severity of the lesions that underline the pathophysiological processes in CA.

Resistin is a cysteine-rich, adipose-derived peptide hormone encoded by the *RETN* gene that is highly expressed in circulating monocytes, macrophages and vascular endothelium [8–10]. It is involved in numerous pathological processes (obesity, disorders of glucose and insulin metabolism, atherosclerosis, malignancies, rheumatic diseases, chronic kidney disease, etc.) [11–14]. Resistin has been suggested as a marker of the severity of myocardial ischemic lesion [8,12] and proposed as a mediator of endothelial dysfunction [8,12,15–17]. Moreover, resistin has been potentially introduced as a marker of proinflammatory status (cytokine-like) in relation to sepsis and in other nonseptic critical pathologies [8,12–14]. In a previous study, we investigated the role of resistin as a biomarker for predicting mortality after CA. The results showed that elevated serum resistin levels were highly predictive of mortality in critically ill patients who survived a CA [14,18].

Taking into account the proposed mechanisms of action of resistin and the pathophysiology of CA, the aim of our study was to investigate the clinical and biological variables that correlate with serum resistin levels in CA survivors.

2. Materials and Methods

A prospective, analytical, longitudinal, observational cohort study included consecutive patients resuscitated after the OHCA and admitted to the ED of County Emergency Hospital Cluj-Napoca between May 2016 and October 2017. Informed consent for inclusion in the study was obtained from patients' proxies in all cases. The study was conducted in accordance with the Declaration of Helsinki, and the protocol was approved by the Ethics Committee of "Iuliu Haţieganu" University of Medicine and Pharmacy, with registration number 59/14.03.2016.

The inclusion criteria were as follows: age between 18–85 years and resuscitated OHCA. The exclusion criteria were as follows: ages under 18 or over 85 years, pregnancy, re-arrest with unsuccessful resuscitation within 6 h from hospital arrival, inmates, absence of informed consent and CA due to trauma, acute bleeding from nontraumatic condition, hypothermia or terminal neoplastic disease.

2.1. *Study Protocol and Laboratory Assays*

The management protocol of the patients admitted to the study, the post-CA shock definition and the lab protocols were previously described [18].

Each patient with out-of-hospital CA admitted to the study was resuscitated by emergency medical team members according to the recommendations of the European Resuscitation Council 2015 [19,20]. Fluids infusion and vasoactive drugs (adrenaline, noradrenaline, dopamine, dobutamine), alone or in combination, were administered in order to maintain mean arterial pressure ≥65 mmHg and urine output ≥0.5 mL/kg/h. For patients remaining comatose after successful resuscitation, able to maintain a systolic blood pressure above 90 mmHg (mean arterial pressure—MAP ≥65 mmHg) and without sepsis, controlled therapeutic hypothermia was administered in the first 24 h, in order to maintain a central temperature with a target between 34–35°C, using ice bags and cooling blanket. Reheating was slow, at a rate of 0.25–0.5 °C/h. According to local protocols which follow current guidelines, hyperthermia, seizures and hyperglycemia were avoided and immediately treated [21,22].

Blood samples were drawn from a peripheral vein where no medication was administered, at 0-time interval (emergency admission), 6, 12, 24, 48 and 72 h following resuscitation. Five-milliliter biochemistry vacutainers with serum separator clot activator were used for blood sample collection. To collect blood samples, we used 5 mL biochemistry vacutainers with serum separator clot activator. The identified hemolyzed samples were excluded and blood samples were immediately repeated. Samples were centrifuged at 3000 rotation/minutes during the first 60 min after collection and were stored at −70 °C. Subsequently, serum concentrations of biomarkers (resistin, S-100B and NSE) were analyzed using a quantitative sandwich immunoassay technique (ELISA; BioVendor, LM, Czech Republic) according to the manufacturer's instructions. After processing, defrosted blood samples were no longer used and underwent destruction.

For every patient, the following data were recorded: demographic (age, gender), clinical (presence of cardiovascular diseases and/or strong risk factors for cardiovascular disease (arterial hypertension, coronary artery disease, valvular heart disease, congestive heart failure, history of stroke, diabetes mellitus and obesity), the rhythm of OHCA, duration of resuscitation, body mass index (BMI), presence of post-CA shock), sequential organ failure assessment (SOFA) score at admission and laboratory data (lactate and glycemia at admission; resistin at 6, 12, 24, 48 and 72 h). Obesity was defined by a body mass index (BMI) ≥30 kg/m^2. The overweight was classified at a BMI between 25 and 29.9 kg/m^2. Post-CA shock was defined as the need to administer vasoactive/inotropic therapy to maintain a MAP >65 mmHg for at least 6 h immediate after return of spontaneous circulation, although fluid therapy was adequate.

2.2. *Statistical Analysis*

Statistical analysis was performed using the MedCalc Statistical Software version 18.11.3 (MedCalc Software bvba, Ostend, Belgium; https://www.medcalc.org; 2019). Quantitative data normality was assessed using the Shapiro–Wilk test, measures of skewness and kurtosis and histograms. Quantitative data were expressed as median and interquartile range (IQR). Qualitative data were characterized by frequency and percentage. For resistin, we calculated the area under the curve (AUC) using the trapezoidal method with measurements from 0 to 12 h, 0 to 24 h, 0 to 48 h and 0 to 72 h. The sample size was calculated from a pilot study (13 patients with post-CA shock and 4 patients without post-CA shock). Calculated AUC for resistin, for 0–12 h measurements, showed a 24 ng × h/mL mean difference between the two groups. For a type 1 (a) error of 0.01 and a type 2 (b) error of 0.05, we calculated a sample size of 34 patients. The power of the study was calculated as 95%. Correlations between quantitative variables were assessed using the Spearman's rank correlation coefficient. The differences between groups were verified with Mann–Whitney test. In order to find out which variables can be independently linked to resistin, we constructed several models using multiple linear regressions. Due to the fact that the resistin values followed a non-normal distribution, we performed a logarithmic transformation. We introduced the variables that were significantly associated with the AUCs for resistin during the univariate analysis. A p-value of less than 0.05 was considered statistically significant.

3. Results

Forty patients admitted to ED who met the inclusion criteria were included in the study. Patient characteristics are described in Table 1. On the first and second day, 12 (30%) patients died, and by the third day there were another three (7.5%) deaths. The 25 survivors after 72 h were followed for 30 days, and we recorded the deaths of 13 of them in this interval. Most of the recorded CA rhythm was asystole. Of the total number of patients admitted in our study, only 11 (28.5%) patients did not develop immediate post-resuscitation shock. Of the total admitted patients, 14 (35%) were obese and 20 (50%) were overweight.

Table 1. Baseline characteristics of the study group.

Characteristics		Eligible Patients with CA (n = 40)
Age, years, median (IQR)		67 (59.2 to 76.0)
Gender, n (%)	**Female**	12 (30.0)
	Male	28 (70.0)
Presenting rhythm, n (%)	**Asystole**	23 (57.5)
	PEA	5 (12.5)
	VF	11 (27.5)
	VT without pulse	1 (2.5)
Duration of CPR, minutes, median (IQR)		15 (7.7 to 28.7)
Current smoking, n (%)		4 (10)
Chronic alcohol consumer, n (%)		5 (12.5)
Medical history, n (%)	**Non-cardiovascular comorbidities**	18 (45.0)
	Cardiovascular comorbidities	26 (65.0)
	Arterial hypertension	23 (57.5)
	Coronary artery disease	17 (42.5)
	Valvular heart disease	8 (20%)
	Congestive heart failure	15 (37.5)
	Stroke	3 (7.5)
	Diabetes mellitus	7 (17.5)
BMI, median (IQR)		28 (26.0 to 31.0)
Obesity, n (%)		14 (35)
SOFA score, median (IQR)		15 (12.0 to 16.0)
Patients with post-CA shock, n (%)		29 (72.5)
Lactate (mmol/L), median (IQR)		10.42 (7.6 to 12.9)
Blood glucose (mg/dL), median (IQR)		249.0 (156.0 to 330.0)

IQR = interquartile range; PEA = pulseless electrical activity; VF = ventricular fibrillation; VT = ventricular tachycardia; CPR = cardiopulmonary resuscitation; BMI = body mass index; SOFA = sequential organ failure assessment score; CA = cardiac arrest.

For serum resistin levels we calculated the AUCs using the trapezoidal method with measurements from 0 to 24 h, 0 to 48 h and 0 to 72 h. Resistin levels and AUCs showed an increase in the first 12 h after admission, followed by a gradual decrease in the next 60 h (Table 2).

Table 2. Median serum levels of resistin and the AUC for resistin during the first 72 h.

Variable		Median (IQR)
Resistin, (ng/mL)	**at 0 h**	7.1 (4.6 to 11.8)
	at 6 h	9.8 (4.4 to 17.7)
	at 12 h	13.5 (5.5 to 21.0)
	at 24 h	12.3 (6.7 to 21.0)
	at 48 h	7.2 (3.5 to 14.6)
	at 72 h	7.4 (3.6 to 11.9)
AUC resistin, (ng × h/mL)	**in the first 12 h**	26.0 (11.5 to 43.2)
	in the first 24 h	25.8 (15.2 to 44.7)
	in the first 48 h	16.6 (10.4 to 35.1)
	in the first 72 h	34.6 (17.9 to 46.5)

AUC = area under the curve; IQR = interquartile range.

We found that SOFA score and serum lactate values at admission were the most important clinical and laboratory parameters associated with serum resistin levels (strong positive correlation to all repeated measurements) (Table 3). The serum resistin levels were not influenced by BMI.

Table 3. Correlations between the AUCs for resistin and the study quantitative variables.

Variable	AUC for 0–12 h		AUC for 0–24 h		AUC for 0–48 h		AUC for 0–72 h	
	r	*p*	r	*p*	r	*p*	r	*p*
Age, years	0.316	0.04	0.360	0.03	0.467	0.01	0.356	0.08
Duration of CPR, minutes	0.364	0.02	0.386	0.02	0.414	0.02	0.357	0.08
BMI	0.039	0.8	−0.148	0.4	−0.183	0.3	−0.141	0.5
SOFA score	0.586	<0.001	0.579	<0.001	0.510	0.006	0.529	0.007
Lactate (mmol/L)	0.499	<0.001	0.592	<0.001	0.501	0.007	0.509	0.009
Blood glucose (mg/dL)	0.185	0.2	0.417	0.01	0.176	0.3	−0.023	0.9

AUC = area under the curve; CPR = cardiopulmonary resuscitation; BMI = body mass index; SOFA = sequential organ failure assessment score; r = correlation coefficient.

The AUCs for resistin were higher in patients who presented asystole or PEA rhythm of CA (especially), cardiovascular comorbidities, history of congestive heart failure, arterial hypertension or post-CA shock (Table 4). We found no associations between AUCs for resistin and history of coronary artery disease, stroke, diabetes mellitus, obesity, smoking or alcoholic beverages.

Several models based on multiple linear regression were used in order to determine the independent association between clinical/laboratory data and the AUCs for resistin. The variables that were significantly linked to the AUCs in the univariate analysis were introduced in the models. Due to the fact that the resistin values followed a non-normal distribution, we performed a logarithmic transformation. When we introduced the history of congestive heart failure or arterial hypertension as separate variables, we found no statistically significant association with the log AUCs for resistin. Post-CA shock or cardiovascular comorbidities were independently associated with the log AUC for resistin for 0–12 h and 0–24 h. The only identified variable independently linked to the log AUC for resistin for 0–48 h and 0–72 h was the presence of post-CA shock (Table 5).

Table 4. Associations between the AUC for resistin and the qualitative variables studied.

Variable		AUC for 0–12 h		AUC for 0–24 h		AUC for 0–48 h		AUC for 0–72 h	
		Median (IQR)	*p*	Median (IQR)	*p*	Median (IQR)	*p*	Median (IQR)	*p*
Gender	Female	26.5 (23.0 to 42.5)	0.4	30.0 (17.4 to 44.1)	0.8	20.6 (13.3 to 49.2)	0.3	25.0 (17.1 to 74.0)	0.7
	Male	23.0 (10.2 to 43.2)		25.2 (13.8 to 44.7)		15.9 (9.3 to 33.8)		35.3 (18.7 to 46.1)	
Presenting rhythm of CA	Asystole/ PEA	30.5 (22.0 to 47.7)	0.002	30.3 (19.9 to 51.4)	0.002	23.5 (14.5 to 38.7)	0.009	37.8 (25.0 to 69.8)	0.01
	VF/VT without pulse	10.5 (4.2 to 22.5)		14.3 (8.0 to 24.1)		12.4 (4.8 to 16.0)		23.4 (13.8 to 31.9)	
Cardiovascular comorbidities	present	29.0 (22.0 to 45.5)	0.03	37.2 (18.3 to 50.2)	0.01	22.7 (14.2 to 38.1)	0.06	37.4 (23.6 to 64.0)	0.08
	absent	16.5 (4.7 to 31.5)		18.8 (11.1 to 25.8)		13.7 (5.3 to 28.4)		27.6 (15.0 to 36.7)	
History of arterial hypertension	present	28 (22 to 45)	0.1	37.2 (18.2 to 49.1)	0.05	22 (14.1 to 39)	0.1	37.8 (22.2 to 67.3)	0.1
	absent	18 (7 to 37)		19.9 (14.3 to 26.4)		14.5 (5.8 to 27.3)		29.3 (15.4 to 36.9)	
History of congestive heart failure	present	30.5 (23 to 46.5)	0.04	38 (29.9 to 49.7)	0.02	34.8 (19.6 to 46.4)	0.02	52.8 (23.5 to 92)	0.04
	absent	18.5 (7.5 to 32.7)		19.3 (9.8 to 31.6)		14.5 (9.2 to 23.9)		27.6 (16.9 to 36.8)	
Post-CA shock	present	31.0 (24.0 to 47.5)	<0.001	30.3 (24.1 to 51.4)	<0.001	30.8 (15.9 to 38.7)	0.002	41.8 (23.4 to 70.8)	0.01
	absent	10.0 (4.0 to 15.0)		13.4 (8.0 to 18.8)		12.4 (4.8 to 15.8)		27.5 (12.1 to 34.6)	

AUC = area under the curve; IQR = interquartile range; PEA = pulseless electrical activity; VF = ventricular fibrillation; VT = ventricular tachycardia; CA = cardiac arrest.

Table 5. Multiple linear regression for the AUCs for resistin.

Variables for the log of AUC for 0–12 h	B	*p*	95.0% CI for B	
			Min	Max
(Constant)	0.784	<0.001	0.581	0.988
Post-CA shock	0.528	<0.001	0.309	0.747
Cardiovascular comorbidities	0.214	0.04	0.009	0.419
Variables for the log of AUC for 0–24 h	**B**	*p*	**95.0% CI for B**	
			Min	**Max**
(Constant)	0.954	<0.001	0.768	1.140
Post-CA shock	0.415	<0.001	0.211	0.619
Cardiovascular comorbidities	0.201	0.04	0.004	0.397
Variables for the log of AUC for 0–48 h	**B**	*p*	**95.0% CI for B**	
			Min	**Max**
(Constant)	0.939	<0.001	0.739	1.139
Post-CA shock	0.470	0.001	0.212	0.727
Variables for the log of AUC for 0–72 h	**B**	*p*	**95.0% CI for B**	
			Min	**Max**
(Constant)	1.321	<0.001	1.154	1.488
Post-CA shock	0.303	0.01	0.079	0.526

AUC = area under the curve; B = standardized beta coefficient; CA = cardiac arrest.

4. Discussions

CA involves the most severe form of circulatory failure. The complex changes produced by disruption of cell morpho-functional integrity during the general ischemia phase do not stop with the return of spontaneous circulation and are subsequently supplemented by those appearing during the reperfusion phase. The release of proinflammatory cytokines with the onset of systemic inflammatory response syndrome and endothelial damage (with coagulation/anticoagulation and fibrinogenesis/fibrinolysis imbalance) are intricate mechanisms that ultimately contribute to organ failures with negative impact prognosis of resuscitated patients [6,8,13,14,23].

In our previous study, we investigated for the first time the serum levels of resistin as a possible predictor of mortality after CA. Our results were promising, showing that high serum values of resistin accurately predicted death at 30 days, making resistin a marker with a high predictive value of survival [14,18].

However, resistin levels can be influenced by a variety of factors, such as the presence of atherosclerosis, obesity or sepsis. In light of this, we investigated the possible correlations of several clinical and biochemical factors with the serum concentration of resistin in patients with CA, for a better understanding of its role in CA [18].

Initially described in 1994 as a way of quantifying organ dysfunction by evaluating respiratory, cardiovascular, hepatic, renal, neurological and coagulation systems [24], the SOFA score remained useful over the years and is now being used with accuracy in quantifying the prognosis of critically ill patients [25]. The ischemia-reperfusion lesion is one of the most important mechanisms that link CA to multiple organ failures, including circulatory and cardiac dysfunction. Our results showed that there is a strong correlation between the severity of the disease (quantified by the SOFA score) and serum levels of resistin, a potential marker that may correctly reflect organ failures.

Over time, elevated levels of resistin have been associated with increased risk of coronary heart disease, especially with myocardial infarction (but not with stroke) [26] and with the degree of heart failure, both responsible for increasing the rate of cardiac events, including the risk of death [26,27]. At the same time, obesity, diabetes, high carbohydrate and unsaturated fat diet and chronic alcohol consumption, but not smoking, were described as cardiovascular risk factors correlated with elevated human serum resistin levels [28–31]. In our study, we found no associations between resistin levels in patients with CA and history of coronary artery disease, stroke, diabetes mellitus, obesity, smoking or alcoholic beverages. This reinforces the idea that in an acute critical illness high levels of resistin (or other adipokines) are mostly due to inflammatory status and not to adipose tissue mass or pre-existing unhealthy lifestyle [32].

At multivariate analysis, we found that the presence of post-CA shock and cardiovascular comorbidities were independently associated with serum resistin levels in the first 24 h after CA.

In fact, the presence of post-CA shock was the only independent variable associated with serum resistin levels at 48 and 72 h following CA. These results show that the elevated serum concentrations of resistin might be influenced by the post-CA shock, rather than by pre-CA cardiovascular comorbidities. The shock that occurs after CA is the result of myocardial dysfunction, vasoplegic shock and systemic inflammatory response [25]. Part of a complex vicious circle, as this shock becomes more refractory to treatment, cardiocirculatory dysfunction evolves in turn into a more severe form, resulting in multiple organ failures responsible for early death. The strong association of resistin with post-CA shock and with the presence of cardiovascular comorbidities may support the theory that serum resistin levels correlate equally with both the amplitude of the inflammatory process and cardiac dysfunction after resuscitation.

In previous studies, increased serum levels of lactate upon admission to the emergency department and intensive care units were associated with the negative prognosis of patients with acute critical illness [18]. Our data revealed that high serum levels of lactate at admission correlate strongly with serum resistin levels. This may support the idea that resistin is directly involved in the process of systemic inflammation in CA pathogenesis, seeing as elevated lactate levels are in fact associated with severe cardiocirculatory dysfunction [33]. However, at multivariate analysis, the aforementioned correlation did not remain statistically significant, suggesting that there were other important factors that interfere in the CA physiopathological sequence.

To our knowledge, this is the first study that evaluated the factors that influence the kinetics of resistin after CA. These results were obtained on a small number of patients, although statistically significant. The high number of measurements present an accurate kinetics of resistin after a CA, with a peak at 12–24 h and a rapid decrease to admission values after 48 h. This is important for future studies on acute events, as it shows that the focus on resistin should be especially in the first 24 h.

In order to strengthen our hypothesis, it is essential that we develop further/future studies on larger groups of patients. Also, they must include other markers of acute inflammation, with a special interest for those reportedly correlated with resistin during acute cardiovascular events: tumor necrosis factor α (TNF-α), interleukin-6 (IL-6), high-sensitivity C-reactive protein (hs-CRP) and other proinflammatory cytokines [34]. Resistin promotes the production of TNF-α, IL-1β, IL-6 and other cytokines [12,35]. There are several drugs that have been shown to reduce the levels of resistin in chronic administration: statins, anti-TNF-α monoclonal antibodies and folic acid [36–38]. Experimental animal or in vitro studies in acute situations with drugs that lower resistin concentration are worth considering.

Other markers that could provide insights into the functions and pathophysiological implications of resistin are the microvesicles (large extracellular vesicles that appear from different cells after apoptosis) [39]. Platelet-derived microvesicles are a source of TNF-α and IL-6, while endothelial-derived microvesicles are stimulated by TNF-α [40]. Elevated levels of endothelial-derived microvesicles were found in acute coronary syndrome patients, but they were not evaluated in patients that survived a CA; one can speculate that investigating this class of micro-vesicles will offer valuable data [41,42].

Markers that evaluate post-cardiac-arrest myocardial dysfunction should be studied in any future research on patients after a successfully resuscitated CA. Left ventricular systolic dysfunction is present in almost 60% of patients resuscitated after CA [33]. The assessment of left ventricle ejection fraction, biomarkers of ventricular dysfunction and the correlation with proinflammatory markers will generate a better understanding of the complexity of PCAS. The N-terminal pro-B-type natriuretic peptide

(NT-proBNP) and marinobufagenin are reliable indicators of ventricular dysfunction and, as such, can serve as excellent candidates for future studies on OHCA [43,44].

Even though the multivariate analysis showed that the post-CA shock was independently associated with higher levels of resistin, an important bias could be the presence of cardiovascular comorbidities. The myocardial systolic and diastolic dysfunctions appear in post-CA shock, even if the patient does not have a prior coronary disease [45]. Future studies should include patients with noncardiac causes of CA, because the presence of cardiac diseases aggravates the left ventricular dysfunction. Other diseases that were proven to have an influence on the resistin concentrations should be excluded (nonalcoholic fatty liver disease, asthma, autoimmune disease, chronic kidney disease) [46]. That could provide a clearer picture about the association between post-CA shock and resistin kinetics.

5. Conclusions

Our findings demonstrate strong independent correlation between high serum resistin levels, cardiac comorbidities and post-CA shock. The impact of the post-CA shock on serum concentration of resistin was greater than that of cardiac comorbidities.

Author Contributions: Conceptualization, R.M.T., Ş.C.V. and D.I.; Data curation, R.M.T., A.G. and R.R.; Formal analysis, R.R., Ş.C.V. and D.I.; Funding acquisition, R.M.T.; Investigation, R.M.T. and A.G.; Methodology, R.M.T. and Ş.C.V.; Supervision, D.I.; Writing—original draft, R.M.T., A.G., Ş.C.V. and D.I. All authors have read and agreed to the published version of the manuscript.

Acknowledgments: The study was partially funded by "Iuliu Hațieganu" University of Medicine and Pharmacy, Cluj-Napoca, through the Doctoral Research Project-2015[No. 7690/42/15.04.2016]. The financial support allocated from the grant was used for the acquisition of biomarkers and laboratory supplies.

References

1. Nolan, J.P.; Soar, J.; Cariou, A.; Cronberg, T.; Moulaert, V.R.; Deakin, C.D.; Bottiger, B.W.; Friberg, H.; Sunde, K.; Sandroni, C. European Resuscitation Council and European Society of Intensive Care Medicine Guidelines for Post-resuscitation Care. *Intensive Care Med.* **2015**, *41*, 2039–2056. [CrossRef] [PubMed]
2. Nolan, J.P.; Neumar, R.W.; Adrie, C.; Aibiki, M.; Berg, R.A.; Bottiger, B.W.; Callaway, C.; Clark, R.S.; Geocadin, R.G.; Jauch, E.C.; et al. Post-cardiac arrest syndrome: Epidemiology, pathophysiology, treatment, and prognostication. A Scientific Statement from the International Liaison Committee on Resuscitation; the American Heart Association Emergency Cardiovascular Care Committee; the Council on Cardiovascular Surgery and Anesthesia; the Council on Cardiopulmonary, Perioperative, and Critical Care; the Council on Clinical Cardiology; the Council on Stroke. *Resuscitation* **2008**, *79*, 350–379. [PubMed]
3. Mongardon, N.; Dumas, F.; Ricome, S.; Grimaldi, D.; Hissem, T.; Pène, F.; Cariou, A. Postcardiac arrest syndrome: From immediate resuscitation to long-term outcome. *Ann. Intensive Care* **2011**, *1*, 45. [CrossRef] [PubMed]
4. Huet, O.; Dupic, L.; Batteux, F.; Matar, C.; Conti, M.; Chereau, C.; Lemiale, V.; Harrois, A.; Mira, J.P.; Vicaut, E.; et al. Postresuscitation syndrome: Potential role of hydroxyl radical-induced endothelial cell damage. *Crit. Care Med.* **2011**, *39*, 1712–1720. [CrossRef]
5. Gando, S.; Nanzaki, S.; Morimoto, Y.; Kobayashi, S.; Kemmotsu, O. Out-of-hospital cardiac arrest increases soluble vascular endothelial adhesion molecules and neutrophil elastase associated with endothelial injury. *Intensive Care Med.* **2000**, *26*, 38–44. [CrossRef]
6. Jou, C.; Shah, R.; Figueroa, A.; Patel, J.K. The role of inflammatory cytokines in cardiac arrest. *J. Intensive Care Med.* **2018**, 885066618817518. [CrossRef]
7. Adrie, C.; Monchi, M.; Laurent, I.; Um, S.; Yan, S.B.; Thuong, M.; Cariou, A.; Charpentier, J.; Dhainaut, J.F. Coagulopathy after successful cardiopulmonary resuscitation following cardiac arrest: Implication of the protein C anticoagulant pathway. *J. Am. Coll. Cardiol.* **2005**, *46*, 21–28. [CrossRef]

8. Mocan Hognogi, L.D.; Goidescu, C.M.; Farcaş, A.D. Usefulness of the adipokines as biomarkers of ischemic cardiac dysfunction. *Dis. Markers* **2018**, *2018*, 8. [CrossRef]
9. Patel, L.; Buckels, A.C.; Kinghorn, I.J.; Murdock, P.R.; Holbrook, J.D.; Plumpton, C.; Macphee, C.H.; Smith, S.A. Resistin is expressed in human macrophages and directly regulated by PPAR gamma activators. *Biochem. Biophys. Res. Commun.* **2003**, *300*, 472–476. [CrossRef]
10. Wang, H.; Chu, W.S.; Hemphill, C.; Elbein, S.C. Human resistin gene: Molecular scanning and evaluation of association with insulin sensitivity and type 2 diabetes in Caucasians. *J. Clin. Endocrinol. Metab.* **2002**, *87*, 2520–2524. [CrossRef]
11. Vlaicu, S.I.; Tatomir, A.; Boodhoo, D.; Vesa, S.; Mircea, P.A.; Rus, H. The role of complement system in adipose tissue-related inflammation. *Immunol. Res.* **2016**, *64*, 653–664. [CrossRef] [PubMed]
12. Filkova, M.; Haluzik, M.; Gay, S.; Senolt, L. The role of resistin as a regulator of inflammation: Implications for various human pathologies. *Clin. Immunol.* **2009**, *133*, 157–170. [CrossRef] [PubMed]
13. Macdonald, S.P.; Stone, S.F.; Neil, C.L.; van Eeden, P.E.; Fatovich, D.M.; Arendts, G.; Brown, S.G. Sustained elevation of resistin, NGAL and IL-8 are associated with severe sepsis/septic shock in the emergency department. *PLoS ONE* **2014**, *9*, e110678. [CrossRef] [PubMed]
14. Koch, A.; Gressner, O.A.; Sanson, E.; Tacke, F.; Trautwein, C. Serum resistin levels in critically ill patients are associated with inflammation, organ dysfunction and metabolism and may predict survival of non-septic patients. *Crit Care* **2009**, *13*, R95. [CrossRef]
15. Chen, C.; Jiang, J.; Lu, J.M.; Chai, H.; Wang, X.; Lin, P.H.; Yao, Q. Resistin decreases expression of endothelial nitric oxide synthase through oxidative stress in human coronary artery endothelial cells. *Am. J. Physiol. Heart Circ. Physiol.* **2010**, *299*, H193–H201. [CrossRef]
16. Hsu, W.Y.; Chao, Y.W.; Tsai, Y.L.; Lien, C.C.; Chang, C.F.; Deng, M.C.; Ho, L.T.; Kwok, C.F.; Juan, C.C. Resistin induces monocyte-endothelial cell adhesion by increasing ICAM-1 and VCAM-1 expression in endothelial cells via p38MAPK-dependent pathway. *J. Cell Physiol.* **2011**, *226*, 2181–2188. [CrossRef]
17. Ciobanu, D.M.; Mircea, P.A.; Bala, C.; Rusu, A.; Vesa, S.; Roman, G. Intercellular adhesion molecule-1 (ICAM-1) associates with 24-h ambulatory blood pressure variability in type 2 diabetes and controls. *Cytokine* **2019**, *116*, 134–138. [CrossRef]
18. Tat, R.M.; Golea, A.; Vesa, S.C.; Ionescu, D. Resistin-Can it be a new early marker for prognosis in patients who survive after a cardiac arrest? A pilot study. *PLoS ONE* **2019**, *14*, e0210666. [CrossRef]
19. Perkins, G.D.; Handley, A.J.; Koster, R.W.; Castrén, M.; Smyth, M.A.; Olasveengen, T.; Monsieurs, K.G.; Raffay, V.; Gräsner, J.T.; Wenzel, V.; et al. European Resuscitation Council Guidelines for Resuscitation 2015: Section 2. Adult basic life support and automated external defibrillation. *Resuscitation* **2015**, *95*, 81–99. [CrossRef]
20. Soar, J.; Nolan, J.P.; Bottiger, B.W.; Perkins, G.D.; Lott, C.; Carli, P.; Pellis, T.; Sandroni, C.; Skrifvars, M.B.; Smith, G.B.; et al. European Resuscitation Council Guidelines for Resuscitation 2015: Section 3. Adult advanced life support. *Resuscitation* **2015**, *95*, 100–147. [CrossRef]
21. Nolan, J.P.; Soar, J.; Cariou, A.; Cronberg, T.; Moulaert, V.R.; Deakin, C.D.; Bottiger, B.W.; Friberg, H.; Sunde, K.; Sandroni, C. European Resuscitation Council and European Society of Intensive Care Medicine Guidelines for Post-resuscitation Care 2015: Section 5 of the European Resuscitation Council Guidelines for Resuscitation 2015. *Resuscitation* **2015**, *95*, 202–222. [CrossRef] [PubMed]
22. Callaway, C.W.; Soar, J.; Aibiki, M.; Böttiger, B.W.; Brooks, S.C.; Deakin, C.D.; Donnino, M.W.; Drajer, S.; Kloeck, W.; Morley, P.T. Part 4: Advanced Life Support: 2015 International Consensus on Cardiopulmonary Resuscitation and Emergency Cardiovascular Care Science With Treatment Recommendations. *Circulation* **2015**, *132*, S84–S145. [CrossRef] [PubMed]
23. Fain, J.N.; Cheema, P.S.; Bahouth, S.W.; Lloyd Hiler, M. Resistin release by human adipose tissue explants in primary culture. *Biochem. Biophys. Res. Commun.* **2003**, *300*, 674–678. [CrossRef]
24. Vincent, J.L.; Moreno, R.; Takala, J.; Willatts, S.; De Mendonca, A.; Bruining, H.; Reinhart, C.K.; Suter, P.; Thijs, L.G. The SOFA (Sepsis-related Organ Failure Assessment) score to describe organ dysfunction/failure. On behalf of the Working Group on Sepsis-Related Problems of the European Society of Intensive Care Medicine. *Intensive Care Med.* **1996**, *22*, 707–710. [CrossRef]
25. Raith, E.P.; Udy, A.A.; Bailey, M.; McGloughlin, S.; MacIsaac, C.; Bellomo, R.; Pilcher, D.V. Prognostic accuracy of the SOFA score, SIRS criteria, and qSOFA score for in-hospital mortality among adults with suspected infection admitted to the intensive care unit. *JAMA* **2017**, *317*, 290–300. [CrossRef]

26. Gencer, B.; Auer, R.; De Rekeneire, N.; Butler, J.; Kalogeropoulos, A.; Bauer, D.C.; Kritchevsky, S.B.; Miljkovic, I.; Vittinghoff, E.; Harris, T.; et al. Association between resistin levels and cardiovascular desease events in older adults: The health, aging and body composition study. *Atherosclerosis* **2016**, *245*, 181–186. [CrossRef]
27. Takeishi, Y.; Niizeki, T.; Arimoto, T.; Nozaki, N.; Hirono, O.; Nitobe, J.; Watanabe, T.; Takabatake, N.; Kubota, I. Serum resistin is associated with high risk in patients with congestive heart failure. *Circ. J.* **2007**, *71*, 460–464. [CrossRef]
28. Lemming, E.W.; Byberg, L.; Stattin, K.; Ahmad, S.; Lind, L.; Elmståhl, S.; Larsson, S.C.; Wolk, A.; Michaëlsson, K. Dietary Pattern Specific Protein Biomarkers for Cardiovascular Disease: A Cross-Sectional Study in 2 Independent Cohorts. *J. Am. Heart Assoc.* **2019**, *8*, e011860.
29. McTernan, P.G.; Fisher, F.M.; Valsamakis, G.; Chetty, R.; Harte, A.; McTernan, C.L.; Clark, P.M.; Smith, S.A.; Barnett, A.H.; Kumar, S. Resistin and type 2 diabetes: Regulation of resistin expression by insulin and rosiglitazone and the effects of recombinant resistin on lipid and glucose metabolism in human differentiated adipocytes. *J. Clin. Endocrinol. Metab.* **2003**, *88*, 6098–6106. [CrossRef]
30. Steppan, C.M.; Bailey, S.T.; Bhat, S.; Brown, E.J.; Banerjee, R.R.; Wright, C.M.; Patel, H.R.; Ahima, R.S.; Lazar, M.A. The hormone resistin links obesity to diabetes. *Nature* **2001**, *409*, 307–312. [CrossRef]
31. Shuldiner, A.R.; Yang, R.; Gong, D.W. Resistin, obesity, and insulin resistance—The emerging role of the adipocyte as an endocrine organ. *N. Engl. J. Med.* **2001**, *345*, 1345–1346. [CrossRef] [PubMed]
32. Koch, A.; Weiskirchen, R.; Krusch, A.; Bruensing, J.; Buendgens, L.; Herbers, U.; Yagmur, E.; Koek, G.H.; Trautwein, C.; Tacke, F. Visfatin serum levels predict mortality in critically ill patients. *Dis. Markers* **2018**, *2018*, 7315356. [CrossRef] [PubMed]
33. Jentzer, J.C.; Chonde, M.D.; Dezfulian, C. Myocardial dysfunction and shock after cardiac arrest. *Biomed. Res. Int.* **2015**, *2015*, 314796. [CrossRef] [PubMed]
34. Liu, X.; Zheng, X.; Su, X.; Tian, W.; Hu, Y.; Zhang, Z. Plasma Resistin Levels in Patients with Acute Aortic Dissection: A Propensity Score-Matched Observational Case-Control Study. *Med. Sci. Monit.* **2018**, *24*, 6431–6437. [CrossRef]
35. Silswal, N.; Singh, A.K.; Aruna, B.; Mukhopadhyay, S.; Ghosh, S.; Ehtesham, N.Z. Human resistin stimulates the pro-inflammatory cytokines TNF-alpha and IL-12 in macrophages by NF-kappaB-dependent pathway. *Biochem. Biophys. Res. Commun.* **2005**, *334*, 1092–1101. [CrossRef]
36. Shyu, K.G.; Chua, S.K.; Wang, B.W.; Kuan, P. Mechanism of inhibitory effect of atorvastatin on resistin expression induced by tumor necrosis factor-alpha in macrophages. *J. Biomed. Sci.* **2009**, *16*, 50. [CrossRef]
37. Gonzalez-Gay, M.A.; Garcia-Unzueta, M.T.; Gonzalez-Juanatey, C.; Miranda-Filloy, J.A.; Vazquez-Rodriguez, T.R.; De Matias, J.M.; Martin, J.; Dessein, P.H.; Llorca, J. Anti-TNF-alpha therapy modulates resistin in patients with rheumatoid arthritis. *Clin. Exp. Rheumatol.* **2008**, *26*, 311–316.
38. Seto, S.W.; Lam, T.Y.; Or, P.M.; Lee, W.Y.; Au, A.L.; Poon, C.C.; Li, R.W.S.; Chan, S.W.; Yeung, J.H.K.; Leung, G.P.H.; et al. Folic acid consumption reduces resistin level and restores blunted acetylcholine-induced aortic relaxation in obese/diabetic mice. *J. Nutr. Biochem.* **2010**, *21*, 872–880. [CrossRef]
39. Słomka, A.; Urban, S.K.; Lukacs-Kornek, V.; Żekanowska, E.; Kornek, M. Large Extracellular Vesicles: Have We Found the Holy Grail of Inflammation? *Front. Immunol.* **2018**, *9*, 2723. [CrossRef]
40. Balvers, K.; Curry, N.; Kleinveld, D.J.; Böing, A.N.; Nieuwland, R.; Goslings, J.C.; Juffermans, N.P. Endogenous microparticles drive the proinflammatory host immune response in severely injured trauma patients. *Shock* **2015**, *43*, 317–321. [CrossRef]
41. Alexy, T.; Rooney, K.; Weber, M.; Gray, W.D.; Searles, C.D. TNF-α alters the release and transfer of microparticle-encapsulated miRNAs from endothelial cells. *Physiol. Genom.* **2014**, *46*, 833–840. [CrossRef] [PubMed]
42. Morel, O.; Pereira, B.; Averous, G.; Faure, A.; Jesel, L.; Germain, P.; Grunebaum, L.; Ohlmann, P.; Freyssinet, J.M.; Bareiss, P.; et al. Increased levels of procoagulant tissue factor-bearing microparticles within the occluded coronary artery of patients with ST-segment elevation myocardial infarction: Role of endothelial damage and leukocyte activation. *Atherosclerosis* **2009**, *204*, 636–641. [CrossRef] [PubMed]
43. Fridman, A.I.; Matveev, S.A.; Agalakova, N.I.; Fedorova, O.V.; Lakatta, E.G.; Bagrov, A.Y. Marinobufagenin, an endogenous ligand of alpha-1 sodium pump, is a marker of congestive heart failure severity. *J. Hypertens.* **2002**, *20*, 1189–1194. [CrossRef] [PubMed]

44. Myhre, P.L.; Tiainen, M.; Pettilä, V.; Vaahersalo, J.; Hagve, T.A.; Kurola, J. NT-proBNP in patients with out-of-hospital cardiac arrest: Results from the FINNRESUSCI Study. *Resuscitation* **2016**, *104*, 12–18. [CrossRef] [PubMed]
45. Laurent, I.; Monchi, M.; Chiche, J.D.; Joly, L.M.; Spaulding, C.; Bourgeois, B.; Cariou, A.; Rozenberg, A.; Carli, P.; Weber, S.; et al. Reversible myocardial dysfunction in survivors of out-of-hospital cardiac arrest. *J. Am. Coll. Cardiol.* **2002**, *40*, 2110–2116. [CrossRef]
46. Jamaluddin, M.S.; Weakley, S.M.; Yao, O.; Chen, C. Resistin: Functional Roles and Therapeutic Considerations for Cardiovascular Disease. *Br. J. Pharmacol.* **2012**, *165*, 622–632. [CrossRef]

11

The Polymorphisms of the Peroxisome-Proliferator Activated Receptors' Alfa Gene Modify the Aerobic Training Induced Changes of Cholesterol and Glucose

Agnieszka Maciejewska-Skrendo [1], Maciej Buryta [1], Wojciech Czarny [2], Pawel Król [2], Michal Spieszny [3], Petr Stastny [4,*], Miroslav Petr [4], Krzysztof Safranow [5] and Marek Sawczuk [6]

1 Department of Molecular Biology, Faculty of Physical Education, Gdansk University of Physical Education and Sport, 80-336 Gdansk, Poland
2 Department of Anatomy and Anthropology, Faculty of Physical Education, University of Rzeszow, 35-310 Rzeszow, Poland
3 Institute of Sports, Faculty of Physical Education, University of Physical Education and Sport, 31-571 Kraków, Poland
4 Department of Sport Games, Faulty of Physical Education and Sport, Charles University, 162-52 Prague, Czech Republic
5 Department of Biochemistry and Medical Chemistry, Pomeranian Medical University, 70-204 Szczecin, Poland
6 Unit of Physical Medicine, Faculty of Tourism and Recreation, Gdansk University of Physical Education and Sport, 80-336 Gdansk, Poland
* Correspondence: stastny@ftvs.cuni.cz

Abstract: Background: PPARα is a transcriptional factor that controls the expression of genes involved in fatty acid metabolism, including fatty acid transport, uptake by the cells, intracellular binding, and activation, as well as catabolism (particularly mitochondrial fatty acid oxidation) or storage. *PPARA* gene polymorphisms may be crucial for maintaining lipid homeostasis and in this way, being responsible for developing specific training-induced physiological reactions. Therefore, we have decided to check if post-training changes of body mass measurements as well as chosen biochemical parameters are modulation by the *PPARA* genotypes. Methods: We have examined the genotype and alleles' frequencies (described in *PPARA* rs1800206 and rs4253778 polymorphic sites) in 168 female participants engaged in a 12-week training program. Body composition and biochemical parameters were measured before and after the completion of a whole training program. Results: Statistical analyses revealed that *PPARA* intron 7 rs4253778 CC genotype modulate training response by increasing low-density lipoproteins (LDL) and glucose concentration, while *PPARA* Leu162Val rs1800206 CG genotype polymorphism interacts in a decrease in high-density lipoproteins (HDL) concentration. Conclusions: Carriers of *PPARA* intron 7 rs4253778 CC genotype and Leu162Val rs1800206 CG genotype might have potential negative training-induced cholesterol and glucose changes after aerobic exercise.

Keywords: human performance; aerobic training; genetic predisposition; lipid metabolism; glucose tolerance; VO_2max; mitochondria activity; cholesterol levels

---

1. Introduction

PPARα is a transcriptional factor that controls the expression of genes involved in fatty acid metabolism, including fatty acid transport, uptake by the cells, intracellular binding, and activation, as well as catabolism (particularly mitochondrial fatty acid oxidation) or storage [1]. PPARα is expressed at moderate levels, mainly in the liver and skeletal muscles, but also in the heart, kidney, brown fat, and large intestine [2–4]. PPARα-dependent transcriptional activity results from a direct interaction of the nuclear receptor with its ligands [5]. The primary natural PPARα ligands are unsaturated fatty acids that directly bind to the PPARα via ligand binding domain (LBD) and enable its heterodimerization with the retinoid X receptor (RXR)-α. Such PPAR:RXR complex binds via PPARα DNA binding domain (DBD) to the PPRE (peroxisome proliferator response element) sequence in the promoter region of target genes [6]. In comparison with the unsaturated fatty acids, saturated fatty acids are poor PPAR ligands [7]. Moreover, synthetic compounds, such as hypolipidemic agents, prostaglandin 12 analogs, leukotriene B4 analogs, leukotriene D4 antagonist, carnitine palmitoyl transferase I (CPT1) inhibitors, fatty acyl-CoA dehydrogenase inhibitors, can activate PPAR [8–10]. It is worth noting that an alternative activation pathway of PPAR:RXR may also occur through ligand binding to RXR [11,12]. In addition to ligand-dependent activation, PPARα may also be regulated by insulin-induced trans-activation that occurs through the phosphorylation of two mitogen-activated protein (MAP) kinase sites at positions 12 and 21 located in the activation function (AF)-1-like domain within PPARα receptor [13].

The *PPARA* gene has been mapped on the human chromosome 22 (locus 22q12-q13.1) and comprises a total of eight exons encoding PPARα protein [14]. Within the entire gene, several polymorphic sites have been identified, with the most studied variant, a missense mutation C/G (rs1800206), resulting in Leu162Val amino acids substitution. This polymorphic site is located in the exon 5 of the *PPARA* gene that encodes the second zinc finger of the DNA binding domain in the PPARα protein. Despite the fact that Leu to Val is a conservative change, this amino acids substitution has functional consequences on protein activity, because the 162 position is next to a cysteine which coordinates the zinc atom and, at the same time, Leu162Val is located upstream of a region determining the specificity and polarity of PPARα binding to different PPREs [15]. In vitro experiments revealed that PPARα isoform with Val in the 162 position has increased PPRE-dependent transcriptional activity compared with the PPARα isoform with Leu in the same position when treated with the PPARα ligand [16]. Interestingly, observed differences were ligand concentration-dependence: At higher concentrations of the ligand, the 162Val variant's transactivation activity was five-fold greater as compared with Leu162 variant [17]. In addition, in vivo observations confirmed that Leu162Val polymorphism exerts an effect on plasma lipoprotein–lipid profile. Carriers of the minor G allele (for Val in the 162 position) compared with homozygotes of the C allele (for Leu162) had significantly higher concentrations of plasma total and low-density lipoproteins (LDL)-apolipoprotein B as well as and LDL cholesterol [18]. In Type II diabetic patients, G allele carriers had higher levels of total cholesterol, high-density lipoproteins (HDL) cholesterol, and apoAI [16]. Moreover, G allele carriers were characterized by a better response to lipid-lowering drugs, showing a greater lowering effect with regard to total cholesterol and non-HDL-cholesterol than C allele homozygotes treated with the same drug [19]. Furthermore, other studies revealed that Leu162Val polymorphism influences the conversion from impaired glucose tolerance to type 2 diabetes [20] as well as being associated with progression of coronary atherosclerosis and the risk of coronary artery disease [21].

The second polymorphic site that has been studied in many contexts is a C/G substitution in *PPARA* intron 7 (rs4253778). It was described for the first time in 2002 in the publications focused on genetic modulators influencing the progression of coronary atherosclerosis and the risk of coronary artery disease [21] as well as left ventricular growth [22]. It has been revealed that *PPARA* rs4253778 polymorphism influences human left ventricular growth observed in response to exercise and hypertension: The C allele carriers had significantly higher left ventricular mass. Moreover, the observed effect was additive: CC homozygotes had a 3-fold greater, and GC heterozygotes had a 2-fold greater increase in left ventricular mass than G allele homozygotes [22]. Taking into account that one of the molecular adaptations described in the hypertrophied heart is reduced PPARα activity [23] and, at the same time, an increase in glucose utilization and a decrease in fatty acid oxidation (FAO) is observed [24,25], it has been hypothesized that the *PPARA* intron 7 C allele affects PPARα function and is connected with downregulation of the expression of mitochondrial FAO enzymes, leading to reduced FAO and impaired cellular lipid homeostasis [22]. Study with diabetic patients has confirmed that C allele carriers are characterized by reduced the lipid-lowering response to fenofibrate treatment in comparison with GG homozygotes [26]. Next, studies with athletes representing different sports disciplines revealed that GG homozygotes were more prevalent in the groups of endurance-type athletes engaged in prolonged aerobic exertion [27,28], while the C allele was frequently observed in power-oriented athletes who were involved in shorter and very intense anaerobic exertion [29]. These results were partly explained by muscle biopsies showing the association between *PPARA* rs4253778 polymorphism and fiber type composition, particularly the correlation between G allele and increased proportion of type I (oxidative) fibers as well as the association of the C allele with the propensity to skeletal muscle hypertrophy, and a facilitation of glucose utilization in response to anaerobic exercise [29].

All the aforementioned facts suggest that *PPARA* polymorphisms may be crucial for maintaining lipid homeostasis and in this way, be responsible for developing specific training-induced physiological reactions. Therefore, we have decided to check if post-training changes of body composition measurements, as well as chosen biochemical parameters (LDL, HDL, glucose), are modulated by the *PPARA* genotypes. To test this hypothesis, we have examined the genotype and alleles' frequencies (described in *PPARA* rs1800206 and rs4253778 polymorphic sites) in female participants engaged in a 12-week training program.

2. Experimental Section

2.1. Ethics Statement

The procedures followed in the study were conducted ethically according to the principles of the World Medical Association Declaration of Helsinki and ethical standards in sport and exercise science research. The study was approved by the Ethics Committee of the Regional Medical Chamber in Szczecin (Approval number 09/KB/IV/2011). All participants were given a consent form and a written information sheet concerning the study, providing all pertinent information (purpose, procedures, risks, and benefits of participation). The experimental procedures were conducted in accordance with the set of guiding principles for reporting the results of genetic association studies defined by the Strengthening the Reporting of Genetic Association studies (STREGA) Statement [30].

2.2. Participants

Out of 201 recruited Polish Caucasian women (range 19–24 years) we have obtained 182 full sets of pre-training and post-training body composition and biochemical data in those who completed a 12-week training program. From these 182 participants, the genetic material was isolated and 168 samples (age 21.6 ± 1.3 years, body mass 60.6 ± 7.6 kg, 21.6 ± 2.4) were successfully genotyped for PPARA rs1800206 and rs4253778. None of the included individuals had engaged in regular physical activity in the previous 6 months. The level of physical activity over the last 6 months has been estimated in every participant according to Global Physical Activity Questionnaire (GPAQ) as well as the individual recording of the subject's own activity, such as direct observation and activity diaries [31]. They had no history of any metabolic or cardiovascular diseases. Participants were nonsmokers and refrained from taking any medications or supplements known to affect metabolism. Before the training phase, all participants were included in a dietary program and had received an individual dietary plan. For every participant, the Basal Metabolic Rate (BMR) as well as the Physical Activity Level (PAL, calculated as the ratio of Total Energy Expenditure (TEE) to BMR), was defined. Every participant was asked to keep a balanced diet customized for the individual's PAL coefficient and body mass according to nutrition standards described for the Polish population [32] during the study and for 2 months before the study. The participants were asked to keep a food diary every day. Weekly consultations were held in which the quality and quantity of meals were analyzed and, if necessary, minor adjustments were made. The nutrition and general lifestyle conditions for all participants during the training phase were considered as similar. During the last weekly session before the 12-week training program, the participants underwent the graded exercise VO_2max test and body composition screen.

2.3. *Training Intervention*

Maximum heart rate (HRmax) was calculated directly in every subject by a continuous graded exercise test on an electronically braked cycle ergometer (Oxycon Pro, Erich JAEGER GmbH, Hoechberg, Germany) which was performed to determine their aerobic capacity (VO2max). The heart rate (HR) at each step of the training program was measured in every subject using HR personal monitoring devices (Polar T31 straps and CE0537 Watches, Lake Success, NY, USA) with customized setup. The training stage was preceded by a week-long familiarization stage, when the examined women exercised 3 times a week for 30 min, at an intensity of about 50% of their HRR (HR Reserve) calculated according to the Karvonen formula. After the week-long familiarization stage, proper training has started. Each training unit consisted of a warm-up routine (10 min), the main aerobic routine (43 min), and stretching and breathing exercise (7 min). The main aerobic routine was a combination of two alternating styles—low and high impact as described by Zarebska et al. [33–35]. Low impact style comprised movements with at least one foot on the floor at all times, whereas high impact styles included running, hopping, and jumping with a variety of flight phases [36]. Music of variable rhythm intensity (tempo) was incorporated into both styles. A 12-week program of low–high impact aerobics was divided as follows: (1) 3 weeks (9 training units), 60 min each, at about 50–60% of HRR, music tempo 135–140 BPM (beats per min), (2) 3 weeks (9 training units), 60 min each, at 55–65% of HRR, music tempo 135–140 BPM, (3) 3 weeks (9 training units), 60 min with the intensity of 60–70% of HRR, music tempo 140–152 BPM, and (4) 3 weeks (9 training units), 60 min with an intensity of 65–75% of HRR, music tempo 140–152 BPM. All 36 training units were administered and supervised by the same instructor.

2.4. *Body Composition Measurements*

Body mass and body composition were assessed by the bioimpedance method (body's inherent resistance to an electrical current) with the use of the electronic scale "Tanita TBF 300M" (Horton Health Initiatives, Orland Park, IL, USA) as described by Zarebska et al. [33]. The device was plugged in and calibrated with the consideration of the weight of the clothes (0.2 kg). Afterward, data regarding age, body height, and sex of the subject were inserted. Then, the subjects stood on the scale with their bare feet on the marked places without leaning any body part. The device analyses body composition based on the differences in the ability to conduct electrical current by body tissues (different resistance) due to different water content. Body mass and body composition measurements were taken with the use of the electronic scale "Tanita" are as follows: total body mass (kg), fat free mass (FFM, kg), fat mass (kg), body mass index (BMI = body mass (kg)/(body height (m))^2, in kg.m^{-2}), tissue impedance (Ohm), total body water (TBW, kg), and basal metabolic rate (BMR, kJ).

2.5. *Biochemical Analyses*

Fasting blood samples were obtained in the morning from the elbow vein before the start of the aerobic fitness training program and repeated at the 12th week of this training program (after the 36th training unit). Compete blood samples (taken before and after 12-week training period) were obtained for 182 participants. The analyses were performed immediately after the blood collection, as described by Leońska-Duniec et al. [37]. Blood samples from each participant were collected in 2 tubes. For biochemical analyses, a 4.9 mL·S-Monovette tube with ethylenediaminetetraacetic acid (K 3 EDTA; 1.6 mg EDTA/mL blood) and separating gel (SARSTEDT AG and Co., Nümbrecht, Germany) were used. Blood samples for biochemical analyses were centrifuged 300× g for 15 min at room temperature to receive blood plasma. All biochemical analyses were conducted using Random Access Automatic Biochemical Analyzer for Clinical Chemistry and Turbidimetry A15 (BIO-SYSTEMS S.A., Barcelona,

Spain). Blood plasma was used to determine lipid profile: triglycerides (TGL), total cholesterol, high-density lipoproteins (HDL) and low-density lipoproteins (LDL) concentrations. Plasma TGL and total cholesterol concentrations were determined using a diagnostic colorimetric enzymatic method according to the manufacturer's protocol (BioMaxima S.A., Lublin, Poland). The manufacturer's declared intra-assay coefficients of variation (CV) of the method were <2.5% and <1.5% for the TGL and total cholesterol determinations, respectively. HDL plasma concentration was determined using the human anti-β-lipoprotein antibody and colorimetric enzymatic method according to the manufacturer's protocol (BioMaxima S.A.). The manufacturer's declared intra-assay CV of the method was <1.5%. Plasma concentrations of LDL were determined using a direct method according to the manufacturer's protocol (PZ Cormay S.A., Lomianki, Poland). The manufacturer's declared intra-assay CV of the method was 4.97%. All analysis procedures were verified with the use of a multi-parametric control serum (BIOLABO S.A.S, Maizy, France), as well as control serum of normal level (BioNormL) and high level (BioPathL) lipid profiles (BioMaxima S.A.).

2.6. Genetic Analyses

The buccal cells donated by the subjects were collected in Resuspension Solution (GenElute Mammalian Genomic DNA Miniprep Kit, Sigma-Aldrich Chemie Gmbh, Munich, Germany) with the use of sterile foam-tipped applicators (Puritan, Holbrook, NY 11741, USA). DNA was extracted from the buccal cells using a GenElute Mammalian Genomic DNA Miniprep Kit (Sigma-Aldrich Chemie Gmbh, Munich, Germany) according to the manufacturer's protocol. DNA isolates were evaluated for quantity, quality, and integrity of DNA using the spectrophotometer BioPhotometer Plus (Eppendorf, Wesseling-Berzdorf, Germany). Only 168 isolates passed the evaluation and were used for subsequent genotyping.

To discriminate *PPARA* I7 rs4253778 (G > C) as well as Leu162Val rs1800206 (C > G) alleles, TaqMan Pre-Designed SNP Genotyping Assays were used (Applied Biosystems, Waltham, MA, USA) (assay IDs: C___2985251_10 and C___8817670_20, respectively) including primers and fluorescently labeled (FAM and VIC) MGBTM TaqMan probes to detect alleles. All samples were genotyped in duplicate on a StepOne Real-Time Polymerase Chain Reaction (RT-PCR) instrument (Applied Biosystems, Waltham, MA, USA) as previously described [37]. PCR products were then subjected to Endpoint-genotyping analysis using an allelic discrimination assay at StepOne Software v2.3 (Applied Biosystems, Carlsbad, CA, USA) to measure the relative amount of allele-specific fluorescence (FAM or VIC), which leads directly to the determination of individual genotypes. Genotypes were assigned using all of the data from the study simultaneously.

2.7. Statistical Analyses

Allele frequencies were determined by gene counting. An χ^2 test was used to test the Hardy–Weinberg equilibrium. To examine the hypothesis that the *PPARA* I7 rs4253778 polymorphism modulate training response, we conducted a repeated measure 2 × 3 ANOVA for genes and 2 × 2 ANOVA for alleles comparison with one between-subject factor (*PPARA* I7 rs4253778 genotype: GG vs. GC vs. CC, GG vs. GC + CC, GG + GC vs. CC) and one within-subject factor (time: before training versus after training) for twelve dependent variables. To examine the hypothesis that *PPARA* Leu162Val rs1800206 modulate training response, we conducted a repeated measure of 2 × 2 ANOVA. Kolmogorov–Smirnov test was used to check for data normality, Mauchly's test for data sphericity, and a post hoc Tukey test was applied when interaction was significant and was used to perform pair-wise comparisons. The effect size (partial eta squared–η^2) of each test was calculated for all analyses and was classified according to Larson-Hall [38], where η^2: 0.01, 0.06, 0.14 were estimated for small, moderate, and large effect, respectively. All statistics were performed in STATISTICA software (version 13; StatSoft, Tulsa, OK, USA) with the level of statistical significance set at $p < 0.05$.

3. Results

PPARA I7 rs4253778, as well as Leu162Val rs1800206 genotypes, conformed to Hardy–Weinberg equilibrium ($p = 0.887$ and $p = 0.572$, respectively) and phenotype outcomes were normally distributed, with no disruption of sphericity (Supplementary File S1). The genotyping error was assessed as 1%, while the call rate (the proportion of samples in which the genotyping provided unambiguous reading) exceeded 95%.

The ANOVA showed genotype × training interactions in *PPARA* I7 rs4253778 for LDL ($F_{1, 165} = 5.12$, $p = 0.025$, $\eta^2 = 0.03$) (Table 1), where post hoc test showed that LDL increased in *PPARA* I7 rs4253778 CC homozygotes after training intervention (79.17 ± 14.16 vs. 95.48 ± 15.35 mg/dL), which did not appear in other genotypes (Figure 1). ANOVA in *PPARA* I7 rs4253778 allele × training interactions showed differences in LDL ($F_{1, 166} = 4.59$, $p = .034$, $\eta^2 = 0.03$), where post hoc analyses showed that CC homozygotes and not G allele carriers increased the LDL concentration after training intervention (Table 1).

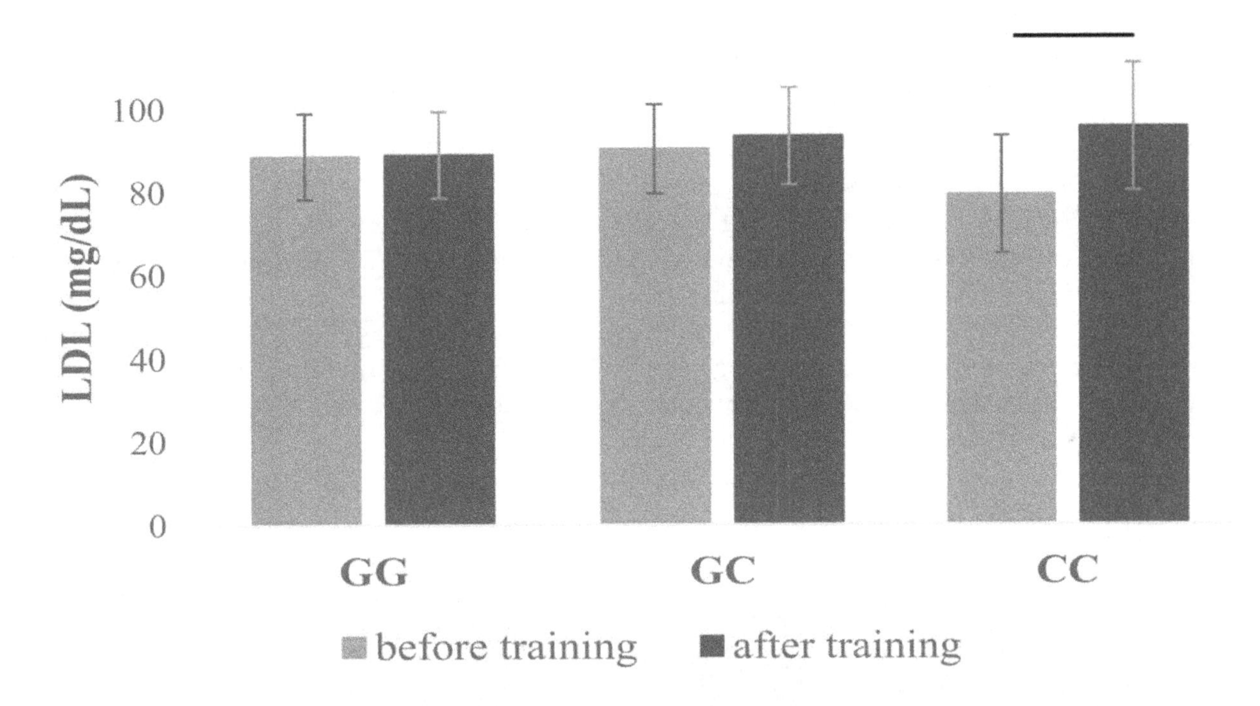

Figure 1. Changes in plasma low-density lipoproteins (LDL) concentrations measured before and after the completion of the 12-week training program in carriers of different *PPARA* I7 rs4253778 genotypes. The values are mean ± SD.

Other *PPARA* I7 rs4253778 genotype × training interactions were found in glucose plasma concentrations ($F_{2, 165} = 3.99$, $p = 0.02$, $\eta^2 = 0.05$) (Table 1), where post hoc showed that carriers of GG and GC genotypes decreased glucose concentration over the period of training (78.83 ± 10.20 vs. 76.44 ± 10.21 and 77.62 ± 8.92 vs. 73.34 ± 9.28, respectively, mg/dL), while for CC homozygotes were characterized by the opposite effect of training and demonstrated a significant increase of glucose concentration (70.50 ± 7.76 vs. 78.17 ± 12.58 mg/dL) (Figure 2) (Table 1). Furthermore, ANOVA in PPARA I7 rs4253778 allele × training interactions showed differences in glucose concentration ($F_{1, 166} = 6.68$, $p = 0.011$, $\eta^2 = 0.06$), where post hoc showed that G allele carriers decreased glucose concentration and CC homozygotes increased glucose concentration (Table 1).

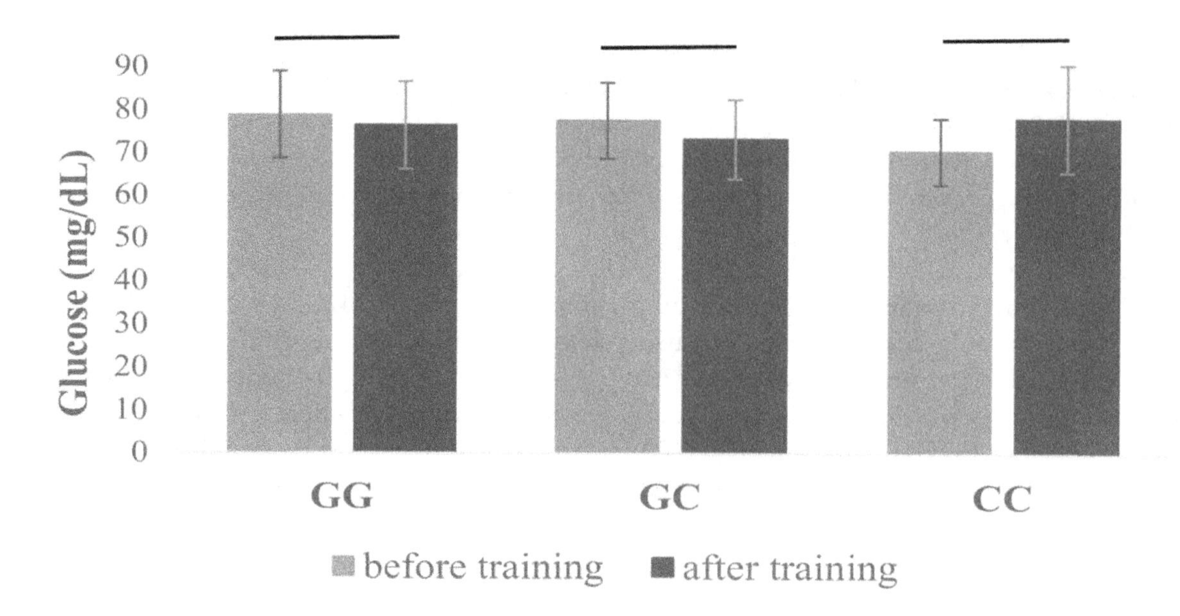

Figure 2. Changes in plasma glucose concentrations measured before and after the completion of the 12-week training program in carriers of different *PPARA* I7 rs4253778 genotypes. The values are mean ± SD.

HDL plasma concentration resulted in statistical differences in *PPARA* Leu162Val rs1800206 genotype ($F_{1,166} = 22.68$, $p < 0.001$, $\eta^2 = 0.12$) and training interactions ($F_{1,166} = 6.30$, $p = 0.013$, $\eta^2 = 0.04$) (Table 2), where post hoc showed that HDL decreased in both *PPARA* Leu162Val rs1800206 genotypes (CC and CG) in the course of training (65.12 ± 13.51 vs. 61.78 ± 13.48 and 64.82 ± 11.83 vs. 54.03 ± 12.08, respectively) (Figure 3) and this training decrease was bigger in CG genotype (only G allele carriers) when compared to CC homozygotes (Table 2). There were no other effects of training or *PPARA* Leu162Val rs1800206 genotypes observed in dependent variables.

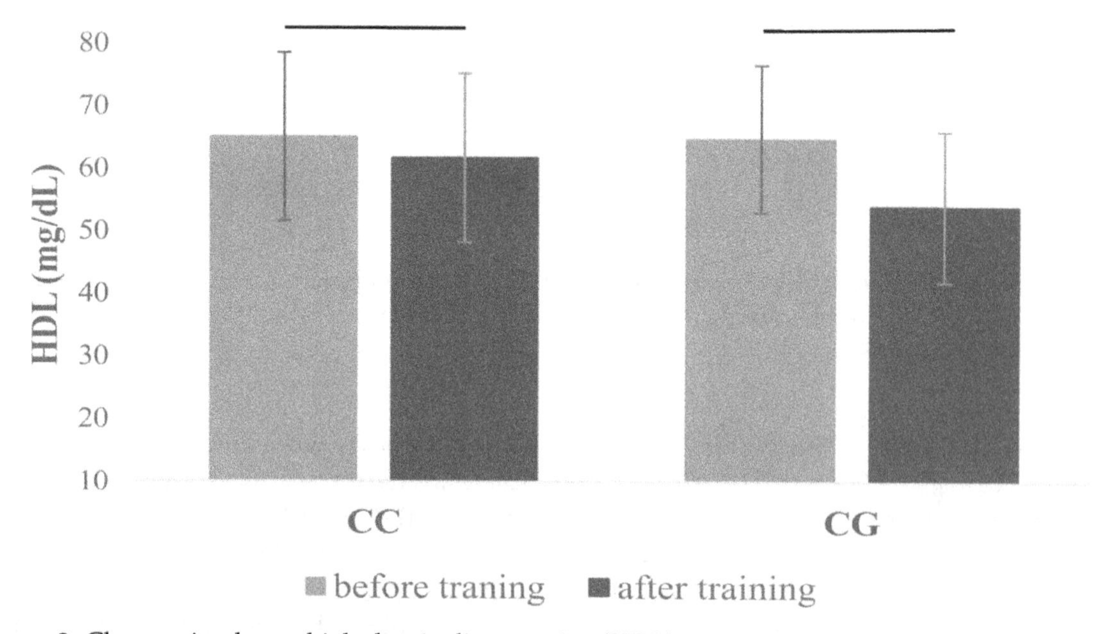

Figure 3. Changes in plasma high-density lipoproteins (HDL) concentrations measured before and after the completion of the 12-week training program in carriers of different *PPARA* Leu162Val rs1800206 genotypes. The values are mean ± SD.

Table 1. The *PPARA* I7 rs4253778 genotypes and response to training.

Variable	GG (n = 109)		GC (n = 53)		CC (n = 6)		p Values for Genotypes		p Values for Allele × Training Interaction	
	Before Training	**After Training**	**Before Training**	**After Training**	**Before Training**	**After Training**	**Genotype**	**Training**	**GG vs. GC+CC**	**GG+GC vs. CC**
Body mass (kg)	59.82 ± 7.45	59.12 ± 7.31	62.35 ± 7.93	61.51 ± 7.86	58.93 ± 6.92	58.27 ± 7.35	0.130	0.859	0.220	0.544
BMI (kg/m^2)	21.36 ± 2.36	21.14 ± 2.30	22.06 ± 2.51	21.82 ± 2.48	21.47 ± 2.85	21.25 ± 2.87	0.226	0.984	0.964	0.510
BMR (kJ)	6027.11 ± 322.75	5988.31 ± 301.69	6117.87 ± 333.88	6087.24 ± 337.16	6035.00 ± 309.97	5970.17 ± 322.14	0.194	0.855	0.889	0.602
Tissue impedance (Ohm)	556.21 ± 64.49	542.09 ± 62.98	536.09 ± 62.33	524.34 ± 62.26	557.17 ± 50.41	543.50 ± 42.88	0.257	0.382	0.643	0.578
FM (kg)	14.42 ± 4.98	13.54 ± 4.97	15.67 ± 5.21	14.59 ± 5.35	14.32 ± 5.15	13.10 ± 5.53	0.565	0.647	0.955	0.979
FFM (kg)	45.38 ± 3.10	45.79 ± 3.06	46.45 ± 3.34	46.91 ± 3.58	44.62 ± 2.57	45.17 ± 2.38	0.084	0.936	0.874	0.491
TBW (kg)	33.32 ± 2.46	33.56 ± 2.28	33.84 ± 2.88	34.32 ± 2.69	32.67 ± 1.88	33.37 ± 1.51	0.229	0.481	0.813	0.429
Total cholesterol (mg/dL)	169.11 ± 22.86	167.16 ± 24.21	172.30 ± 29.33	170.53 ± 33.83	165.00 ± 10.18	172.67 ± 10.65	0.671	0.549	0.983	0.076
TGL (mg/dL)	81.90 ± 35.08	85.27 ± 36.75	76.15 ± 24.53	81.55 ± 32.75	85.50 ± 38.52	73.50 ± 15.54	0.825	0.475	0.679	0.414
HDL (mg/dL)	64.09 ± 12.29	61.21 ± 12.65	66.75 ± 15.18	60.86 ± 15.46	68.80 ± 14.95	62.28 ± 12.26	0.059	0.211	0.085	0.481
LDL (mg/dL)	88.54 ± 20.31	88.91 ± 20.34	90.26 ± 25.69	93.32 ± 29.70	79.17 ± 14.16	95.48 ± 15.35	0.648	**0.025**	0.171	**0.033**
Glucose (mg/dL)	78.83 ± 10.20	76.44 ± 10.21	77.62 ± 8.92	73.34 ± 9.28	70.50 ± 7.76	78.17 ± 12.58	0.298	**0.020**	0.101	**0.011**

The values are mean ± SD; p values (analyzed by two-way mixed ANOVA test) for main effects (genotype and training) genotype × training interaction; bold p values-statistically significant differences ($p < 0.05$); BMI–body mass index; BMR–basal metabolic rate; FM–fat mass; FFM–fat free mass; TBW–total body water; TGL–triglycerides; HDL–high-density lipoproteins; LDL–low-density lipoproteins.

Table 2. The *PPARA* Leu162Val rs18000206 genotypes and response to training.

Variable	CC (n = 154)		CG (n = 14)		p Values for Main Effects	
	Before Training	After Training	Before Training	After Training	Genotype	Training
Body mass (kg)	60.57 ± 7.69	59.90 ± 7.58	60.77 ± 7.37	59.21 ± 7.13	0.063	0.052
BMI (kg/m^2)	21.55 ± 2.46	21.34 ± 2.39	22.03 ± 2.16	21.58 ± 2.39	0.0.64	0.099
BMR (kJ)	6055.80 ± 328.86	6021.35 ± 317.31	6058.43 ± 304.72	5991.64 ± 304.76	0.064	0.303
Tissue impedance (Ohm)	548.23 ± 62.99	535.32 ± 62.33	568.21 ± 71.46	549.93 ± 64.19	0.233	0.582
FM (kg)	14.73 ± 5.09	13.85 ± 5.10	15.63 ± 4.89	13.98 ± 5.34	0.098	0.163
FFM (kg)	45.77 ± 3.19	46.20 ± 3.25	44.79 ± 3.20	45.24 ± 3.15	0.716	0.090
TBW (kg)	33.52 ± 2.60	33.86 ± 2.41	32.81 ± 2.36	33.13 ± 2.32	0.096	0.950
Total cholesterol (mg/dL)	170.99 ± 24.67	169.36 ± 27.58	158.78 ± 23.55	158.07 ± 21.24	0.690	0.876
TGL (mg/dL)	80.86 ± 32.29	85.12 ± 35.55	73.14 ± 31.12	67.71 ± 22.64	0.900	0.294
HDL (mg/dL)	65.12 ± 13.51	61.78 ± 13.48	64.82 ± 11.83	54.03 ± 12.08	**0.001**	**0.013**
LDL (mg/dL)	89.60 ± 21.69	90.55 ± 23.39	79.43 ± 23.59	90.43 ± 26.16	0.259	0.587
Glucose (mg/dL)	78.41 ± 9.74	75.32 ± 10.02	75.36 ± 10.59	77.71 ± 10.67	0.795	0.053

The values are mean ± SD; p values (analyzed by two-way mixed ANOVA test) for genotype × training interaction; BMI–body mass index; BMR–basal metabolic rate; FM–fat mass; FFM–fat free mass; TBW–total body water; TGL–triglycerides; HDL–high-density lipoproteins; LDL–low-density lipoproteins.

Our statistical analyses revealed that *PPARA* intron 7 rs4253778 polymorphism modulate training response in reference to plasma LDL and glucose concentration, while *PPARA* Leu162Val rs1800206 polymorphism interacts with HDL concentration. Taken together, our results supply additional information about the potential role played by genetic variants described in the *PPARA* gene in training-induced biochemical changes.

4. Discussion

This study aimed to check if post-training changes of body mass measurements, as well as chosen biochemical parameters observed in physically active women, are modulated by specific genotypes. The verified hypothesis assumed that in the presence of specific genotypes and alleles in the *PPARA* gene would influence the post-training response observed in biochemical parameter changes in the course of the 12-week training program. Taking onto account *PPARA* intron 7 (rs4253778) genotype × training interactions, there were two statistically significant effects: for LDL and glucose plasma concentrations. For all genotypes, a slight increase in LDL level was observed. However, the rise of LDL concentration reached the highest point in intron 7 CC homozygotes when compared to G allele carriers. Moreover, the CC homozygotes were characterized by an unexpected increase in glucose plasma concentration, while in GC and GG participants, the reverse trend of decreasing glucose concentration was noted. It is commonly expected that LDL, as well as glucose plasma levels, would decrease after regular physical activity [39]. However, more detailed analyses revealed that beneficial changes of the lipid profile are achieved only when the intensity of training is moderate (the exercises are performed below the anaerobic threshold), while the training above the anaerobic threshold intensity may not lead to such healthy effects; what is more it may even reverse these beneficial trends in the context of plasma lipid concentrations [40]. A meta-analysis of studies on the impact of aerobic training on plasma HDL concentration revealed that the minimum duration of aerobic exercises necessary for achieving the beneficial effect of HDL level elevation is about 120 minutes per week, which is an equivalent of 900 kcal energy expenditure [41]. In the exercise protocol used in our study, we had about 180 min exercises per week, and the intensity of the exercises was gradually increased from 50% to 60% to 65% to 75% heart rate reserve. Each training unit consisted of a warm-up, the main aerobic routine, and the ending phase, including stretching and a breathing exercise [33–35]. The structure of the main routine that was a combination of two alternating styles of low and high intensity may resemble interval training, in which the high-intensity workouts are similar to anaerobic exercises, while low-intensity sets correspond to a restitution phase. The summary volume of aerobic exercises probably was not enough to achieve the expected beneficial changes in the lipid profile and glucose level, especially in *PPARA* intron 7 CC homozygotes.

The functional role of *PPARA* intron 7 polymorphism was suggested for the first time in the prospective study of healthy middle-aged men in the United Kingdom [21] as well as in the study of male British Army recruits undergoing a 10-week physical training program [22]. It has been demonstrated that intron 7 C allele is associated with progression of atherosclerosis [21] and is positively correlated with left ventricular growth in response to exercise [22]. Based on the results of the studies showing that hypertrophied heart is characterized by reduced PPARα activity [23] and, in the same time, downregulation of the expression of mitochondrial FAO enzymes [25] with accompanying increases in expression of genes encoding glycolytic enzymes [24], it has been speculated that intron 7 C allele is responsible for lowering the expression of the *PPARA* gene and in this way, is indirectly connected with downregulation of the expression of key metabolic enzymes, leading to impairment of cellular lipid and glucose homeostasis. Another issue is, of course, the question of how the polymorphism located in the non-coding region influences the gene's expression. One possible answer could be that *PPARA* intron 7 alleles are not direct casual variants, but are rather in linkage disequilibrium with an unidentified polymorphism (within the *PPARA* gene or in its regulatory region) that alters encoded protein levels and, as a consequence, may change the expression of PPARα target genes [27,29,42,43]. There is also a hypothesis that, considering this SNP location, the *PPARA* intron 7 polymorphism may change and disrupt a microRNA site [44].

Considering that the proper expression of the *PPARA* gene, necessary for maintaining the appropriate level of PPARα protein, is crucial for regulation of carbohydrate/lipid metabolism, and that the intron 7 C allele may affect this expression process, it is may be expected that the lipid profile and glucose levels would be altered in C allele carriers. Indeed, our results seem to confirm this assumption because we have observed that LDL and glucose levels in CC homozygotes were different from the normal range, with the surprising effect of a post-training increase of plasma glucose concentration as well as the highest rise of LDL levels observed in CC participants. These results suggest that *PPARA* intron 7 CC genotype may be in the group of disadvantageous factors responsible for developing unexpected post-training effects. Probably the CC homozygotes should undergo a different training program with increased volume of aerobic exercises to achieve the expected beneficial results.

When *PPARA* Leu162Val (rs1800206) genotype × training interactions were taken into account, only one statistically significant effect was observed: for post-training changes of HDL levels. In the case of both recorded measurements in these SNP genotypes (CC and CG) we have observed a slight decrease of HDL levels. However, this lowering effect was more pronounced in G allele carriers, in which at least half of the PPARα protein amount comprised the Val amino acid in the 162 position. It is worth noting that rs1800206 GG homozygotes are very rare in the human population, in our study, there were no such individuals in the whole study group.

The C→G substitution, described as *PPARA* rs1800206 polymorphism, is placed within the coding region of the gene, what makes it functional "by definition", causing an amino acid change in the 162 position (Leu162Val) that is located within DNA binding domain (DBD) of the PPARα protein [18]. DBD is directly involved in the interaction between the PPARα transcription factor and PPRE sequences in the promoter region of target genes [6]. Detailed in vitro analyses revealed that PPARα constructs with Val amino acid in the 162 position is activated by the endogenous ligands to a lesser extent when compared with "wild type" PPARα with Leu amino acid residue in the same localization [45]. The PPARα Leu form, that is produced in CC homozygotes, is considered as an active form of this transcriptional factor, displaying a higher transcriptional activity [45] and being able to stimulate the expression of the genes encoding β-oxidation enzymes more efficiently, which cause the shift of the metabolic balance toward catabolic pathways [46,47].

In vivo studies have shown that Leu162Val polymorphism is associated with total plasma cholesterol [16,48,49], LDL [18,49], HDL [16], as well as apolipoprotein B (apoB) [18,48,49], apolipoprotein A-I (apoA-I) [16], and apolipoprotein C-III (apoC-III) [49] concentrations. Moreover, Leu162Val is involved in diabetes and arteriosclerosis progression [16,20,21]. To be more specific, the studies of diabetic patients and non-diabetic subjects revealed that the rs1800206 G allele (also designed as the 162Val allele) carriers were characterized by higher levels of plasma total cholesterol, LDL, and apoB levels in comparison with CC homozygotes [18]. The large population-based study confirmed that the presence of the rs1800206 G allele is correlated with higher levels of total cholesterol, LDL, apoB, and apoC [49]. Moreover, the study of men with metabolic syndrome showed that the frequency of the rs1800206 G allele was higher in subjects having simultaneously abdominal obesity, hypertriglyceridemia, and low HDL levels. The same study demonstrated that carriers of the G allele were characterized by higher plasma apoB and triglyceride (TG) levels and the presence of G allele was associated with components of metabolic syndrome [50]. In another relative large-scale study of middle-aged whites, the G allele was also correlated with an increase in fasting levels of serum lipids [51]. In a controlled dietary intervention trial, in which saturated fat was replaced with either monounsaturated fat or carbohydrate in isoenergetic diets, the effects of *PPARA* Leu162Val genotypes in the determination of plasma lipid concentrations were assessed. The results of this study revealed that Leu162Val variants influence plasma LDL cholesterol concentration, especially being a determinant of small dense LDL (sdLDL) [52]. It has been confirmed in several independent studies showing that rs1800206 CC homozygotes are characterized by a larger LDL particle with reduced density and by an increased general proportion of large LDL particles in the total cholesterol pool [53,54]. Such larger and more buoyant LDL particles are less prone to oxidation processes which create protecting conditions in case of atherosclerosis progression, while small dense LDLs are considered as risk factors of atherosclerosis and coronary artery disease [55,56]. Studies in patients demonstrated that fibrate ligands of PPARα can reduce production of sdLDL, so in carriers of the less active PPARα Val form (that is produced in rs1800206 G allele carriers), activation by dietary ligands could result in a shift to a higher proportion of sdLDL [47,57].

All the aforementioned studies led us to the suggestion that the *PPARA* rs1800206 G allele (producing PPARα protein with Val amino acid in the 162 position) may be associated with developing in its carriers the adverse effects in the context of lipid metabolism. Our results, at least in part, confirm this hypothesis, because the unfavorable post-training effects expressed by an increase of the HDL level was pointed out most firmly in GC heterozygotes, while in CC homozygotes these disadvantageous changes were significantly restricted.

We are aware that our study has some limitations. The first issue of almost every genetic association study has a proper number of participants in the study group. In our case, this could also be a problem, and we see the need for replicating our results in another, preferably larger, population. Especially, *PPARA* I7 rs4253778 CC genotype was rare ($n = 6$) and might cause statistical bias. On the other hand, this rs4253778 CC genotype has been rare in previous studies on the Caucasian population, where it was shown to influence physical condition level [58,59]. The second question is whether the analyzed *PPARA* polymorphisms are true causative factors or perhaps only in linkage disequilibrium with variants directly engaged in developing a specific trait. This problem has been brought up in many studies, and in most cases, the conclusion is that the variation within the *PPARA* gene does not influence any physiological traits alone. Thus, it should be underlined that *PPARA* diversity probably accounts for only a small portion of phenotypic variability, due to the polygenic character of the traits connected with body mass and biochemical parameters measured in our experiment, implying that multiple gene-environment interactions may contribute to the observed differential effects.

5. Conclusions

The results obtained in the current study support our initial hypothesis and suggest that *PPARA* intron 7 rs4253778, as well as Leu162Val rs1800206 variants, play a role in differentiating the beneficial effects of physical activity between the specific genotype carriers. We have demonstrated that harboring a specific *PPARA* intron 7 rs4253778 as well as Leu162Val rs1800206 genotypes may be associated with different post-training changes of measured biochemical parameters. We have observed the surprising effect of a post-training increase of plasma glucose concentration as well as the highest rise of LDL levels in rs4253778 CC participants, which led us to the suggestion that rs4253778 C allele may affect the lipid profile and glucose levels. On the other hand, we have also indicated that some individuals may benefit from being an rs1800206 CC homozygote because in such participants the unfavorable training effects were significantly restricted.

The information obtained in this study can be used as an additional source of precise information about a person undertaking physical effort, determining at the molecular level its inherent metabolic characteristics. Potentially, such information may help design individualized forms of training and more effective optimization and control of the obtained post-training or other treatment effects. Due to the importance of the polymorphic forms analyzed in *PPARA* gene in the etiology of many human diseases, they can be used as a molecular tool of pro-health prophylaxis, helpful in estimating the risk of disorders, such as obesity.

Author Contributions: A.M.-S., P.S., M.B., M.P., and M.S. conceived and designed the experiments; A.M.-S., W.C., P.K., M.S., M.B. and K.S. performed the experiments; A.M.-S., P.S., M.B., M.P., W.C., P.K., M.S. and M.S., K.S. analyzed the data; A.M.-S. and M.S. contributed reagents/materials/analysis tools; A.M.-S., P.S., M.B., M.P., and M.S. wrote the paper.

Acknowledgments: This experiment was supported by Grant UM0-2012/07/B/NZ7/ 01155 founded by the Polish Ministry of Science and Higher Education (http://www.nauka.gov.pl/). This article was written during a scientific training session in the Faculty of Physical Education and Sport of Charles University in Prague (Czech Republic), and the study was supported by a research grant from Charles University UNCE\HUM\032. The funders had no role in study design, data collection, and analysis, decision to publish, or preparation of the paper. The experiments comply with the current laws of the country in which they were performed. The authors would like to thank all participants who decided to spend time to take part in their study and make the research possible.

References

1. Desvergne, B.; Wahli, W. Peroxisome proliferator-activated receptors: Nuclear control of metabolism. *Endocr. Rev.* **1999**, *20*, 649–688. [PubMed]
2. Auboeuf, D.; Rieusset, J.; Fajas, L.; Vallier, P.; Frering, V.; Riou, J.P.; Staels, B.; Auwerx, J.; Laville, M.; Vidal, H. Tissue distribution and quantification of the expression of mRNAs of peroxisome proliferator–activated receptors and liver X receptor-α in humans: No alteration in adipose tissue of obese and NIDDM patients. *Diabetes* **1997**, *46*, 1319–1327.
3. Mukherjee, R.; Jow, L.; Croston, G.E.; Paterniti, J.R. Identification, characterization, and tissue distribution of human peroxisome proliferator-activated receptor (PPAR) isoforms PPARγ2 versus PPARγ1 and activation with retinoid X receptor agonists and antagonists. *J. Biol. Chem.* **1997**, *272*, 8071–8076. [CrossRef] [PubMed]
4. Palmer, C.N.; Hsu, M.-H.; Griffin, K.J.; Raucy, J.L.; Johnson, E.F. Peroxisome proliferator activated receptor-α expression in human liver. *Mol. Pharm.* **1998**, *53*, 14–22. [CrossRef]
5. Willson, T.M.; Wahli, W. Peroxisome proliferator-activated receptor agonists. *Curr. Opin. Chem. Biol.* **1997**, *1*, 235–241. [CrossRef]
6. Dowell, P.; Peterson, V.J.; Zabriskie, T.M.; Leid, M. Ligand-induced peroxisome proliferator-activated receptor α conformational change. *J. Biol. Chem.* **1997**, *272*, 2013–2020. [CrossRef] [PubMed]
7. Kliewer, S.A.; Sundseth, S.S.; Jones, S.A.; Brown, P.J.; Wisely, G.B.; Koble, C.S.; Devchand, P.; Wahli, W.; Willson, T.M.; Lenhard, J.M.; et al. Fatty acids and eicosanoids regulate gene expression through direct interactions with peroxisome proliferator-activated receptors α and γ. *Proc. Natl. Acad. Sci. USA* **1997**, *94*, 4318–4323. [CrossRef] [PubMed]

8. Brown, P.J.; Smith-Oliver, T.A.; Charifson, P.S.; Tomkinson, N.C.; Fivush, A.M.; Sternbach, D.D.; Wade, L.E.; Orband-Miller, L.; Parks, D.J.; Blanchard, S.G.; et al. Identification of peroxisome proliferator-activated receptor ligands from a biased chemical library. *Chem. Biol.* **1997**, *4*, 909–918. [CrossRef]
9. Henke, B.R.; Blanchard, S.G.; Brackeen, M.F.; Brown, K.K.; Cobb, J.E.; Collins, J.L.; Harrington, W.W., Jr.; Hashim, M.A.; Hull-Ryde, E.A.; Kaldor, I.; et al. N-(2-benzoylphenyl)-L-tyrosine PPARγ agonists. 1. Discovery of a novel series of potent antihyperglycemic and antihyperlipidemic agents. *J. Med. Chem.* **1998**, *41*, 5020–5036. [CrossRef]
10. Lehmann, J.M.; Moore, L.B.; Smith-Oliver, T.A.; Wilkison, W.O.; Willson, T.M.; Kliewer, S.A. An antidiabetic thiazolidinedione is a high affinity ligand for peroxisome proliferator-activated receptor γ (PPARγ). *J. Biol. Chem.* **1995**, *270*, 12953–12956. [CrossRef]
11. Gearing, K.; Göttlicher, M.; Teboul, M.; Widmark, E.; Gustafsson, J.-A. Interaction of the peroxisome-proliferator-activated receptor and retinoid X receptor. *Proc. Natl. Acad. Sci. USA* **1993**, *90*, 1440–1444. [CrossRef]
12. Keller, H.R.; Dreyer, C.; Medin, J.; Mahfoudi, A.; Ozato, K.; Wahli, W. Fatty acids and retinoids control lipid metabolism through activation of peroxisome proliferator-activated receptor-retinoid X receptor heterodimers. *Proc. Natl. Acad. Sci. USA* **1993**, *90*, 2160–2164. [CrossRef] [PubMed]
13. Juge-Aubry, C.E.; Hammar, E.; Siegrist-Kaiser, C.; Pernin, A.; Takeshita, A.; Chin, W.W.; Burger, A.G.; Meier, C.A. Regulation of the transcriptional activity of the peroxisome proliferator-activated receptor α by phosphorylation of a ligand-independent trans-activating domain. *J. Biol. Chem.* **1999**, *274*, 10505–10510. [CrossRef] [PubMed]
14. Sher, T.; Yi, H.F.; McBride, O.W.; Gonzalez, F.J. cDNA cloning, chromosomal mapping, and functional characterization of the human peroxisome proliferator activated receptor. *Biochemistry* **1993**, *32*, 5598–5604. [CrossRef] [PubMed]
15. Hsu, M.-H.; Palmer, C.N.; Song, W.; Griffin, K.J.; Johnson, E.F. A carboxyl-terminal extension of the zinc finger domain contributes to the specificity and polarity of peroxisome proliferator-activated receptor DNA binding. *J. Biol. Chem.* **1998**, *273*, 27988–27997. [CrossRef]
16. Flavell, D.; Torra, I.P.; Jamshidi, Y.; Evans, D.; Diamond, J.; Elkeles, R.; Bujac, S.R.; Miller, G.; Talmud, P.J.; Staels, B.; et al. Variation in the PPARα gene is associated with altered function in vitro and plasma lipid concentrations in Type II diabetic subjects. *Diabetologia* **2000**, *43*, 673–680. [CrossRef] [PubMed]
17. Sapone, A.; Peters, J.M.; Sakai, S.; Tomita, S.; Papiha, S.S.; Dai, R.; Friedman, F.K.; Gonzalez, F.J. The human peroxisome proliferator-activated receptor α gene: identification and functional characterization of two natural allelic variants. *Pharm. Genom* **2000**, *10*, 321–333. [CrossRef]
18. Vohl, M.-C.; Lepage, P.; Gaudet, D.; Brewer, C.G.; Bétard, C.; Perron, P.; Houde, G.; Cellier, C.; Faith, J.M.; Després, J.P.; et al. Molecular scanning of the human PPARα gene: Association of the L162V mutation with hyperapobetalipoproteinemia. *J. Lipid Res.* **2000**, *41*, 945–952.
19. Elkeles, R.S.; Diamond, J.R.; Poulter, C.; Dhanjil, S.; Nicolaides, A.N.; Mahmood, S.; Richmond, W.; Mather, H.; Sharp, P.; Feher, M.D.; et al. Cardiovascular outcomes in type 2 diabetes: A double-blind placebo-controlled study of bezafibrate: The St. Mary's, Ealing, Northwick Park Diabetes Cardiovascular Disease Prevention (SENDCAP) Study. *Diabetes Care* **1998**, *21*, 641–648. [CrossRef]
20. Andrulionytė, L.; Kuulasmaa, T.; Chiasson, J.-L.; Laakso, M. Single Nucleotide Polymorphisms of the Peroxisome Proliferator–Activated Receptor-α Gene (PPARA) Influence the Conversion From Impaired Glucose Tolerance to Type 2 Diabetes: The STOP-NIDDM Trial. *Diabetes* **2007**, *56*, 1181–1186. [CrossRef]
21. Flavell, D.M.; Jamshidi, Y.; Hawe, E.; Pineda Torra, I.S.; Taskinen, M.-R.; Frick, M.H.; Nieminen, M.S.; Kesäniemi, Y.A.; Pasternack, A.; Staels, B.; et al. Peroxisome proliferator-activated receptor α gene variants influence progression of coronary atherosclerosis and risk of coronary artery disease. *Circulation* **2002**, *105*, 1440–1445. [CrossRef]
22. Jamshidi, Y.; Montgomery, H.E.; Hense, H.-W.; Myerson, S.G.; Torra, I.P.; Staels, B.; World, M.J.; Doering, A.; Erdmann, J.; Hengstenberg, C.; et al. Peroxisome proliferator–activated receptor α gene regulates left ventricular growth in response to exercise and hypertension. *Circulation* **2002**, *105*, 950–955. [CrossRef] [PubMed]
23. Barger, P.M.; Brandt, J.M.; Leone, T.C.; Weinheimer, C.J.; Kelly, D.P. Deactivation of peroxisome proliferator–activated receptor-α during cardiac hypertrophic growth. *J. Clin. Investig.* **2000**, *105*, 1723–1730. [CrossRef] [PubMed]

24. Allard, M.; Schonekess, B.; Henning, S.; English, D.; Lopaschuk, G.D. Contribution of oxidative metabolism and glycolysis to ATP production in hypertrophied hearts. *Am. J. Physiol. Heart Circ. Physiol.* **1994**, *267*, H742–H750. [CrossRef] [PubMed]
25. Sack, M.N.; Rader, T.A.; Park, S.; Bastin, J.; McCune, S.A.; Kelly, D.P. Fatty acid oxidation enzyme gene expression is downregulated in the failing heart. *Circulation* **1996**, *94*, 2837–2842. [CrossRef] [PubMed]
26. Foucher, C.; Rattier, S.; Flavell, D.M.; Talmud, P.J.; Humphries, S.E.; Kastelein, J.J.; Ayyobi, A.; Pimstone, S.; Frohlich, J.; Ansquer, J.C.; et al. Response to micronized fenofibrate treatment is associated with the peroxisome–proliferator-activated receptors alpha G/C intron7 polymorphism in subjects with type 2 diabetes. *Pharmacogenetics* **2004**, *14*, 823–829. [CrossRef]
27. Maciejewska, A.; Sawczuk, M.; Cieszczyk, P. Variation in the PPARalpha gene in Polish rowers. *J. Sci. Med. Sport* **2011**, *14*, 58–64. [CrossRef] [PubMed]
28. Eynon, N.; Meckel, Y.; Sagiv, M.; Yamin, C.; Amir, R.; Sagiv, M.; Goldhammer, E.; Duarte, J.A.; Oliveira, J. Do PPARGC1A and PPARalpha polymorphisms influence sprint or endurance phenotypes? *Scand. J. Med. Sci. Sports* **2010**, *20*, e145–e150. [CrossRef]
29. Ahmetov, I.I.; Mozhayskaya, I.A.; Flavell, D.M.; Astratenkova, I.V.; Komkova, A.I.; Lyubaeva, E.V.; Tarakin, P.P.; Shenkman, B.S.; Vdovina, A.B.; Netreba, A.I.; et al. PPARalpha gene variation and physical performance in Russian athletes. *Eur. J. Appl. Physiol.* **2006**, *97*, 103–108. [CrossRef]
30. Little, J.; Higgins, J.P.; Ioannidis, J.P.; Moher, D.; Gagnon, F.; Von Elm, E.; Khoury, M.J.; Cohen, B.; Davey-Smith, G.; Grimshaw, J.; et al. STrengthening the REporting of Genetic Association studies (STREGA)—An extension of the STROBE statement. *Genet. Epidemiol.* **2009**, *33*, 581–598. [CrossRef]
31. Hills, A.P.; Mokhtar, N.; Byrne, N.M. Assessment of physical activity and energy expenditure: An overview of objective measures. *Front. Nutr.* **2014**, *16*, 5. [CrossRef]
32. Jarosz, M. *Normy żywienia dla Populacji Polski*; Institut Żywności I Żywienia: Warszawa, Poland, 2017.
33. Zarebska, A.; Jastrzebski, Z.; Cieszczyk, P.; Leonska-Duniec, A.; Kotarska, K.; Kaczmarczyk, M.; Sawczuk, M.; Maciejewska-Karlowska, A. The Pro12Ala polymorphism of the peroxisome proliferator-activated receptor gamma gene modifies the association of physical activity and body mass changes in Polish women. *PPAR Res.* **2014**, *2014*, 1–7. [CrossRef] [PubMed]
34. Zarebska, A.; Jastrzebski, Z.; Kaczmarczyk, M.; Ficek, K.; Maciejewska-Karlowska, A.; Sawczuk, M.; Leońska-Duniec, A.; Krol, P.; Cieszczyk, P.; Zmijewski, P.; et al. The GSTP1 c. 313A> G polymorphism modulates the cardiorespiratory response to aerobic training. *Biol. Sport* **2014**, *31*, 261–266. [CrossRef] [PubMed]
35. Zarębska, A.; Jastrzębski, Z.; Moska, W.; Leońska-Duniec, A.; Kaczmarczyk, M.; Sawczuk, M.; Maciejewska-Skrendo, A.; Zmijewski, P.; Ficek, K.; Trybek, G.; et al. The AGT gene M235T polymorphism and response of power-related variables to aerobic training. *J. Sports Sci. Med.* **2016**, *15*, 616–624.
36. De Angelis, M.; Vinciguerra, G.; Gasbarri, A.; Pacitti, C. Oxygen uptake, heart rate and blood lactate concentration during a normal training session of an aerobic dance class. *Eur. J. Appl. Physiol. Occup. Physiol.* **1998**, *78*, 121–127. [CrossRef] [PubMed]
37. Leońska-Duniec, A.; Jastrzębski, Z.; Zarębska, A.; Maciejewska, A.; Ficek, K.; Cięszczyk, P. Assessing effect of interaction between the FTO A/T polymorphism (rs9939609) and physical activity on obesity-related traits. *J. Sport Health Sci.* **2018**, *7*, 459–464. [CrossRef] [PubMed]
38. Larson-Hall, J. A Guide to Doing Statistics in Second Language Research Using SPSS. *Ibérica* **2010**, *20*, 167–204.
39. Fikenzer, K.; Fikenzer, S.; Laufs, U.; Werner, C. Effects of endurance training on serum lipids. *Vasc. Pharm.* **2018**, *101*, 9–20. [CrossRef]
40. Aellen, R.; Hollmann, W.; Boutellier, U. Effects of aerobic and anaerobic training on plasma lipoproteins. *Int. J. Sports Med.* **1993**, *14*, 396–400. [CrossRef]
41. Kodama, S.; Tanaka, S.; Saito, K.; Shu, M.; Sone, Y.; Onitake, F.; Suzuki, E.; Shimano, H.; Yamamoto, S.; Kondo, K.; et al. Effect of aerobic exercise training on serum levels of high-density lipoprotein cholesterol: A meta-analysis. *Arch. Intern. Med.* **2007**, *167*, 999–1008. [CrossRef]
42. Chen, E.S.; Mazzotti, D.R.; Furuya, T.K.; Cendoroglo, M.S.; Ramos, L.R.; Araujo, L.Q.; Burbano, R.R.; Smith Mde, A. Association of PPARα gene polymorphisms and lipid serum levels in a Brazilian elderly population. *Exp. Mol. Pathol.* **2010**, *88*, 197–201. [CrossRef]

43. Doney, A.S.; Fischer, B.; Lee, S.P.; Morris, A.D.; Leese, G.; Palmer, C.N. Association of common variation in the PPARA gene with incident myocardial infarction in individuals with type 2 diabetes: A Go-DARTS study. *Nucl. Recept.* **2005**, *3*, 4. [CrossRef]
44. Cresci, S.; Jones, P.G.; Sucharov, C.C.; Marsh, S.; Lanfear, D.E.; Garsa, A.; Courtois, M.; Weinheimer, C.J.; Wu, J.; Province, M.A.; et al. Interaction between PPARA genotype and β-blocker treatment influences clinical outcomes following acute coronary syndromes. *Pharmacogenomics* **2008**, *9*, 1403–1417. [CrossRef] [PubMed]
45. Rudkowska, I.; Verreault, M.; Barbier, O.; Vohl, M.-C. Differences in Transcriptional Activation by the Two Allelic (L162V Polymorphic) Variants of PPAR after Omega-3 Fatty Acids Treatment. *Ppar. Res.* **2009**, *2009*, 369602. [CrossRef] [PubMed]
46. Berneis, K.; Rizzo, M. LDL size: Does it matter? *Swiss. Med. Wkly.* **2004**, *134*, 720–724. [PubMed]
47. Caslake, M.; Packard, C.; Gaw, A.; Murray, E.; Griffin, B.; Vallance, B.; Shepherd, J. Fenofibrate and LDL metabolic heterogeneity in hypercholesterolemia. *Arter. Thromb* **1993**, *13*, 702–711. [CrossRef]
48. Lacquemant, C.; Lepretre, F.; Torra, I.P.; Manraj, M.; Charpentier, G.; Ruiz, J.; Staels, B.; Froguel, P. Mutation screening of the PPARalpha, gene in type 2 diabetes associated with coronary heart disease. *Diabetes Metab.* **2000**, *26*, 393–402. [PubMed]
49. Tai, E.; Demissie, S.; Cupples, L.; Corella, D.; Wilson, P.; Schaefer, E.; Ordovas, J.M. Association between the PPARA L162V polymorphism and plasma lipid levels: the Framingham Offspring Study. *Arter. Thromb. Vasc. Biol.* **2002**, *22*, 805–810. [CrossRef]
50. Robitaille, J.; Brouillette, C.; Houde, A.; Lemieux, S.; Pérusse, L.; Tchernof, A.; Gaudet, D.; Vohl, M.-C. Association between the PPARα-L162V polymorphism and components of the metabolic syndrome. *J. Hum. Gen.* **2004**, *49*, 482.
51. Sparsø, T.; Hussain, M.S.; Andersen, G.; Hainerova, I.; Borch-Johnsen, K.; Jørgensen, T.; Hansen, T.; Pedersen, O. Relationships between the functional PPARα Leu162Val polymorphism and obesity, type 2 diabetes, dyslipidaemia, and related quantitative traits in studies of 5799 middle-aged white people. *Mol. Genet. Metab.* **2007**, *90*, 205–209. [CrossRef]
52. AlSaleh, A.; Frost, G.S.; Griffin, B.A.; Lovegrove, J.A.; Jebb, S.A.; Sanders, T.A.; O'Dell, S.D.; RISCK Study Investigators. PPARγ2 gene Pro12Ala and PPARα gene Leu162Val single nucleotide polymorphisms interact with dietary intake of fat in determination of plasma lipid concentrations. *J. Nutr. Nutr.* **2011**, *4*, 354–366. [CrossRef]
53. Bouchard-Mercier, A.; Godin, G.; Lamarche, B.; Pérusse, L.; Vohl, M.-C. Effects of peroxisome proliferator-activated receptors, dietary fat intakes and gene–diet interactions on peak particle diameters of low-density lipoproteins. *J. Nutr. Nutr.* **2011**, *4*, 36–48. [CrossRef] [PubMed]
54. Egert, S.; Kratz, M.; Kannenberg, F.; Fobker, M.; Wahrburg, U. Effects of high-fat and low-fat diets rich in monounsaturated fatty acids on serum lipids, LDL size and indices of lipid peroxidation in healthy non-obese men and women when consumed under controlled conditions. *Eur. J. Nutr.* **2011**, *50*, 71–79. [CrossRef] [PubMed]
55. Lamarche, B.; Lemieux, I.; Despres, J. The small, dense LDL phenotype and the risk of coronary heart disease: Epidemiology, patho-physiology and therapeutic aspects. *Diabetes Metab.* **1999**, *25*, 199–212.
56. Berneis, K.K.; Krauss, R.M. Metabolic origins and clinical significance of LDL heterogeneity. *J. Lipid Res.* **2002**, *43*, 1363–1379. [CrossRef] [PubMed]
57. Jakob, T.; Nordmann, A.J.; Schandelmaier, S.; Ferreira-González, I.; Briel, M. Fibrates for primary prevention of cardiovascular disease events. *Cochrane Database Syst. Rev.* **2016**, *11*, CD009753. [CrossRef] [PubMed]
58. Stastny, P.; Lehnert, M.; De Ste Croix, M.; Petr, M.; Svoboda, Z.; Maixnerova, E.; Varekova, R.; Botek, M.; Petrek, M.; Kocourkova, L.; et al. Effect of COL5A1, GDF5, and PPARA Genes on a Movement Screen and Neuromuscular Performance in Adolescent Team Sport Athletes. *J. Strength Cond. Res.* **2019**. [CrossRef] [PubMed]
59. Petr, M.; Stastny, P.; Pecha, O.; Šteffl, M.; Šeda, O.; Kohlíková, E. PPARA intron polymorphism associated with power performance in 30-s anaerobic Wingate Test. *PLoS ONE* **2014**, *9*, e107171. [CrossRef]

12

Neopterin is Associated with Disease Severity and Outcome in Patients with Non-Ischaemic Heart Failure

Lukas Lanser [1], Gerhard Pölzl [2], Dietmar Fuchs [3], Günter Weiss [1] and Katharina Kurz [1,*]

[1] Department of Internal Medicine II, Medical University of Innsbruck, 6020 Innsbruck, Austria; lukas.lanser@i-med.ac.at (L.L.); guenter.weiss@i-med.ac.at (G.W.)
[2] Department of Internal Medicine III, Medical University of Innsbruck, 6020 Innsbruck, Austria; gerhard.poelzl@tirol-kliniken.at
[3] Division of Biological Chemistry, Biocenter, Medical University of Innsbruck, 6020 Innsbruck, Austria; dietmar.fuchs@i-med.ac.at
* Correspondence: katharina.kurz@tirol-kliniken.at

Abstract: Inflammation and immune activation play an important role in the pathogenesis of cardiac remodelling in patients with heart failure. The aim of this study was to assess whether biomarkers of inflammation and immune activation are linked to disease severity and the prognosis of heart failure patients. In 149 patients (65.8% men, median age 49.7 years) with heart failure from nonischaemic cardiomyopathy, the biomarkers neopterin and C-reactive protein were tested at the time of diagnosis. Patients were followed-up for a median of 58 months. During follow-up, nineteen patients died, five had a heart transplantation, two needed a ventricular assistance device, and twenty-one patients had to be hospitalised because of heart failure decompensation. Neopterin concentrations correlated with N-terminal prohormone of brain natriuretic peptide (NT-proBNP) concentrations (rs = 0.399, $p < 0.001$) and rose with higher New York Heart Association (NYHA) class (I: 5.60 nmol/L, II: 6.90 nmol/L, III/IV: 7.80 nmol/L, $p = 0.033$). Higher neopterin levels were predictive for an adverse outcome (death or hospitalisation due to HF decompensation), independently of age and sex and of established predictors in heart failure such as NYHA class, NT-proBNP, estimated glomerular filtration rate (eGFR), and left ventricular ejection fraction (LV-EF) (HR 2.770; 95% CI 1.419–5.407; $p = 0.003$). Patients with a neopterin/eGFR ratio ≥ 0.133 (as a combined marker for immune activation and kidney function) had a more than eightfold increased risk of reaching an endpoint compared to patients with a neopterin/eGFR ratio ≤ 0.065 (HR 8.380; 95% CI 2.889–24.308; $p < 0.001$). Neopterin is associated with disease severity and is an independent predictor of prognosis in patients with heart failure.

Keywords: Neopterin; inflammation; heart failure; adverse outcome

---

1. Introduction

Activation and down-regulation of the immune response are important mechanisms to control tissue damage, initiate the healing process, and to remove dead cells and debris after a harmful stimulus [1]. However, prolonged immune activation promotes local and systemic inflammatory processes, thereby contributing to tissue damage and organ failure over time. This has also been shown in patients with chronic heart failure (CHF) [2], where increased concentrations of circulating cytokines and biomarkers of inflammation were associated with a poor outcome [3–5]. Therefore, the balance of physiological and pathological immune activation contributes to heart failure (HF) progression and determines the outcomes of these patients [2]. Immune activation in CHF is driven by several factors:

pro-inflammatory cells are found in the failing myocardium itself [3] but systemic immune activation also plays a role [6]. In fact, low-grade immune activation has been established to greatly contribute to atherogenesis [7]. Additionally, circulating endotoxins, which translocate from the intestinal tract into the systemic circulation [8], as well as the hypoxia of body tissues [9–11] and central inhibition of the parasympathetic nervous system appear to be involved [6].

Elevated parameters of inflammation have been shown to predict an unfavourable clinical course of patients with cardiovascular diseases [12–14]. Several studies have demonstrated that the pteridine neopterin is a good prognostic marker for an adverse outcome in patients with clinically inapparent atherosclerosis [12,15], chronic stable angina pectoris [16–18], and acute coronary syndrome [19].

Neopterin is produced by activated monocytes, macrophages and dendritic cells (DCs) upon stimulation with interferon gamma (IFN-γ). Therefore, neopterin levels reflect the extent of T-helper cell type 1 (Th1) immune activation. Monocytes stimulated by IFN-γ also produce reactive oxygen species (ROS) [20] concomitantly with neopterin, thus inducing oxidative stress, which also plays a key role in the progress of HF [21–23]. Neopterin was demonstrated to correlate with cardiac dysfunction following cardiac surgery [24] and cardiac remodelling in patients with CHF [25]. In addition, neopterin concentrations correlated with the severity of heart failure in patients with preserved ejection fraction (HFpEF) and the probability of future cardiovascular events [26].

The aim of this study was to assess the relationship between the inflammatory biomarkers, C-reactive protein (CRP), neopterin, and disease severity, as well as to evaluate the predictive value of these parameters for the outcome of HF patients with nonischaemic cardiomyopathy (CMP).

2. Experimental Section

2.1. Study Population

We retrospectively analysed the data of 475 caucasian patients with HF caused by nonischaemic CMP. Patients with more than mild-to-moderate valve disease as well as ischaemic cardiomyopathy were not included in the study, since there are studies describing significant differences in immune activation between patients with ischemic and non-ischemic cardiomyopathy [27]. At our department, specific investigations such as echocardiography, coronary angiography (CAG), right heart catheterization, and endomyocardial biopsy (EMB) were performed in patients with nonischaemic CAG. These investigations took place between 2009 and 2014 over the course of an elective hospitalisation, and only patients with compensated HF were investigated. All patients were diagnosed and treated according to prevailing guidelines at the cardiology department at Innsbruck University Hospital. Data of all HF patients with available neopterin and C-reactive protein concentrations (n = 149) were analysed. The final study population consisted of 98 men and 51 women. The study conformed to the ethical principles outlined in the Declaration of Helsinki and was approved by the ethics committee of the Innsbruck Medical University (ID of the ethical votum: UN4280, session number 298/4.11). All patients gave written informed consent to participate in this study.

2.2. Follow-Up Analysis

Patients were followed up until May 2017. For the outcome analysis, we defined the event-free survival as time between invasive diagnosis and laboratory testing, and the occurrence of the combined endpoint. Components of the combined event were death or hospitalisation for cardiac decompensation, whatever came first. Information about patients' events was obtained from the clinical information system (KIS), the local mortality registry, from the patients' relatives or from the patients themselves.

2.3. Measurements

Blood samples were taken from all patients at their first hospitalisation and stored at −80°C. Concentrations of all laboratory variables were measured at the central laboratory of the Innsbruck University Hospital, which undergoes regular internal and external quality control and evaluation.

Neopterin was measured by an enzyme-linked immunosorbent assay (IBL International GmbH, Hamburg, Germany). C-reactive protein (CRP) was detected with an immunoturbidimetry test (Roche, Mannheim, Germany). In order to estimate the glomerular filtration rate (eGFR), we used the IDMS-traceable MDRD study equation (eGFR(mL/min/1.73 m2) = 175 × (serum creatinine) − 1.154 × age − 0.203 (×0.742 if female)).

Hemodynamic parameters were measured in the course of a right and left heart catheterisation, while the left ventricular ejection fraction (LV-EF) was measured during an echocardiography.

2.4. Statistical Analysis

Quantitative variables are presented as medians (25th, 75th percentile) because there was no Gaussian distribution given. Categorical variables are presented as prevalence and percentage. The Kolmogorov-Smirnov test was used to evaluate the normal distribution of the measured data. To test for differences between two or more groups, Mann-Whitney-U test (two unpaired groups), Kruskal-Wallis test (more than two unpaired groups) and Pearson chi-square test were used. Spearman rank correlation was used to assess cross-sectional relations between neopterin, HF severity and kidney function. We used proportional hazard regression analysis to analyse the potential risk factors for an adverse outcome and logarithmised parameters that showed a skewed distribution. All tests used were two-tailed and p-values < 0.05 were considered as statistically significant. The statistical analysis was performed with SPSS Statistics Version 24.0 for Macintosh (IBM Corporation, Armonk, NY, USA).

3. Results

Demographic and clinical characteristics, laboratory measurements, and haemodynamic parameters of the whole population and separately for patients with and without an event within five years are depicted in Table 1.

Table 1. Patient characteristics.

Variable	Total	No Event *	Event *	Significance
	n = 149	n = 115	n = 34	*p*-Value
	Median (IQR)	Median	Median	
Demographic and clinical characteristics				
Age (years)	49.7 (38.5–61.7)	48.9	51.4	0.074
BMI (kg/m^2)	24.81 (22.00–27.74)	25.25	23.55	0.025
Heart rate (bpm)	70 (60–82)	70	73	0.220
Diast. BP (mmHg)	80 (70–85)	80	77	0.751
Syst. BP (mmHg)	120 (110–132)	120	115	0.193
Hypertension	45.2%	45.5%	44.1%	0.884
Atrial fibrillation	9.7%	9.7%	9.4%	0.952
NYHA class, overall	-	-	-	0.072
NYHA class I	22.4%	26.3%	9.1%	-
NYHA class II	44.2%	43.9%	45.5%	-
NYHA class III/IV	33.3%	29.8%	45.5%	-
Laboratory measurements				
Neopterin (nmol/L)	6.90 (5.00–9.70)	6.50	10.00	<0.001
CRP (mg/L)	0.20 (0.10–0.63)	0.20	0.20	0.966
eGFR (mL/min/1.73m^2)	74.11 (58.39–90.47)	78.29	65.57	0.001
Neopterin/eGFR ratio	0.097 (0.057–0.148)	0.082	0.162	<0.001
NT-proBNP (ng/L)	1340 (501–3266)	1025	3835	<0.001
Hemodynamics				
LV-EF (%)	37.0 (25.7–49.7)	36.0	46.0	0.052
Cardiac index (L/min/m^2)	1.93 (1.68–2.45)	2.01	1.78	0.003
mean PAP (mmHg)	26.0 (19.0–33.0)	24.0	32.5	0.001
PCWP (mmHg)	17 (11–25)	15	24	<0.001
RAP (mmHg)	9 (6–12)	8	11	0.003

Table 1. *Cont.*

Variable	Total	No Event *	Event *	Significance
	n = 149	n = 115	n = 34	*p*-Value
	Median (IQR)	Median	Median	
Medication and Treatment				
ACE inhibitor/ARB	77.7%	79.8%	70.6%	0.256
Beta-blocker	74.8%	78.8%	61.8%	0.045
MRA	34.5%	33.3%	38.2%	0.598
Diuretics	57.8%	52.6%	75.8%	0.018
Cardiac glycosides	2.0%	1.8%	2.9%	0.666
Pacemaker	3.4%	3.5%	2.9%	0.872

Data from 149 patients are presented as medians (interquartile range). (*) Event within five years. Parameters that differed significantly are printed in italic letters. IQR = interquartile range; BMI = body mass index; BP = blood pressure; NYHA = New York Heart Association; CRP = C-reactive protein; eGFR = estimated glomerular filtration rate; NT-proBNP = N-terminal prohormone of brain natriuretic peptide; RAP = right atrial pressure; mean PAP = mean pulmonary artery pressure; PCWP = pulmonary capillary wedge pressure; LV-EF = left ventricular ejection fraction; ACE = angiotensin converting enzyme; ARB = angiotensin II receptor blocker; MRA = mineralocorticoid receptor antagonist.

The percentage of patients with reduced LV-EF <40% was 63.4% (66.3% of men, 58.0% of women, $p = 0.323$). Reduced kidney function (eGFR $\leq$ 60 mL/min/1.73m^2) was found in 40 patients (26.8%) but only seven of them (4.7%) were presented with advanced renal insufficiency (eGFR $\leq$ 45 mL/min/1.73m^2).

3.1. Inflammation Correlates With HF Severity and Cardiac Function

Inflammatory parameters (CRP and/or neopterin) were elevated in 72 patients (48.3%). Out of these, 25 patients (16.8%) showed elevated CRP concentrations (>0.5 mg/L), 27 patients (18.1%) elevated neopterin concentrations (>8.7 nmol/L), and 20 patients (13.4%) showed both elevated CRP and neopterin concentrations.

Neopterin concentrations were positively correlated with CRP concentrations (rs = 0.343, $p < 0.001$; Figure 1A). Additionally, significant correlations were found between neopterin concentrations and NT-proBNP concentrations (rs = 0.399, $p < 0.001$, Figure 1B), cardiac index (rs = −0.287, $p = 0.001$), right atrial pressure (RAP, rs = 0.170, $p = 0.043$), pulmonary artery mean pressure (mean PAP, rs = 0.227, p = 0.007) and pulmonary capillary wedge pressure (PCWP, rs = 0.244, $p = 0.004$) were found. Neopterin progressively increased with higher NYHA class (I: 5.60 nmol/L, II: 6.90 nmol/L, III/IV: 7.80 nmol/L, $p = 0.033$, Figure 1C).

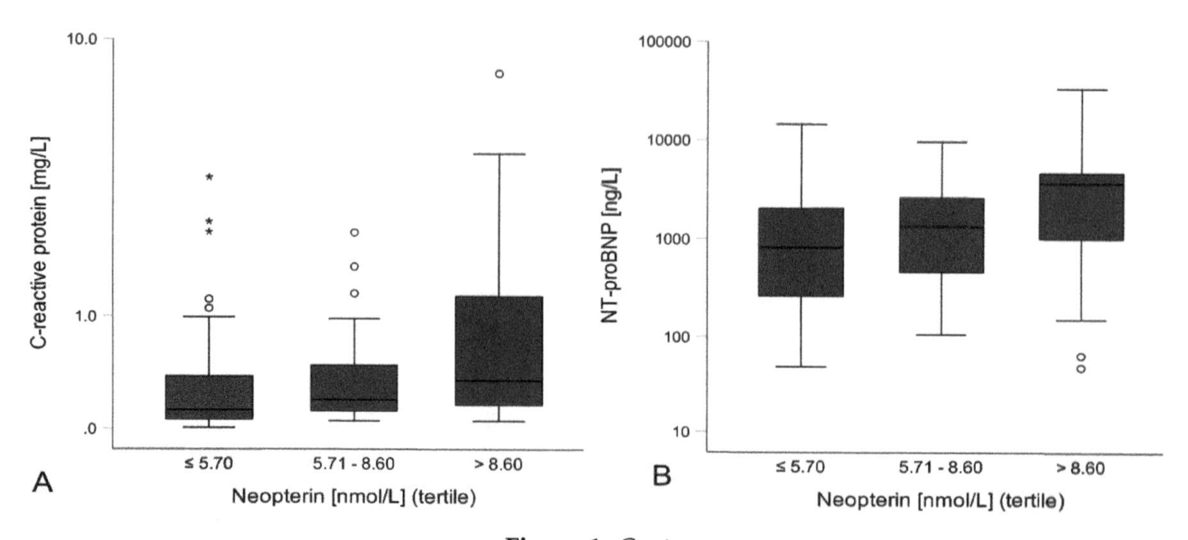

Figure 1. *Cont.*

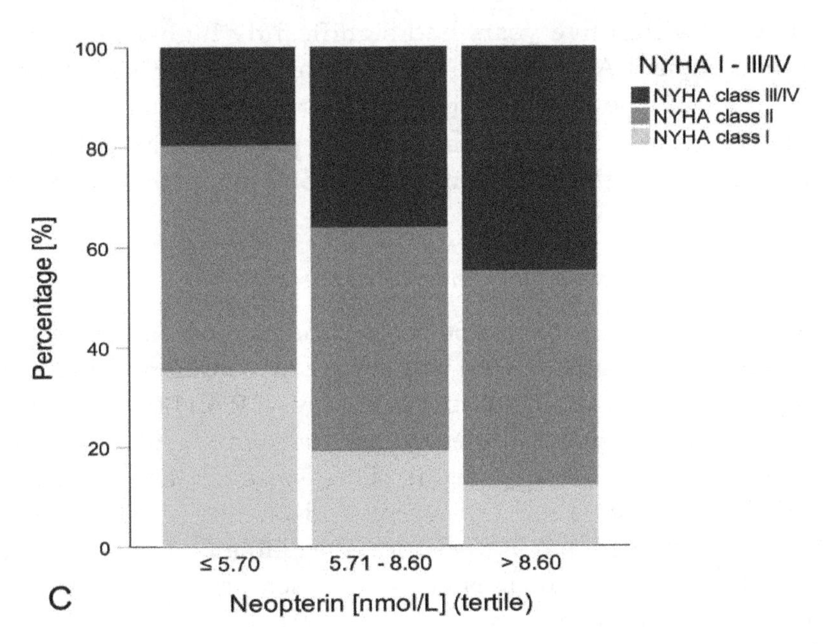

Figure 1. Inflammation and HF severity: Higher neopterin concentrations were associated with higher CRP (**A**) and NT-proBNP concentrations (**B**). Patients with higher neopterin concentrations also had higher NYHA classes (**C**).

CRP concentrations also correlated significantly with NT-proBNP concentrations (rs = 0.232, $p = 0.006$) and showed a positive dose-response relationship with increasing NYHA class (I: 0.16 mg/L, II: 0.17 mg/L, III/IV: 0.25 mg/L, $p = 0.030$).

3.2. Neopterin/eGFR Ratio and HF Severity

As patients with reduced eGFR (≤60 mL/min/1.73m^2) had significantly higher neopterin concentrations than patients with preserved kidney function (8.90 nmol/L vs. 6.00 nmol/L, $p < 0.001$), we adjusted neopterin concentrations for the kidney function and calculated a neopterin/eGFR ratio. Correlation analysis showed a highly significant correlation of the neopterin/eGFR ratio with NT-proBNP concentrations (rs = 0.438, $p < 0.001$), cardiac index (rs = −0.383, $p < 0.001$), right atrial pressure (RAP, rs = 0.172, $p = 0.041$), pulmonary artery mean pressure (mean PAP, rs = 0.281, $p = 0.001$) and pulmonary capillary wedge pressure (PCWP, rs = 0.302, $p < 0.001$). Patients with a higher NYHA class showed a significant higher neopterin/eGFR ratio (I: 0.060, II: 0.098, III/IV: 0.131, $p = 0.003$).

3.3. Neopterin/eGFR Ratio and Left Ventricular Ejection Fraction

The LV-EF was reduced (<40%) in 49.7% of our patients (Heart Failure with reduced Ejection Fraction—HFrEF), while 22.1% had a preserved LV-EF ≥ 50% (Heart Failure with preserved Ejection Fraction—HFpEF) and 21.5% a LV-EF between 40%–49.9% (Heart Failure with mid-range Ejection Fraction—HFmrEF). Patients with HFmrEF had the lowest neopterin concentrations (5.35 nmol/L, $p = 0.021$) and the highest eGFR (84.28 mL/min/1.73m2, $p = 0.003$) compared to patients with HFrEF and HFpEF (Appendix A, Table A1). Interestingly enough, neopterin concentrations did not differ significantly between patients with HFrEF and HFpEF (7.00 nmol/L vs. 7.40 nmol/L, $p = 0.235$), while patients with HFpEF had a significantly lower eGFR compared to patients with HFrEF (66.15 mL/min/1.73m2 vs. 76.48 mL/min/1.73m2, $p = 0.026$).

3.4. Laboratory Parameters and Event-Free Survival

The median follow-up of patients in this study was 58 months (0–98). A total of 40 patients reached the combined endpoint: 19 patients (12.8%) died and 21 patients (14.1%) were hospitalised for cardiac decompensation.

Patients with an event within five years had significantly higher neopterin and NT-proBNP concentrations, as well as a higher RAP and were found to have a higher NYHA class, while the cardiac index and eGFR were significantly lower compared to patients without an event. Interestingly enough, CRP concentrations, LV-EF, or age did not differ between patients with or without an event, while patients with an event showed a higher BMI compared to patients with no event (Table 1).

3.5. *Neopterin is a Predictor for an Adverse Outcome in Patients with HF*

Patients with neopterin concentrations >8.60 nmol/L (highest tertile) had a fourfold higher risk of reaching an endpoint compared to patients with neopterin concentrations ≤5.70 nmol/L (lowest tertile) in Cox regression analysis sex-stratified and adjusted for age (HR 4.118; 95% CI 1.727–9.820; $p = 0.001$; Figure 2A). The cumulative five-year event rates for the neopterin tertiles were 8.4% (≤5.70 nmol/L), 20.0% (5.71–8.60 nmol/L) and 46.6% (≥8.61 nmol/L). This was even independent of kidney function since a higher neopterin/eGFR ratio (logarithmised) was also predictive for future adverse events in Cox regression analysis sex-stratified and adjusted for age (Table 2). Patients with a neopterin/eGFR ratio ≥ 0.133 had a more than eightfold increased risk of reaching an endpoint compared to patients with a neopterin/eGFR ratio ≤ 0.065 (HR 8.380; 95% CI 2.889–24.308; $p < 0.001$, Figure 2B).

Table 2. Cox regression analysis.

Variable	Univariate Model			Multivariate Model		
	HR	95% CI	*p*-Value	HR	95% CI	*p*-Value
Neopterin (nmol/L) _Ln *	2.874	1.663–4.966	<0.001	2.770	1.419–5.407	0.003
eGFR (mL/min/1.73m²) _Ln	0.321	0.174–0.593	<0.001	2.723	0.936–7.926	0.066
NT-proBNP (ng/L) _Ln	1.665	1.253–2.214	<0.001	1.368	0.972–1.926	0.072
NYHA class II vs. I	2.542	0.852–7.578	0.094	3.200	0.830–12.329	0.091
NYHA class III/IV vs. I	3.245	1.070–9.840	0.038	3.126	0.751–13.006	0.117
LV-EF (%) _Ln	2.245	0.989–5.096	0.053	2.884	1.096–7.589	0.032
Neopterin/eGFR ratio _Ln	1.748	1.420–2.152	<0.001			
Cardiac index (L/min/m²) _Ln	0.250	0.062–1.008	0.051			
mean PAP (mmHg) _Ln	2.979	1.168–7.599	0.022			
PCWP (mmHg)_Ln	2.453	1.203–5.002	0.014			
RAP (mmHg) _Ln	3.536	1.584–7.894	0.002			
BMI (kg/m²) _Ln	0.188	0.032–1.114	0.066			

Univariate and multivariate Cox regression analyses models are adjusted for age and stratified for sex. * Neopterin levels were also adjusted for the eGFR in the univariate model. Variables showing a skewed distribution were logarithmised with the natural logarithm and marked with "_Ln". HR = hazard ratio; CI = confidence interval; eGFR = estimated glomerular filtration rate; NT-proBNP = N-terminal prohormone of brain natriuretic peptide; NYHA = New York Heart Association; LV-EF = left ventricular ejection fraction; mean PAP = pulmonary artery mean pressure; PCWP = pulmonary capillary wedge pressure; RAP = right atrial pressure; BMI = body mass index.

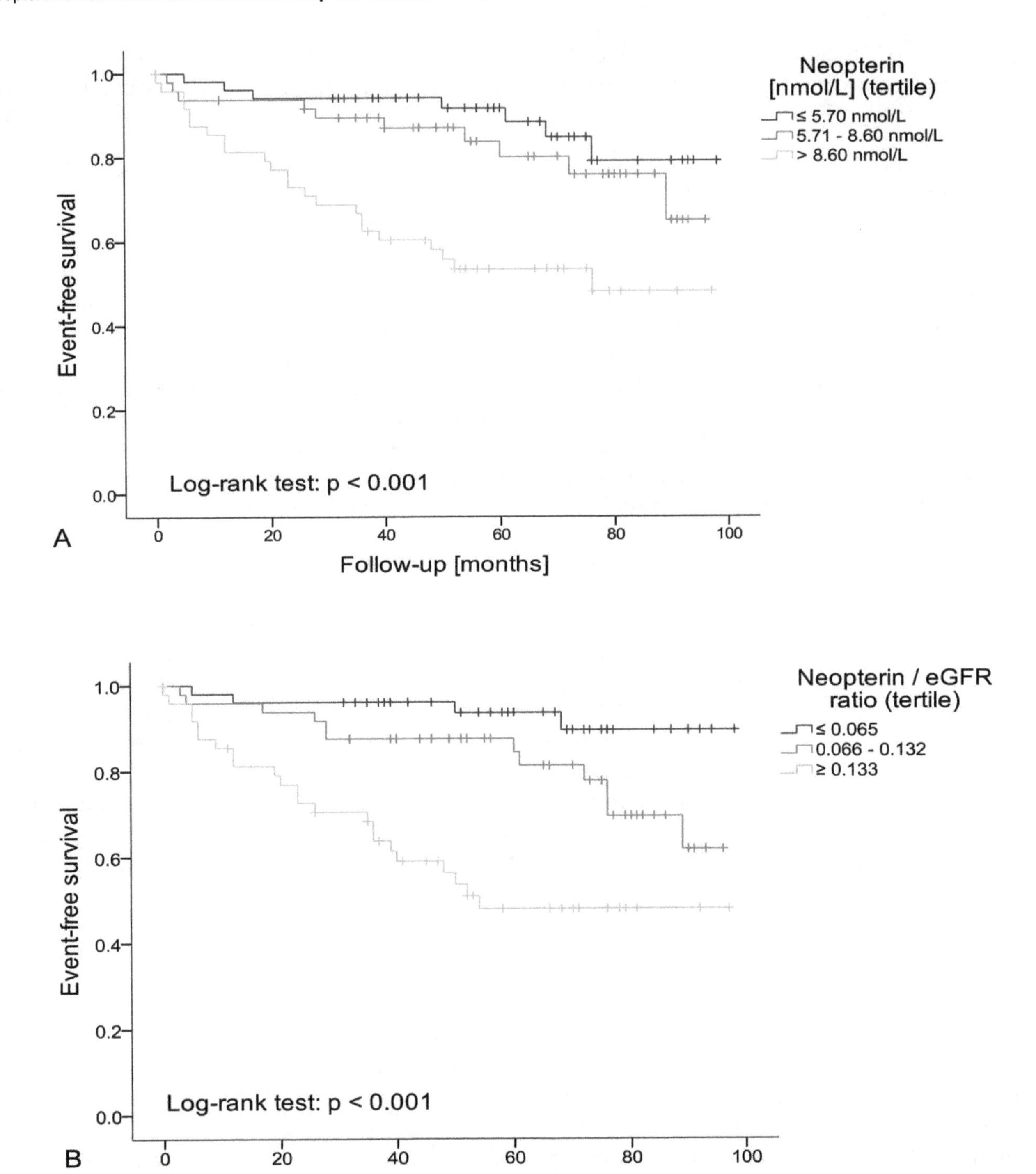

Figure 2. (**A**) Patients with higher neopterin levels (Neopterin > 8.60 nmol/L) had a fourfold higher risk of reaching an endpoint compared to patients within neopterin levels ≤5.70 nmol/L in Cox regression analysis sex-stratified and adjusted for age ($p = 0.001$); (**B**) The same was also true for patients with a higher neopterin/eGFR ratio: Patients with a neopterin/eGFR ratio ≥ 0.133 had a more than eight-fold increased risk of reaching an endpoint compared to patients with a neopterin/eGFR ratio ≤ 0.065 ($p < 0.001$).

A multivariate regression model stratified for sex was calculated with neopterin, age, eGFR, NT-proBNP, NYHA functional class, and LV-EF as co-variates that were considered clinically meaningful. Multivariate Cox regression analysis showed that baseline neopterin levels were associated with the combined endpoint, independently of established and widely available predictors of HF such as eGFR,

NT-proBNP, NYHA class and LV-EF (Table 2). Neopterin was also an independent predictor for an unfavourable outcome when correcting for co-medications (ACE inhibitor/ARB, beta-blocker, MRA, diuretics or cardiac glycosides) in Cox regression analysis. Patients with diuretics had significantly higher neopterin concentrations than those without (7.50 nmol/L vs. 5.80 nmol/L, $p = 0.001$).

4. Discussion

This study demonstrates that serum neopterin concentrations are linked to disease severity and can predict a worse outcome in patients with HF caused by non-ischaemic CMP. We also show that calculation of the neopterin/eGFR ratio is very useful to predict a worse outcome of patients and might be well suited as a "combined" marker for immune activation and decreased kidney function.

Recent studies have proposed a key role of inflammation in the determination of cardiovascular risk [28]. Levels of inflammatory cytokines are elevated in HF patients and related to an adverse outcome [29]. Activation of the immune system following cardiac injury is, per se, a protective (i.e., physiological) mechanism. Several studies have demonstrated that a short-term low-grade expression of stress-activated proinflammatory cytokines within the failing heart has beneficial consequences [30–32]. These cytokines induce the upregulation of so-called protective proteins in the heart that are part of the myocardial stress response such as cardiac hypertrophy, cardiac remodeling, and cardiac repair. However, the sustained or excessive expression of proinflammatory cytokines can cause tissue injury, consequently leading to progressive LV dysfunction and adverse LV remodeling [1,5,30]. Accordingly, patients with chronic inflammatory disease including rheumatoid arthritis [33], systemic lupus erythematosus [34] or atopic dermatitis [35] were shown to have an increased cardiovascular risk.

Our data show that higher neopterin concentrations, which originate from activated monocytes and macrophages upon stimulation with the proinflammatory cytokine IFN-γ, are associated with an impaired cardiac function: Elevated neopterin concentrations were found in patients with higher NYHA class, lower cardiac index, and increased NT-proBNP concentrations.

The association of neopterin concentrations with the combined endpoint was independent of age or sex and established predictors in HF such as NT-proBNP, NYHA class, eGFR, and LV-EF. Interestingly enough, CRP concentrations were not associated with the outcome in our population, although CRP is regarded as a powerful predictor of adverse outcome in cardiovascular disease (CVD) and HF [36]. While CRP is an acute phase protein and synthesised by the liver mainly upon IL-6 [37], neopterin is a more specific marker reflecting the interaction of T-cells (IFN-γ signalling) and monocytes/macrophages within Th1 immune activation. While CRP was shown earlier to be elevated in patients with acute cardiac events (unstable angina pectoris, non-ST-elevation myocardial infarction, or ST-elevation myocardial infarction), neopterin did not differ between these patients, but was predictive for a higher risk of an adverse long-term outcome in patients with coronary artery disease compared to high CRP concentrations [12].

There are only few studies in which CRP and neopterin levels were tested in parallel in large populations: In all these trials, neopterin was predictive for an increased cardiovascular mortality, but also for the overall mortality, independent of other established risk factors [12,14,19], and also independent of the acute phase marker CRP. Hazard ratios for adverse outcomes were higher for elevated neopterin concentrations as compared with high CRP concentrations in the LURIC study (patients with different kinds of cardiovascular diseases) [12,38], and neopterin was also predictive of an adverse outcome after adjusting for NT-ProBNP values, while CRP was not. Contrarily, in the HUSK study (population-based study in West Norway) CRP seemed slightly better for the prediction of CVD mortality, while IFN-γ-mediated inflammatory markers (neopterin and tryptophan degradation) better predicted non-CVD mortality [14]. Unfortunately, testing for neopterin is not performed in most routine labs, while the measurement of CRP is easily available everywhere.

Previous studies have also shown that neopterin, but not CRP, is associated with LV dysfunction [16] and predicts an increased cardiovascular risk [18] in patients with stable angina pectoris. On the other hand, elevated CRP levels are an established cardiovascular risk factor [39], which has also been used recently in the CANTOS trial, which assessed the effect of anti-inflammatory treatment with the monoclonal antibody Canakinumab (targeting interleukin-1β) in patients with prior myocardial infarction and elevated CRP [40]. Canakinumab was very effective in preventing adverse cardiac events and decreasing CRP concentrations in patients, indicating that the downregulation of chronic inflammatory processes is able to improve patient outcomes.

Considering this possible role of immune activation in the pathogenesis of cardiovascular disease, the determination of other inflammatory markers like neopterin appears to be a promising strategy to assess the actual risk of HF patients for a cardiovascular event. In particular, it may also serve as decision-making tool for anti-inflammatory therapy to decide if immune activation is over-whelming or within the normal range. In our population, the neopterin/eGFR ratio was also correlated with all relevant risk markers as well as with HF severity and it was predictive for a worse outcome. Calculation of the neopterin/eGFR ratio might in fact allow an even better risk stratification of patients with HF, as it combines the information from two risk factors (inflammation and decreased renal function). Thus, it would certainly be interesting to investigate the predictive power of this combined marker in future HF trials with a higher number of patients.

Still, it has to be emphasised that there are also other very important factors that contribute importantly to the development of inflammation. Moreover, the interaction between genetic and environmental factors might play a prominent role and significantly modulates inflammatory processes [41]. In patients with HF other mechanisms such as transthyretin amyloidosis or HF with preserved ejection fraction should also be investigated in more detail [42]. Further studies examining the effects of an impaired cholesterol efflux, which is linked to an increased CV risk, might provide interesting new data [43]. Last but not least, the role of diet should be evaluated in more detail in patients with CVD and HF. A very interesting recent study reviewed the impact of diet on inflammation, and in fact, the change of diet might represent a relatively easy and reasonable strategy to reduce the risk of CVD [41].

Strengths and Limitations

This study shows the clinical potential of neopterin and neopterin/eGFR ratio for the prediction of the course of CHF. Unfortunately, neopterin and CRP were not available in all patients who were initially included in the study, which resulted in a smaller sample size. This must be taken into account when interpreting the results of multivariate Cox regression analysis. The fact that the study was carried out with patients with non-ischemic CMP does not allow for a sweeping generalisation about all HF patients. The collection of event data, including patients questioning themselves and relative driven information, also represents a certain bias.

5. Conclusions

This study indicates that Th_1 immune activation, reflected by neopterin concentrations, plays a crucial role in the pathogenesis of HF caused by nonischaemic CMP. Neopterin concentrations as well as the neopterin/eGFR ratio are linked to disease severity and are associated with disease progression and an adverse outcome for patients with HF. Further longitudinal studies with a higher number of patients are needed to prove the role of neopterin in HF.

Author Contributions: Conceptualization, G.W. and G.P.; methodology, G.W. and G.P.; software, L.L. and K.K.; validation, L.L., G.P., D.F., G.W., and K.K.; formal analysis, L.L. and K.K.; investigation, L.L. and K.K.; data curation, L.L. and K.K.; writing—original draft preparation, L.L. and K.K.; writing—review and editing, G.W., G.P. and D.F.; visualization, L.L.

Appendix A

Table A1. Heart failure classification, demographic and clinical characteristics and laboratory measurements.

Variable	HFrEF, LV-EF < 40%	HFmrEF, LV-EF 40–49.9%	HFpEF, LV-EF ≥ 50%	Sig.
	n = 74 Median (IQR)	n = 32 Median (IQR)	n = 33 Median (IQR)	p-Value
Demographic and clinical characteristics				
Age (years)	46.3 (36.2–55.8)	46.3 (35.3–55.8)	55.6 (48.2–69.2)	0.005
BMI (kg/m^2)	24.00 (21.60–27.30)	24.76 (22.35–28.05)	24.40 (22.00–28.90)	0.516
Heart rate (bpm)	72 (63–85)	69 (60–79)	70 (60–81)	0.385
Syst. BP (mmHg)	115 (110 – 140)	126 (110–140)	126 (120–150)	0.003
Laboratory measurements				
Neopterin (nmol/L)	7.00 (5.20–9.20)	5.35 (3.95–8.10)	7.40 (5.90–11.50)	0.021
CRP (mg/L)	0.24 (0.13–0.63)	0.25 (0.07–0.63)	0.15 (0.10–0.25)	0.120
eGFR (mL/min/1.73m^2)	76.48 (58.09–94.34)	84.28 (71.12–101.40)	66.15 (54.16–74.23)	0.003
Neopterin/eGFR ratio	0.104 (0.059–0.144)	0.061 (0.046–0.103)	0.126 (0.082–0.190)	0.005
NT-proBNP (ng/L)	2072 (949–3681)	198 (96–745)	1989 (703–4644)	<0.001

Data from 149 patients are presented as medians (interquartile range). Parameters that differed significantly are printed in italic letters. HFrEF = Heart failure with reduced Ejection Fraction; HFmrEF = Heart failure with mid-range Ejection Fraction; HFpEF = Heart Failure with preserved Ejection Fraction; IQR = interquartile range; BMI = body mass index; Syst. BP = systolic blood pressure; CRP = C-reactive protein; eGFR = estimated glomerular filtration rate; NT-proBNP = N-terminal prohormone of brain natriuretic peptide; RAP = right atrial pressure; mean PAP = mean pulmonary artery pressure.

References

1. Medzhitov, R. Inflammation 2010: New adventures of an old flame. *Cell* **2010**, *140*, 771–776. [CrossRef]
2. Dick, S.A.; Epelman, S. Chronic heart failure and inflammation: What do we really know? *Circ. Res.* **2016**, *119*, 159–176. [CrossRef] [PubMed]
3. Torre-Amione, G.; Kapadia, S.; Lee, J.; Durand, J.B.; Bies, R.D.; Young, J.B.; Mann, D.L. Tumor necrosis factor-alpha and tumor necrosis factor receptors in the failing human heart. *Circulation* **1996**, *93*, 704–711. [CrossRef] [PubMed]
4. Vasan, R.S.; Sullivan, L.M.; Roubenoff, R.; Dinarello, C.A.; Harris, T.; Benjamin, E.J.; Sawyer, D.B.; Levy, D.; Wilson, P.W.; D'Agostino, R.B.; et al. Inflammatory markers and risk of heart failure in elderly subjects without prior myocardial infarction: The Framingham Heart Study. *Circulation* **2003**, *107*, 1486–1491. [CrossRef]
5. Mann, D.L. Innate immunity and the failing heart: The cytokine hypothesis revisited. *Circ. Res.* **2015**, *116*, 1254–1268. [CrossRef] [PubMed]
6. Jankowska, E.A.; Ponikowski, P.; Piepoli, M.F.; Banasiak, W.; Anker, S.D.; Poole-Wilson, P.A. Autonomic imbalance and immune activation in chronic heart failure—pathophysiological links. *Cardiovasc. Res.* **2006**, *70*, 434–445. [CrossRef]
7. Libby, P.; Lichtman, A.H.; Hansson, G.K. Immune effector mechanisms implicated in atherosclerosis: From mice to humans. *Immunity* **2013**, *38*, 1092–1104. [CrossRef]
8. Niebauer, J.; Volk, H.D.; Kemp, M.; Dominguez, M.; Schumann, R.R.; Rauchhaus, M.; Poole-Wilson, P.A.; Coats, A.J.; Anker, S.D. Endotoxin and immune activation in chronic heart failure: A prospective cohort study. *Lancet* **1999**, *353*, 1838–1842. [CrossRef]
9. Hasper, D.; Hummel, M.; Kleber, F.X.; Reindl, I.; Volk, H.D. Systemic inflammation in patients with heart failure. *Eur. Heart J.* **1998**, *19*, 761–765. [CrossRef]
10. Suzuki, K.; Nakaji, S.; Yamada, M.; Totsuka, M.; Sato, K.; Sugawara, K. Systemic inflammatory response to exhaustive exercise. Cytokine kinetics. *Exerc. Immunol. Rev.* **2002**, *8*, 6–48.
11. Shephard, R.J. Sepsis and mechanisms of inflammatory response: Is exercise a good model? *Br. J. Sports Med.* **2001**, *35*, 223–230. [CrossRef] [PubMed]
12. Grammer, T.B.; Fuchs, D.; Boehm, B.O.; Winkelmann, B.R.; Maerz, W. Neopterin as a predictor of total and cardiovascular mortality in individuals undergoing angiography in the Ludwigshafen Risk and Cardiovascular Health study. *Clin. Chem.* **2009**, *55*, 1135–1146. [CrossRef] [PubMed]

13. Fuchs, D.; Avanzas, P.; Arroyo-Espliguero, R.; Jenny, M.; Consuegra-Sanchez, L.; Kaski, J.C. The role of neopterin in atherogenesis and cardiovascular risk assessment. *Curr. Med. Chem.* **2009**, *16*, 4644–4653. [CrossRef] [PubMed]
14. Zuo, H.; Ueland, P.M.; Ulvik, A.; Eussen, S.J.; Vollset, S.E.; Nygård, O.; Midttun, Ø.; Theofylaktopoulou, D.; Meyer, K.; Tell, G.S. Plasma biomarkers of inflammation, the kynurenine pathway, and risks of all-cause, cancer, and cardiovascular disease mortality: The Hordaland health study. *Am. J. Epidemiol.* **2016**, *183*, 249–258. [CrossRef] [PubMed]
15. Weiss, G.; Willeit, J.; Kiechl, S.; Fuchs, D.; Jarosch, E.; Oberhollenzer, F.; Reibnegger, G.; Tilz, G.P.; Gerstenbrand, F.; Wachter, H. Increased concentrations of neopterin in carotid atherosclerosis. *Atherosclerosis* **1994**, *106*, 263–271. [CrossRef]
16. Estévez-Loureiro, R.; Recio-Mayoral, A.; Sieira-Rodríguez-Moret, J.A.; Trallero-Araguás, E.; Kaski, J.C. Neopterin levels and left ventricular dysfunction in patients with chronic stable angina pectoris. *Atherosclerosis* **2009**, *207*, 514–518. [CrossRef]
17. Avanzas, P.; Arroyo-Espliguero, R.; Quiles, J.; Roy, D.; Kaski, J.C. Elevated serum neopterin predicts future adverse cardiac events in patients with chronic stable angina pectoris. *Eur. Heart J.* **2005**, *26*, 457–463. [CrossRef]
18. Bjørnestad, E.; Borsholm, R.A.; Svingen, G.F.T.; Pedersen, E.R.; Seifert, R.; Midttun, Ø.; Ueland, P.M.; Tell, G.S.; Bønaa, K.H.; Nygård, O. Neopterin as an effect modifier of the cardiovascular risk predicted by total homocysteine: A prospective 2-cohort study. *J. Am. Heart Assoc.* **2017**, *6*, e006500. [CrossRef]
19. Ray, K.K.; Morrow, D.A.; Sabatine, M.S.; Shui, A.; Rifai, N.; Cannon, C.P.; Braunwald, E. Long-term prognostic value of neopterin: A novel marker of monocyte activation in patients with acute coronary syndrome. *Circulation* **2007**, *115*, 3071–3078. [CrossRef]
20. Nathan, C.F.; Murray, H.W.; Wiebe, M.E.; Rubin, B.Y. Identification of interferon-gamma as the lymphokine that activates human macrophage oxidative metabolism and antimicrobial activity. *J. Exp. Med.* **1983**, *158*, 670–689. [CrossRef]
21. Eisenhut, M. Neopterin in diagnosis and monitoring of infectious diseases. *J. Biomark.* **2013**, *2013*, 196432. [CrossRef] [PubMed]
22. Wirleitner, B.; Reider, D.; Ebner, S.; Böck, G.; Widner, B.; Jaeger, M.; Schennach, H.; Romani, N.; Fuchs, D. Monocyte-derived dendritic cells release neopterin. *J. Leukoc. Biol.* **2002**, *72*, 1148–1153. [PubMed]
23. Gostner, J.M.; Becker, K.; Fuchs, D.; Sucher, R. Redox regulation of the immune response. *Redox. Rep.* **2013**, *18*, 88–94. [CrossRef] [PubMed]
24. Berg, K.S.; Stenseth, R.; Pleym, H.; Wahba, A.; Videm, V. Neopterin predicts cardiac dysfunction following cardiac surgery. *Interact. Cardiovasc. Thorac. Surg.* **2015**, *21*, 598–603. [CrossRef] [PubMed]
25. Caruso, R.; De Chiara, B.; Campolo, J.; Verde, A.; Musca, F.; Belli, O.; Parolini, M.; Cozzi, L.; Moreo, A.; Frigerio, M.; et al. Neopterin levels are independently associated with cardiac remodeling in patients with chronic heart failure. *Clin. Biochem.* **2013**, *46*, 94–98. [CrossRef] [PubMed]
26. Yamamoto, E.; Hirata, Y.; Tokitsu, T.; Kusaka, H.; Tabata, N.; Tsujita, K.; Yamamuro, M.; Kaikita, K.; Watanabe, H.; Hokimoto, S.; et al. The clinical significance of plasma neopterin in heart failure with preserved left ventricular ejection fraction. *ESC Heart Fail.* **2016**, *3*, 53–59. [CrossRef]
27. Karabacak, M.; Doğan, A.; Varol, E.; Uysal, B.A.; Yıldız, İ. Comparison of Inflammatory Markers in Patients with Ischemic and Non-ischemic Heart Failure. *J. Am. Coll. Cardiol.* **2013**, *62*, C137–C138. [CrossRef]
28. Sorriento, D.; Iaccarino, G. Inflammation and cardiovascular diseases: The most recent findings. *Int. J. Mol. Sci.* **2019**, *20*, 3879. [CrossRef]
29. Fiordelisi, A.; Iaccarino, G.; Morisco, C.; Coscioni, E.; Sorriento, D. NFkappaB is a key player in the crosstalk between inflammation and cardiovascular diseases. *Int. J. Mol. Sci.* **2019**, *20*, 1599. [CrossRef]
30. Mann, D.L. Stress-activated cytokines and the heart: From adaptation to maladaptation. *Annu. Rev. Physiol.* **2003**, *65*, 81–101. [CrossRef]
31. Samsonov, M.; Fuchs, D.; Reibnegger, G.; Belenkov, J.N.; Nassonov, E.L.; Wachter, H. Patterns of serological markers for cellular immune activation in patients with dilated cardiomyopathy and chronic myocarditis. *Clin. Chem.* **1992**, *38*, 678–680. [PubMed]
32. Rudzite, V.; Skards, J.I.; Fuchs, D.; Reibnegger, G.; Wachter, H. Serum kynurenine and neopterin concentrations in patients with cardiomyopathy. *Immunol. Lett.* **1992**, *32*, 125–129. [CrossRef]

33. England, B.R.; Thiele, G.M.; Anderson, D.R.; Mikuls, T.R. Increased cardiovascular risk in rheumatoid arthritis: Mechanisms and implications. *BMJ* **2018**, *361*, k1036. [CrossRef] [PubMed]
34. Sinicato, N.A.; da Silva Cardoso, P.A.; Appenzeller, S. Risk factors in cardiovascular disease in systemic lupus erythematosus. *Curr. Cardiol. Rev.* **2013**, *9*, 15–19. [CrossRef] [PubMed]
35. Silverwood, R.J.; Forbes, H.J.; Abuabara, K.; Ascott, A.; Schmidt, M.; Schmidt, S.A.J.; Smeeth, L.; Langan, S.M. Severe and predominantly active atopic eczema in adulthood and long term risk of cardiovascular disease: Population based cohort study. *BMJ* **2018**, *361*, k1786. [CrossRef] [PubMed]
36. Araújo, J.P.; Lourenço, P.; Azevedo, A.; Friões, F.; Rocha-Gonçalves, F.; Ferreira, A.; Bettencourt, P. Prognostic value of high-sensitivity C-reactive protein in heart failure: A systematic review. *J. Card. Fail.* **2009**, *15*, 256–266. [CrossRef] [PubMed]
37. Abrams, J. C-reactive protein, inflammation, and coronary risk: An update. *Cardiol. Clin.* **2003**, *21*, 327–331. [CrossRef]
38. Avanzas, P.; Arroyo-Espliguero, R.; Kaski, J.C. Neopterin—marker of coronary artery disease activity or extension in patients with chronic stable angina? *Int. J. Cardiol.* **2010**, *144*, 74–75. [CrossRef]
39. Fonseca, F.A.; Izar, M.C. High-sensitivity C-reactive protein and cardiovascular disease across countries and ethnicities. *Clinics* **2016**, *71*, 235–242. [CrossRef]
40. Ridker, P.M.; Everett, B.M.; Thuren, T.; MacFadyen, J.G.; Chang, W.H.; Ballantyne, C.; Fonseca, F.; Nicolau, J.; Koenig, W.; Anker, S.D.; et al. Antiinflammatory therapy with canakinumab for atherosclerotic disease. *N. Engl. J. Med.* **2017**, *377*, 1119–1131. [CrossRef]
41. Gambardella, J.; Santulli, G. Integrating diet and inflammation to calculate cardiovascular risk. *Atherosclerosis* **2016**, *253*, 258–261. [CrossRef] [PubMed]
42. Michels da Silva, D.; Langer, H.; Graf, T. Inflammatory and molecular pathways in heart failure-ischemia, HFpEF and transthyretin cardiac amyloidosis. *Int. J. Mol. Sci.* **2019**, *20*, 2322. [CrossRef] [PubMed]
43. Riggs, K.A.; Joshi, P.H.; Khera, A.; Singh, K.; Akinmolayemi, O.; Ayers, C.R.; Rohatgi, A. Impaired HDL metabolism links GlycA, A novel inflammatory marker, with incident cardiovascular events. *J. Clin. Med.* **2019**, *8*, 2137. [CrossRef] [PubMed]

13

Depressed Myocardial Energetic Efficiency Increases Risk of Incident Heart Failure: The Strong Heart Study

Maria-Angela Losi [1,2], Raffaele Izzo [1,2], Costantino Mancusi [1,2], Wenyu Wang [3], Mary J. Roman [4], Elisa T. Lee [5], Barbara V. Howard [6], Richard B. Devereux [4] and Giovanni de Simone [1,2,4,*]

1 Hypertension Research Center, University Federico II of Naples, I-80131 Naples, Italy
2 Department of Advanced Biomedical Sciences, University Federico II of Naples, I-80131 Naples, Italy
3 College of Public Health, University of Oklahoma Health Sciences Center, Oklahoma City, OK 73104, USA
4 Department of Medicine, Weill Cornell Medical College, New York, NY 10065, USA
5 Center for American Indian Health Research, University of Oklahoma Health Sciences Center, Oklahoma City, OK 73126, USA
6 Medstar Health Research Institute, and Georgetown-Howard Universities Center for Translational Sciences, Washington, DC 20057, USA
* Correspondence: simogi@unina.it

Abstract: An estimation of myocardial mechano-energetic efficiency (MEE) per unit of left ventricular (LV) mass (MEEi) can significantly predict composite cardiovascular (CV) events in treated hypertensive patients with normal ejection fraction (EF), after adjustment for LV hypertrophy (LVH). We have tested whether MEEi predicts incident heart failure (HF), after adjustment for LVH, in the population-based cohort of a "Strong Heart Study" (SHS) with normal EF. We included 1912 SHS participants (age 59 ± 8 years; 64% women) with preserved EF (≥50%) and without prevalent CV disease. MEE was estimated as the ratio of stroke work to the "double product" of heart rate times systolic blood pressure. MEEi was calculated as MEE/LV mass, and analyzed in quartiles. During a follow-up study of 9.2 ± 2.3 years, 126 participants developed HF (7%). HF was preceded by acute myocardial infarction (AMI) in 94 participants. A Kaplan-Meier plot, in quartiles of MEEi, demonstrated significant differences, substantially due to the deviation of the lowest quartile ($p < 0.0001$). Using AMI as a competing risk event, sequential models of Cox regression for incident HF (including significant confounders), demonstrated that low MEEi predicted incident HF not due to AMI ($p = 0.026$), after adjustment for significant effect of age, LVH, prolonged LV relaxation, diabetes, and smoking habits with negligible effects for sex, hypertension, antihypertensive therapy, obesity, and hyperlipemia. Low LV mechano-energetic efficiency per unit of LVM, is a predictor of incident, non-AMI related, HF in subjects with initially normal EF.

Keywords: left ventricular hypertrophy; heart failure with preserved ejection fraction; population study; stroke volume; heart rate; echocardiography

---

1. Introduction

Heart failure (HF) is predominantly a disease of the elderly, with nearly 50% of patients having preserved (p) left ventricular (LV) ejection fraction (EF) [1]. Although mechanisms for HFpEF remain incompletely understood, diastolic dysfunction, because it underlies myocardial hypertrophy and fibrosis, is thought to play a dominant role [2]. However, diastolic dysfunction also occurs in systolic HF (HFrEF) and is also common in elderly hypertensive individuals without HF [3]. Thus, abnormalities other than diastolic function are likely to be involved in HFpEF, especially in the presence of LV hypertrophy (LVH) [4].

There is evidence that pressure-overload LVH preserves EF as a measure of LV systolic function at the chamber level, even when contractility is reduced at the level of cardiomyocytes [5]. However, when paralleling the magnitude of LV chamber dimensions, even at normal values of LV systolic chamber function, important differences can occur in the magnitude of stroke volume (SV, i.e. LV pump performance), heart rate (HR), and blood pressure (BP) [6]. As a consequence, at a given EF, hemodynamic workload might differ substantially [6] and, in fact, SV is more predictive of incident HF than EF [7].

A new parameter of LV performance has been recently proposed as a surrogate measure of myocardial mechano-energetic efficiency (MEE), which is the ratio between produced external systolic work (stroke work, SW) and an estimate of myocardial oxygen consumption (MVO2) [8]. MEE per unit of LV mass (MEEi) has been demonstrated to predict composite adverse cardiovascular (CV) events in treated hypertensive patients after adjustment for LVH [9].

One unexplored issue is whether MEEi can also help explain incidence of HF, after adjustment for LVH, in the presence of initial normal EF in population studies. Accordingly, this analysis has been designed to assess whether MEEi can improve the identification of phenotypes at high risk of incident HF in members of the "Strong Heart Study" (SHS) cohort who were free of prevalent cardiovascular (CV) disease and initially had normal EF.

2. Methods

2.1. Participants

We analyzed data from the SHS, a population-based cohort study of CV risk factors and disease in American Indians. Detailed descriptions of the study design and methods have been previously reported [10]. At time of enrollment, a total of 4549 American Indian men and women, aged 45 to 74 years, from communities in Arizona, southwestern Oklahoma, and South and North Dakota participated in the first SHS examination, conducted from 1989 to 1991 (phase 1). The cohort was followed and re-examined twice and has been under continuous yearly surveillance for CV events. The second examination evaluated 89% of all surviving members of the original cohort, who also underwent standard Doppler echocardiography. Thus, the second SHS examination was used as baseline for the present analysis.

From the population of 2794 participants available for the analysis, we excluded 441 participants with prevalent CV (220 with a history of myocardial infarction or cardiac ischemic disease, 44 with a history of stroke and 177 with chronic heart failure) and 94 for low ejection fraction (i.e <50%), 14 because of serum triglycerides (>750 mg/dL), and 333 participants because of incomplete echocardiographic assessment. Thus, for the present study, we included 1912 SHS participants (age 59 ± 8 years; 64% women) with baseline preserved EF and without prevalent CV disease. Institutional review boards of the participating institutions and the participating tribes approved the study and submission of the manuscript.

2.2. Measurements and Definitions

The SHS used standard methodology and strict quality control at each clinical examination [11], which included a personal interview, physical examination with anthropometric and blood pressure measurement, and morning blood sample collection after a 12-hour fast. Exams were performed at local community settings and Indian Health Service clinics by trained study staff.

Arterial hypertension was defined as blood pressure ≥140/90 mmHg or current antihypertensive treatment. Obesity was classified as body mass index ≥30 kg/m^2. Diabetes was defined as fasting glucose ≥126 mg/dL or use of antidiabetic medication. Hyperlipemia was defined as total cholesterol

>200 mg/dL and/or triglyceridemic value >150 mg/dL. Smoking habits were defined as non-smoker, former smoker, and current smoker.

2.3. Echocardiography

Echocardiograms were performed using phased-array machines, with M-mode, two-dimensional, and Doppler capabilities, as previously reported [12]. Echocardiograms were evaluated in the Core Laboratory at the Weill Cornell Medical College in New York by expert readers blinded to the participant's clinical details, using a computerized review station (Digisonics, Inc., Houston, TX, USA) equipped with digitizing tablets and monitor screen overlays for calibration and performance of each needed measurement. Reproducibility of echocardiographic measures was tested in the Weill Cornell adult echocardiography laboratory in an ad hoc designed study [13].

LV internal dimensions and wall thickness were measured as end-diastole and end-systole, respectively, as previously reported [12]. Relative wall thickness, LV mass, and LV mass index (by normalization for height in $m^{2.7}$) were also estimated [6]. LVH was defined with LV mass index >47 $g/m^{2.7}$ for both sexes, a validated population-specific cut-point, maximizing the population risk attributable to LVH [14]. SV was calculated as the difference between LV end-diastolic and end-systolic volumes by the z-derived method [6,15]. EF was obtained by the ratio of SV to end-diastolic volume. Midwall fractional shortening was measured as previously described [16].

The ratio of early to late peak diastolic velocities (E/A ratio) was measured as previously described [17]. Based on previous analyses in the SHS, the E/A ratio was categorized as "normal" when it was between 0.6 and 1.5, in "prolonged relaxation" when it was <0.6 and in "restrictive physiology" when it was >1.5 [17].

To assess MEE, we estimated SW as the product of systolic BP times SV (mmHg × mL). Myocardial oxygen consumption (MVO2) could be estimated using the "double product" (DP) of systolic BP × heart rate [18]. Using this second method, MEE may be estimated in mL/s:

$$MEE = \frac{SW}{DP} \approx \frac{mmHg \times mL}{mmHg \times bpm} = \frac{mL}{bpm \times 60^{-1}} = \frac{mL}{s} \quad (1)$$

Because of the reportedly close dependence of MEE on LV mass, normalization for LV mass was done to estimate energetic expenditure per unit of myocardial mass (MEEi in mL/s/g) [9].

2.4. Outcome

CV events were recorded and adjudicated as previously reported using standardized criteria. [10]. The end-point of the present study was the first occurrence of HF, defined by the Framingham criteria for HF, as previously described [7]. Due to the potential interference with the analyzed outcome, occurrence of acute myocardial infarction (AMI) prior to HF was also censored for analysis as a competing risk event.

2.5. Statistical Analysis

Data were analyzed using IBM-SPSS-statistics (version 23.0; SPSS, New Jersey), and expressed as mean ± 1SD. MEEi was categorized in quartiles and analyzed in exploratory analyses, using linear contrast for trend analysis for age and Kendall's tau as a test for monotonic trends with categorical variables. Cumulative incidences of HF in quartiles of MEEi were analyzed using a Kaplan-Meier plot. Further analyses were focused on the lowest MEEi (corresponding to 25th percentile of the distribution).

We calculated hazard ratios and 95% confidence intervals (CI) of incident HF, using three sequential models of Cox regression. In the first Cox model, the outcome was analyzed in relation to LVH and patterns of E/A ratio, adjusting for age and sex. In the second model, low MEEi, hypertension and anti-hypertensive therapy (no/yes) were forced into the model. In the third model, obesity and diabetes were added to explore how the previous models could be changed by the co-presence of additional CV risk factors. Since the end-point of the present analysis, HF, can also be a consequence of a preceding AMI, a Cox regression was run using AMI preceding HF as a competing risk event. Thus, we censored AMI occurring before HF, in competition with the primary predictor, MEEi [19].

3. Results

Among 1912 SHS participants with normal EF and without prevalent CV disease included in this analysis, prevalence of arterial hypertension, obesity, and diabetes were 27, 51, and 40%, respectively.

Table 1 shows that while age was similar among quartiles of MEEi, the proportion of women was progressively lower with decreasing quartiles of MEEi, and concentric LV geometry and LVH were progressively higher (all p for trend <0.0001), paralleling the progressive increase in prevalent hypertension, obesity, and diabetes (all p for trend <0.0001). There was a significant trend for mitral E/A ratios of <0.6 to sharply increase in the lowest quartile of MEEi, whereas mitral E/A ratios of >1.5 progressively decreased with decreasing quartiles of MEEi (all p for trend <0.0001). Hyperlipemia and smoking habits were not different within quartiles of MEEi.

Table 1. Characteristics of quartiles of LV mass-normalized myocardial mechano-energetic efficiency (MEEi).

		Quartiles of Indexed Myocardial Mechano-Energetic Efficiency			
	Whole Population (n = 1912)	**≥0.45 (n = 478)**	**0.40–0.44 (n = 477)**	**0.35–0.39 (n = 479)**	**≤0.34 (n = 478)**
Age (years)	59 ± 8	59 ± 8	60 ± 8	59 ± 8	60 ± 8
Hypertension (%) [a]	27%	22%	25%	29%	34%
Proportion of women (%) [a]	64%	68%	69%	65%	55%
Concentric LV geometry (%) [a]	4%	0.2 %	1%	2%	11%
LV Hypertrophy (%) [a]	23%	9%	18%	23%	40%
Mitral E/A ratio <0.6 (%) [a]	4.1	2.1	2.5	1.3	10.5
Mitral E/A ratio >1.5 (%) [a]	2.6	4.5	3.4	1.5	1.1
Obesity (%) [a]	51%	40%	51%	57%	58%
Diabetes (%) [a]	40%	25%	37%	41%	57%
Hyperlipemia (%)	58	57	55	59	62
Former smoker (%)	35	33	34	36	38
Current smoker	36	39	35	34	35

LV = left ventricular; [a] Kendall's τ-b: all $p < 0.0001$.

Although only patients with initially normal EF were included in this study, 12% of variability of EF was explained by MEEi, but the explained variability rises to 42% when LV systolic function was evaluated by midwall shortening.

During follow-up studies (median 9.9 years, inter-quartile range 9.3–10.4 years), 126 (7%) participants developed HF, 94 of them after AMI. A Kaplan-Meier cumulative hazard plot demonstrated a significant log-rank, substantially due to the marked deviation of the lowest quartiles of MEEi (Figure 1).

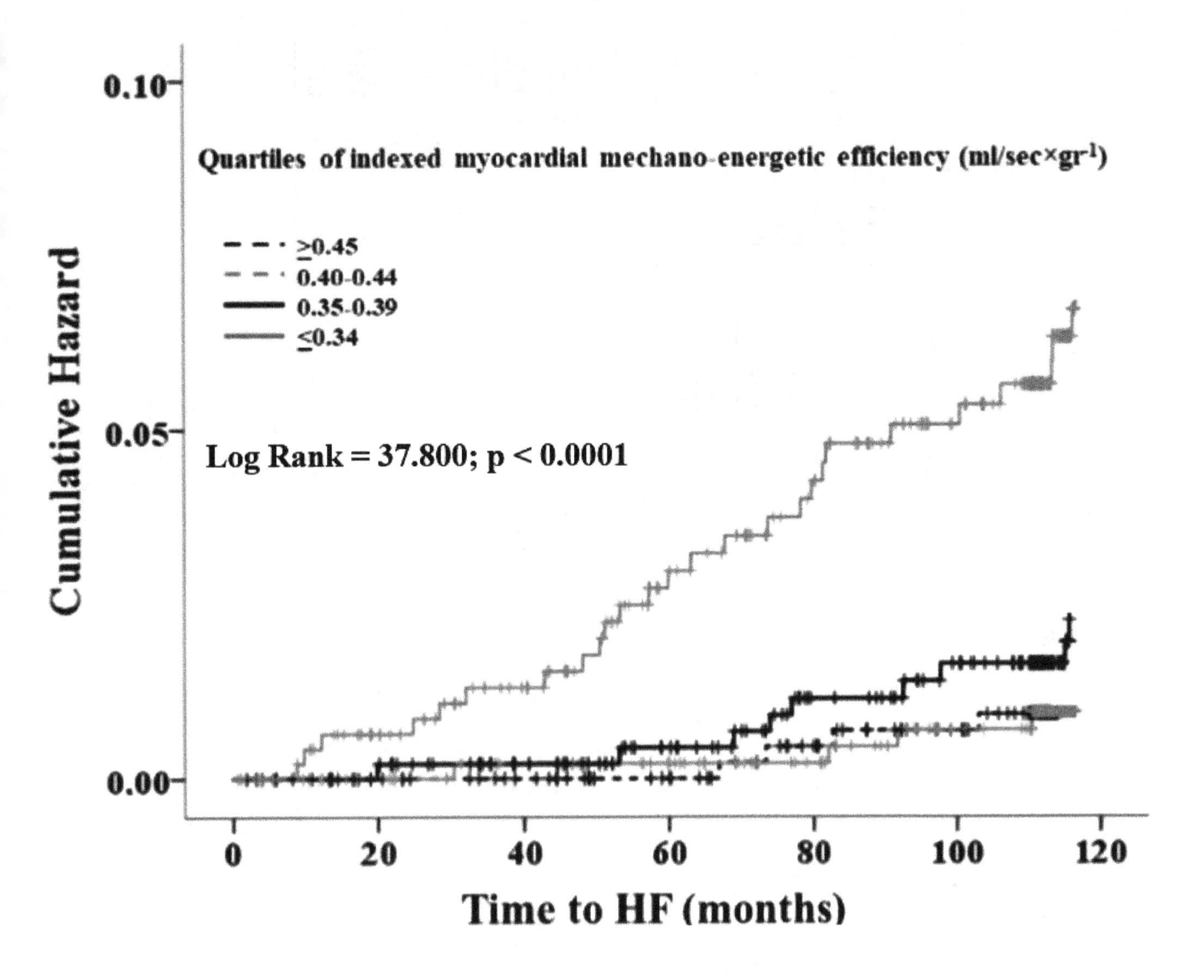

Figure 1. Cumulative hazard of incident heart failure (HF) for quartiles of myocardial mechano-energetic efficiency per unit of left ventricular mass (MEEi). Continuous grey line represents the lowest MEEi quartile.

As seen in Figure 1, we compared the lowest MEEi quartile (i.e. ≤ 0.34 mL $\times$ s^{-1} $\times$ g^{-1}) with all others, defined for convenience as "normal MEEi". Low MEEi was present in 47% of the subgroup, compared to 24% in the subgroup without incident HF ($p < 0.0001$). Table 2 shows sequential models of Cox regressions for incident HF. Low MEEi predicted incident HF after adjustment for LVH and prolonged relaxation. The impact of low MEEi was reduced after the inclusion of diabetes and smoking habits into the model.

The Cox models were also run using continuous variables for systolic blood pressure, body mass index, MEEi, and LV mass index instead of categories, without modifications, and compared to what has been reported in Table 2. Specifically, for each unit of increasing MEEi, there was a significant 2% reduction of hazard of incident-adverse CV events (hazard ratio (HR)= 0.02; 95% CI 0.002–0.347; $p < 0.006$).

A multicollinearity test was performed using all covariates of model 3 to calculate the variance inflation factor (VIF). The value of VIF was always <1.9, demonstrating optimal performance of the model and the low level of multicollinearity between LVH and low MEEi.

Table 2. Sequential models of proportional hazard analysis of incident heart failure (HF) in relation to low MEEi.

Predictors	Model 1			Model 2			Model 3		
	p	HR	95%CI	*p*	HR	95%CI	*p*	HR	95%CI
Age (years)	0.004	1.04	1.01–1.06	0.007	1.04	1.01–1.06	0.001	1.05	1.02–1.08
Female sex	0.666	0.93	0.62–1.38	0.846	0.96	0.63–1.46	0.833	1.05	0.68–1.61
LV Hypertrophy	<0.0001	2.51	1.70–3.73	0.001	2.01	1.37–3.10	0.004	1.89	1.23–2.91
E/A <0.6	<0.0001	3.72	1.99–6.98	0.002	2.85	1.48–5.51	0.004	2.60	1.35–5.05
E/A >1.5	0.612	0.60	0.08–4.33	0.629	0.61	0.09–4.43	0.800	0.77	0.11–5.60
Low MEEi				0.005	1.83	1.21–2.79	0.026	1.61	1.06–2.44
Hypertension				0.484	1.27	0.66–2.45	0.672	1.15	0.60–2.23
Anti-hypertensive therapy (y/n)				0.012	2.28	1.20–4.35	0.094	1.75	0.91–3.35
Diabetes							<0.0001	3.11	2.01–4.80
Obesity							0.191	0.76	0.50–1.15
Hyperlipemia							0.832	0.96	0.64–1.43
Former smoker							0.006	2.11	1.24–3.60
Current Smoker							0.003	2.38	1.35–4.17

LV = left ventricular; MEEi = indexed myocardial mechano-energetic efficiency; HR = hazard ratio.

4. Discussion

Our analysis demonstrates that in a population-based study with initially normal left ventricular ejection fraction (LVEF), reduced myocardial mechano-energetic efficiency for each g of myocardial mass is a strong predictor of incident HF after adjustment for LVH, prolonged relaxation, and associated CV risk factors, including hypertension, obesity, diabetes, and smoking habits. Our analysis merged CV risk factors with markers of preclinical CV disease. The causative effect of primary risk factors was largely offset by their direct effects on the CV system. The only risk factor that could not be fully offset by CV phenotype was diabetes, which in fact remains a potent risk factor for HF, even after adjustment for CV phenotype, as we have previously demonstrated [20].

In our analysis, we provided an estimation of myocardial energetic efficiency using a very simple method on the basis of a simple assumption, which has been already used in different circumstances [5,18], i.e., that MVO2 consumption mainly depends on developed pressure and frequency of contraction. More complex models of estimating myocardial oxygen consumption have been proposed, with strong rationale, but are likely less suitable for a clinical use [21].

4.1. The Conundrum of Development of HF

It is not surprising that a condition of low myocardial mechano-energetic efficiency per unit of myocardial mass significantly contributes to identifying a CV phenotype at risk of developing HF. The link between alterations of myocardial energy balance and HF should merit more attention, especially in the setting of HFpEF. Although we do not have follow-up echocardiograms to compare, we may postulate that incident HFpEF is frequent in our population sample, because our hazard analysis was controlled for incident, intercurrent AMI as a competing risk factor for incident HF, indirectly minimizing the chance that post-ischemic systolic HF could play a substantial role in our findings. Given the frustrating results related to the attempt to improve outcomes in HFpEF [22] and related to the insufficient understanding of its mechanisms, shifting the attention from hemodynamics and cardiac mechanics to the process of production and utilization of energy might be productive [23].

Although increased LV mass is in fact a critical marker of risk, considerable heterogeneity can be found, especially in the setting of HFpEF. In clinical trials and contemporary registries, approximately one-third to two-thirds of patients with HFpEF do not exhibit clear-cut LVH [24]. A proportion of HFpEF patients exhibit eccentric LVH rather than the more usual concentric pattern [24]. Even more intriguing is the evidence that approximately 50% of patients with HFpEF and normal LV mass do not have hypertension [24].

Furthermore, it is noteworthy that in this population with normal EF at baseline, MEEi could explain as much as 42% of midwall shortening variability, compared to the expected negligible correlation with ejection fraction. This finding is physiologically consistent with the assumption that LV systolic chamber function is only a very rough indicator of the status of myocardial mechanics.

Other pathogenetic mechanisms should be investigated.

4.2. Diastolic Dysfunction

Diastolic dysfunction is considered especially important in the context of HFpEF [24]. However, in echocardiographic sub-studies, one-third of patients randomized in controlled trials of HFpEF exhibited normal diastolic function, and a further 20% to 30% only had mild or grade 1 diastolic dysfunction [24]. In addition, a recent study of elderly subjects (age 67 to 90 years) without HF found that 96% of them had abnormal diastolic function, according to guideline-based definitions. In a condition in which diastolic dysfunction has been considered a definite pathophysiologic feature ("diastolic heart failure"), it is unclear whether the absence of diastolic dysfunction in HFpEF reflects a limitation of echocardiography, at least at the light of the present recommendations, or suggests pathophysiological mechanisms that are independent of diastolic function in a substantial proportion of patients. But, perhaps even more importantly, HF is always characterized by increased filling pressure (and therefore real diastolic dysfunction), no matter whether or not EF is reduced.

4.3. LV Production, Delivery, and Utilization of Energy

The evidence of impaired myocardial energy balance adds pathophysiological rationale to the strong effect of increased LV mass function as a marker of risk for HF. The index presented in this and in previous longitudinal analyses [9] allows a concentration of attention on physiological mechanisms more related to the production, delivery, and utilization of energy. While normal hearts mainly oxidize fatty acids to produce energy (ATP), hearts with stage B HF require a shift of production of energy (ATP) toward the most convenient glucose-pyruvate oxidation, a shift that implies adequate insulin sensitivity [25].

An important possible mechanism reducing myocardial efficiency is in fact insulin resistance [26]. The emerging evidence that this index is influenced by conditions of insulin resistance [25] is an indirect validation of our physiologic postulate. This is evident in the present and previous analyses in which diabetes exhibits a substantial importance as a predictor of HF, even more than hypertension (confirmed in the present analysis, as seen in Table 2). The progressive decline of MEEi with the increasing prevalence of diabetes and obesity was demonstrated previously in our Italian registry of hypertensive patients [9,25]. Insulin resistance, typical of type 2 diabetes, results in difficulty in the utilization of glucose [27], increasing reliance on fatty acid oxidation for up to 80–90% of acetyl CoA, at the expense of glucose and lactate oxidation [28]. This increase in fatty acid oxidation is the main determinant of the increased MVO2 at zero work, because of the lower oxygen efficiency for ATP synthesis using fatty acids as substrates [29].

Due to the above considerations and given the ethnic specificity of the SHS, and the particular high prevalence of diabetes and obesity, our findings are not necessarily generalizable and might need to be clarified in other populations with different genetic and environmental backgrounds, especially because algorithms for risk prediction might be substantially affected by prevalence and distribution of individual risk factors [30].

4.4. Final Considerations

Despite the strong association with incident HF, many unconsidered factors could have an impact on the progression of HF, potentially reducing the impact of baseline low myocardial mechano-energetic efficiency during follow-up. Among them, the control of diabetes or blood pressure during follow-up could have a significant impact on the progression of diastolic dysfunction and precipitation of HF. Further studies should help clarifying pathophysiological mechanisms linking myocardial mechano-energetic efficiency to diastolic dysfunction and control of blood pressure and diabetes.

5. Conclusions

This study demonstrated that depressed LV mechano-energetic efficiency per unit of LV mass, computed by using a simple approach comparing external work with the estimated oxygen consumption, is a powerful predictor of incident HF after adjustment for LVH and other confounders in an unselected population-based cohort of American Indians with normal baseline EF. Our results might serve as a hypothesis when testing for a better evaluation of pathophysiology of HFpEF.

Author Contributions: Conceptualization, M.A.L., R.I. and G.d.S.; Data curation, W.W., M.J.R., E.T.L., B.V.H. and R.B.D.; Formal analysis, M.A.L., R.I., C.M., R.B.D. and G.d.S.; Methodology, C.M., W.W., M.J.R., E.T.L., B.V.H. and R.B.D.; Validation C.M., W.W., M.J.R., E.T.L., B.V.H. and R.B.D.; Writing—original draft, M.A.L.; Writing—review & editing, M.A.L. and G.d.S.

References

1. Vasan, R.S.; Larson, M.G.; Benjamin, E.J.; Evans, J.C.; Reiss, C.K.; Levy, D. Congestive heart failure in subjects with normal versus reduced left ventricular ejection fraction: prevalence and mortality in a population-based cohort. *J. Am. Coll. Cardiol.* **1999**, *33*, 1948–1955. [CrossRef]
2. Zile, M.R.; Brutsaert, D.L. New concepts in diastolic dysfunction and diastolic heart failure: Part II: causal mechanisms and treatment. *Circulation* **2002**, *105*, 1503–1508. [CrossRef] [PubMed]
3. Kitzman, D.W. Diastolic dysfunction in the elderly. Genesis and diagnostic and therapeutic implications. *Cardiol. Clin.* **2000**, *18*, 597–617. [CrossRef]
4. Kawaguchi, M.; Hay, I.; Fetics, B.; Kass, D.A. Combined ventricular systolic and arterial stiffening in patients with heart failure and preserved ejection fraction: implications for systolic and diastolic reserve limitations. *Circulation* **2003**, *107*, 714–720. [CrossRef] [PubMed]
5. Laine, H.; Katoh, C.; Luotolahti, M.; Kantola, I.; Jula, A.; Takala, T.O.; Ruotsalainen, U.; Iida, H.; Haaparanta, M.; Nuutila, P.; et al. Myocardial Oxygen Consumption Is Unchanged but Efficiency Is Reduced in Patients With Essential Hypertension and Left Ventricular Hypertrophy. *Circulation* **1999**, *100*, 2425–2430. [CrossRef]
6. de Simone, G.; Izzo, R.; Aurigemma, G.P.; De Marco, M.; Rozza, F.; Trimarco, V.; Stabile, E.; De Luca, N.; Trimarco, B. Cardiovascular risk in relation to a new classification of hypertensive left ventricular geometric abnormalities. *J. Hypertens.* **2015**, *33*, 745–754. [CrossRef] [PubMed]
7. De Marco, M.; Gerdts, E.; Mancusi, C.; Roman, M.J.; Lonnebakken, M.T.; Lee, E.T.; Howard, B.V.; Devereux, R.B.; de Simone, G. Influence of Left Ventricular Stroke Volume on Incident Heart Failure in a Population With Preserved Ejection Fraction (from the Strong Heart Study). *Am. J. Cardiol.* **2017**, *119*, 1047–1052. [CrossRef]
8. de Simone, G.; Chinali, M.; Galderisi, M.; Benincasa, M.; Girfoglio, D.; Botta, I.; D'Addeo, G.; de Divitiis, O. Myocardial mechano-energetic efficiency in hypertensive adults. *J. Hypertens.* **2009**, *27*, 650–655. [CrossRef]
9. de Simone, G.; Izzo, R.; Losi, M.A.; Stabile, E.; Rozza, F.; Canciello, G.; Mancusi, C.; Trimarco, V.; De Luca, N.; Trimarco, B. Depressed myocardial energetic efficiency is associated with increased cardiovascular risk in hypertensive left ventricular hypertrophy. *J. Hypertens.* **2016**, *34*, 1846–1853. [CrossRef]
10. Howard, B.V.; Lee, E.T.; Cowan, L.D.; Devereux, R.B.; Galloway, J.M.; Go, O.T.; Howard, W.J.; Rhoades, E.R.; Robbins, D.C.; Sievers, M.L.; et al. Rising Tide of Cardiovascular Disease in American Indians. *Circulation* **1999**, *99*, 2389–2395. [CrossRef]
11. Ferrara, L.A.; Capaldo, B.; Mancusi, C.; Lee, E.T.; Howard, B.V.; Devereux, R.B.; de Simone, G. Cardiometabolic risk in overweight subjects with or without relative fat-free mass deficiency: The Strong Heart Study. *Nutr. Metab. Cardiovasc. Dis.* **2014**, *24*, 271–276. [CrossRef] [PubMed]
12. Devereux, R.B.; Roman, M.J.; Liu, J.E.; Lee, E.T.; Wang, W.; Fabsitz, R.R.; Welty, T.K.; Howard, B.V. An appraisal of echocardiography as an epidemiological tool. The Strong Heart Study. *Ann. Epidemiol.* **2003**, *13*, 238–244. [CrossRef]
13. Palmieri, V.; Dahlof, B.; DeQuattro, V.; Sharpe, N.; Bella, J.N.; de Simone, G.; Paranicas, M.; Fishman, D.; Devereux, R.B. Reliability of echocardiographic assessment of left ventricular structure and function: The PRESERVE study. Prospective Randomized Study Evaluating Regression of Ventricular Enlargement. *J. Am. Coll. Cardiol.* **1999**, *34*, 1625–1632. [CrossRef]
14. de Simone, G.; Kizer, J.R.; Chinali, M.; Roman, M.J.; Bella, J.N.; Best, L.G.; Lee, E.T.; Devereux, R.B. Strong Heart Study Investigators. Normalization for body size and population-attributable risk of left ventricular hypertrophy: The Strong Heart Study. *Am. J. Hypertens.* **2005**, *18*, 191–196. [CrossRef] [PubMed]
15. de Simone, G.; Devereux, R.B.; Ganau, A.; Hahn, R.T.; Saba, P.S.; Mureddu, G.F.; Roman, M.J.; Howard, B.V. Estimation of left ventricular chamber and stroke volume by limited M-mode echocardiography and validation by two-dimensional and Doppler echocardiography. *Am. J. Cardiol.* **1996**, *78*, 801–807. [CrossRef]
16. de Simone, G.; Devereux, R.B.; Koren, M.J.; Mensah, G.A.; Casale, P.N.; Laragh, J.H. Midwall left ventricular mechanics. An independent predictor of cardiovascular risk in arterial hypertension. *Circulation* **1996**, *93*, 259–265. [CrossRef] [PubMed]
17. Bella, J.N.; Palmieri, V.; Roman, M.J.; E Liu, J.; Welty, T.K.; Lee, E.T.; Fabsitz, R.R.; Howard, B.V.; Devereux, R.B. Mitral ratio of peak early to late diastolic filling velocity as a predictor of mortality in middle-aged and elderly adults: the Strong Heart Study. *Circulation* **2002**, *105*, 1928–1933. [CrossRef]

18. Vanoverschelde, J.L.; Wijns, W.; Essamri, B.; Bol, A.; Robert, A.; LaBar, D.; Cogneau, M.; Michel, C.; Melin, J.A. Hemodynamic and mechanical determinants of myocardial O_2 consumption in normal human heart: Effects of dobutamine. *Am. J. Physiol. Circ. Physiol.* **1993**, *265*, H1884–H1892. [CrossRef]
19. Losi, M.A.; Izzo, R.; De Marco, M.; Canciello, G.; Rapacciuolo, A.; Trimarco, V.; Stabile, E.; Rozza, F.; Esposito, G.; De Luca, N.; et al. Cardiovascular ultrasound exploration contributes to predict incident atrial fibrillation in arterial hypertension: The Campania Salute Network. *Int. J. Cardiol.* **2015**, *199*, 290–295. [CrossRef]
20. de Simone, G.; Devereux, R.B.; Roman, M.J.; Chinali, M.; Barac, A.; Panza, J.A.; Lee, E.T.; Galloway, J.M.; Howard, B.V. Does cardiovascular phenotype explain the association between diabetes and incident heart failure? The Strong Heart Study. *Nutr. Metab. Cardiovasc. Dis.* **2013**, *23*, 285–291. [CrossRef]
21. Devereux, R.B.; Bang, C.N.; Roman, M.J.; Palmieri, V.; Boman, K.; Gerdts, E.; Nieminen, M.S.; Papademetriou, V.; Wachtell, K.; Hille, D.A.; et al. Left Ventricular Wall Stress-Mass-Heart Rate Product and Cardiovascular Events in Treated Hypertensive Patients: LIFE Study. *Hypertension* **2015**, *66*, 945–953. [CrossRef] [PubMed]
22. Massie, B.M.; Carson, P.E.; McMurray, J.J.; Komajda, M.; McKelvie, R.; Zile, M.R.; Anderson, S.; Donovan, M.; Iverson, E.; Staiger, C.; et al. Irbesartan in Patients with Heart Failure and Preserved Ejection Fraction. *New Engl. J. Med.* **2008**, *359*, 2456–2467. [CrossRef] [PubMed]
23. Wende, A.R.; Brahma, M.K.; McGinnis, G.R.; Young, M.E. Metabolic Origins of Heart Failure. *JACC Basic Transl. Sci.* **2017**, *2*, 297–310. [CrossRef] [PubMed]
24. Lewis, G.A.; Schelbert, E.B.; Williams, S.G.; Cunnington, C.; Ahmed, F.; McDonagh, T.A.; Miller, C.A. Biological Phenotypes of Heart Failure With Preserved Ejection Fraction. *J. Am. Coll. Cardiol.* **2017**, *70*, 2186–2200. [CrossRef] [PubMed]
25. Mancusi, C.; Losi, M.A.; Izzo, R.; Canciello, G.; Manzi, M.V.; Sforza, A.; De Luca, N.; Trimarco, B.; de Simone, G. Effect of diabetes and metabolic syndrome on myocardial mechano-energetic efficiency in hypertensive patients. The Campania Salute Network. *J. Hum. Hypertens.* **2017**, *31*, 395–399. [CrossRef]
26. Kolwicz, S.C., Jr.; Purohit, S.; Tian, R. Cardiac metabolism and its interactions with contraction, growth, and survival of cardiomyocytes. *Circ. Res.* **2013**, *113*, 603–616. [CrossRef]
27. Ferrannini, E. Insulin Resistance versus Insulin Deficiency in Non-Insulin-Dependent Diabetes Mellitus: Problems and Prospects. *Endocr. Rev.* **1998**, *19*, 477–490. [CrossRef]
28. Aasum, E.; Hafstad, A.D.; Severson, D.L.; Larsen, T.S. Age-Dependent Changes in Metabolism, Contractile Function, and Ischemic Sensitivity in Hearts From db/db Mice. *Diabetes* **2003**, *52*, 434–441. [CrossRef]
29. Hinkle, P.C. P/O ratios of mitochondrial oxidative phosphorylation. *Biochim. Biophys. Acta* **2005**, *1706*, 1–11. [CrossRef]
30. Ferrario, M.M.; Chiodini, P.; E Chambless, L.; Cesana, G.; Vanuzzo, D.; Panico, S.; Sega, R.; Pilotto, L.; Palmieri, L.; Giampaoli, S. Prediction of coronary events in a low incidence population. Assessing accuracy of the CUORE Cohort Study prediction equation. *Int. J. Epidemiol.* **2005**, *34*, 413–421. [CrossRef]

14

Inositol 1,4,5-Trisphosphate Receptors in Human Disease

Jessica Gambardella [1,2,3], Angela Lombardi [1,4], Marco Bruno Morelli [1,5], John Ferrara [1] and Gaetano Santulli [1,2,3,5,*]

1 Department of Medicine, Einstein-Mount Sinai Diabetes Research Center (ES-DRC), Fleischer Institute for Diabetes and Metabolism, Albert Einstein College of Medicine, New York, NY 10461, USA; jessica.gambardella@einsteinmed.org (J.G.); angela.lombardi@einsteinmed.org (A.L.); marco.morelli@einstein.yu.edu (M.B.M.); j.ferraraeastchester@gmail.com (J.F.)
2 International Translational Research and Medical Education Consortium (ITME), 80100 Naples, Italy
3 Department of Advanced Biomedical Sciences, "Federico II" University, 80131 Naples, Italy
4 Department of Microbiology and Immunology, Albert Einstein College of Medicine, New York, NY 10461, USA
5 Department of Molecular Pharmacology, Wilf Family Cardiovascular Research Institute, Albert Einstein College of Medicine, New York, NY 10461, USA
* Correspondence: gsantulli001@gmail.com

Abstract: Inositol 1,4,5-trisphosphate receptors (ITPRs) are intracellular calcium release channels located on the endoplasmic reticulum of virtually every cell. Herein, we are reporting an updated systematic summary of the current knowledge on the functional role of ITPRs in human disorders. Specifically, we are describing the involvement of its loss-of-function and gain-of-function mutations in the pathogenesis of neurological, immunological, cardiovascular, and neoplastic human disease. Recent results from genome-wide association studies are also discussed.

Keywords: Alzheimer; ataxia; autoimmune disease; cancer; cardiovascular disease; diabetes; GWAS; IP3 Receptors; ITPRs; mutations

---

1. Introduction

Since their discovery in the 1970s, several studies have provided substantial evidence that inositol 1,4,5-trisphosphate receptors (ITPRs) play a pleiotropic role in the regulation of cellular functions. Indeed, their ability to regulate calcium handling poses ITPRs at the heart of molecular networks underlying cellular homeostasis: From proliferation, apoptosis, and differentiation to metabolism and neurotransmission.

ITPR was identified for the first time as a large membrane protein called P400 [1,2] that was able to regulate intracellular calcium spikes [1–3]. After protein purification and cDNA isolation, it became clear that P400 was a channel releasing calcium from the endoplasmic reticulum (ER) [4–6]. Later, ITPR was shown to be a rather peculiar channel, as two-second messengers are needed for its activation: IP3 and calcium [7–12].

Three isoforms of ITPR have been identified (ITPR13) in mammals, which, albeit produced by different genes, show 70% of homology in the primary protein sequence [13]. The similarity in amino acid sequence also reflects the resemblance in protein conformation and spatial organization. All three isoforms consist of five domains: Suppressor domain (SD), IP3 binding core domain (IBC), regulatory domain, transmembrane domain (TD), and C-terminus domain (CTD) [14–17]. These domains are organized in a complex tetrameric "mushroom-like" structure (Figure 1), with the stalk inserted in the ER membrane and the cap exposed to the cytosol [18]. The stalk is mainly represented by the transmembrane TM domain, with its six-helices forming the ion-conducting pore [16]. All the other domains are in the "cap", exposed to the cytosol. This organization makes the IBC domain available to IP3 binding, and the regulatory domain to the many interactions and post-transcriptional modifications that regulate the receptor activity, including phosphorylation and oxidation [16].

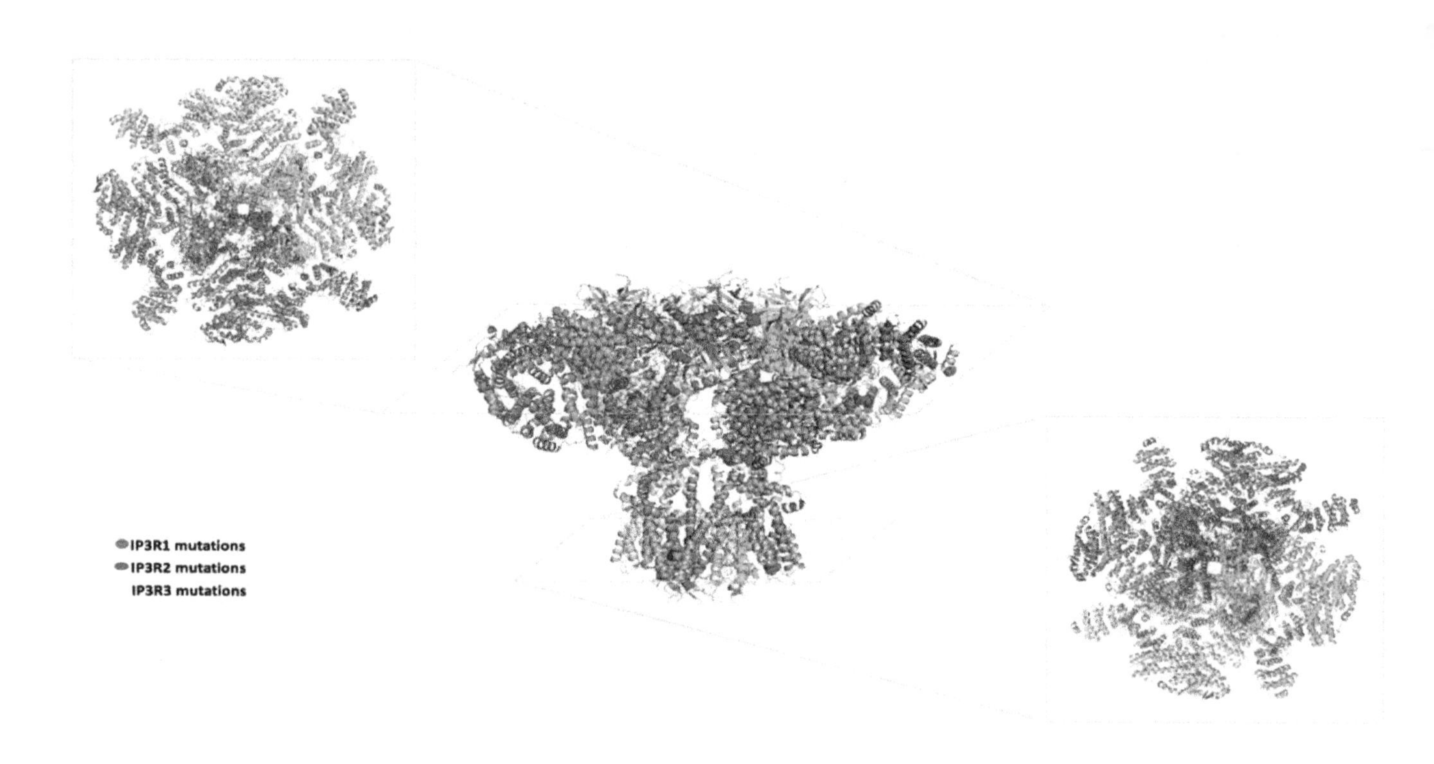

Figure 1. Representative structure of inositol 1,4,5-trisphosphate receptors (ITPRs) (1-3) showing disease-related mutations. In the middle, representative "mushroom-like structure" of ITPRs. For clarity, only the crystal of human isoform 3 is shown. Top left corner: View from the top; bottom right corner: View from the bottom. The residues in red, blue, and yellow indicate the mutations in ITPR1, 2, and 3, respectively, that have been hitherto reported in humans.

Nevertheless, the information on the ITPR molecular organization is still not sufficient for a complete mechanistic definition of its structure–function relationship [10,19]. If the central calcium conducting pore is similar to other ion channels, as suggested by the 4.7 Å structure of ITPR [16], the spatial arrangement of the cytosolic C-terminus is quite unique for ITPR; in particular, these carboxyl tails have the ability to interact with the N-terminal domains of the near subunits, suggesting a mechanism of allosteric regulation dictated by intracellular signals [16]. The feature of ITPR of being prone to modulation by nearby signals gives an idea of the complexity of the ITPR-interactome. In other words, ITPRs have the structural complexity to participate in and regulate a dense network of cellular processes. ITPRs are differently expressed in human tissues, as reported in Table 1, obtained with data retrieved from the Human Protein Atlas [20]. The effects of ITPRs have been extensively studied in preclinical models [21–29]. Here, we offer an overview of the human pathologies where ITPR alterations have a clear causative role. Moreover, we summarize the information derived from innovative studies of the disease-genome profile association, which also suggests the potential, under-investigated role of ITPR in several human pathologies.

Table 1. Protein expression levels of IP3Rs in different human tissues and organs.

Tissue	IP3R1	IP3R2	IP3R3
Cerebral cortex	XX	XX	X
Cerebellum	XX	X	XXX
Hippocampus	XX		
Caudate	XX	X	
Thyroid gland		X	X
Parathyroid gland		XXX	
Adrenal gland		XX	X
Nasopharynx		X	XX
Bronchus		XX	XX
Lung	X	X	XX
Oral mucosa		X	XX
Salivary gland		XX	
Esophagus		X	XX
Stomach	X	XX	XX
Duodenum		XX	XX
Small intestine		XX	XXX
Colon		XX	XX
Rectum		XX	XX
Liver		XX	XX
Gallbladder		XX	X
Pancreas		XX	X
Kidney	X	XXX	X
Urinary bladder		X	XX
Testis	X	XX	XXX
Epididymis	X	XX	X
Seminal vesicle	X	X	X
Prostate	X		X
Vagina			XX
Ovary		X	
Fallopian tube		XX	X
Endometrium		XX	XXX
Cervix, uterine		X	XX
Placenta		X	X
Breast	X	XXX	XX
Heart	X	XX	
Smooth muscle		XX	
Skeletal muscle		XX	
Soft tissue			
Adipose tissue		XX	
Skin		XX	XX
Appendix		XX	XX
Spleen	X		
Lymph node	X		X
Tonsil	X	X	XXX
Bone marrow		X	

X: Low, XX: Medium, XXX: High protein expression level.

2. ITPRs and Neurological Disorders

The function of ITPR has been historically assessed in the neurological field. Indeed, the first identification of P400 protein occurred in Purkinje cells and the neurological signs were the first to be studied in mice [30]. The highest number of ITPR human mutations has been identified in neurological disorders, in particular affecting the isoform 1. Indeed, ITPR1 is the most abundant isoform in the brain, regulating important functions including memory and motor coordination [31].

2.1. *Spinocerebellar Ataxia*

Spinocerebellar ataxia (SCA) is a term referring to a group of hereditary ataxias characterized by degenerative alterations in the part of the brain related to the movement control (cerebellum) and sometimes in the spinal cord. Van de Leemput was the first to identify the deletion of a 5′ portion of ITPR1 in British and Australian families with type 15 SCA [32]. Thereafter, the deletion of exons 1-48 of ITPR1 was identified in other populations, demonstrating that the haploinsufficiency of ITPR1 is involved in SCA15-16 [33,34]. Missense mutations in the ITPR1 gene have been later associated with SCA15: P1059L and P1074L in a Japanese family, and V494I in an Australian family [35,36].

Another form of SCA, SCA29, characterized by an early-onset motor delay, hypotonia, and gait ataxia, is one of the forms more frequently associated with ITPR1 mutations [37]. The missense mutations V1553M and N602D, identified by Huang et al. [38], are among the first mutations observed; G2547A was identified as a de novo mutation but only in one case [39]. In a cohort study on a population of 21 patients with SCA29, Zambonin et al. identified six novel mutations in the ITPR1 gene [40]: Three mutations in the IP3 binding domain (R269G, K279E, K418ins), two mutations in the transmembrane domain (G2506R, I2550T), and one in the regulatory domain (T1386M); no specific genotype–phenotype correlations were observed, but the recurrence in affected subjects suggested the pathogenic role of these mutations.

SCA has been generally associated with a loss of function of ITPR1, however, Casey et al. recently identified a gain-of-function pathogenic mutation [41], detecting a R36C missense variant in three SCA29 affected members of the same family. The resultant ITPR1 mutant displayed a higher IP3 binding affinity than the wild type counterpart, converting the pattern of intracellular calcium release from transient to sigmoidal. This evidence supports the idea that the enhancement of calcium release can contribute to SCA29 pathogenesis. In addition to missense mutations of the ITPR1 gene, a splicing variant was also associated with SCA29: The c.1207-2A-T transition was identified in exon 14 of ITPR1 in four SCA29 patients and was not found in unaffected members of the same family [42].

Notably, all the mutations described above are autosomal dominant variants; however, a missense mutation in the ITPR1 gene was similarly associated with autosomal recessive SCA: In a family with congenital SCA history, the homozygous missense mutation L1787P was identified in all affected individuals, while the heterozygous carriers were asymptomatic [43]. The ability of this mutation to alter the receptor function is only predictive, but the concerned residue is highly conserved and the transition of leucine to proline can affect the protein stability with a high probability. Moreover, missense mutations (T267M, T594I, S277I, T267R) were observed in sporadic infantile-onset SCA [44,45], in congenital ataxias (R269W, R241K, A280D, E512K) [46], and in another subtype of ataxia, ataxic cerebral palsy (S1493D) [47]; other mutations have been reported [48–51] in molecularly unassigned SCA forms (V2541A, T2490M) and in rare forms of cerebellar hypoplasia (T2552P, I2550N).

Intriguingly, there are SCA variants not directly associated with ITPR1 gene mutations, but involving genes functionally close to ITPR1 and its signaling. A good example comes from SCA2 and SCA3, where the causative mutations are alterations in ataxin-2 and -3, respectively. In both cases, the mutant forms of ATXs are able to bind ITPR1 increasing the sensitivity of the channel for IP3 and enhancing channel gating [52,53]. Of interest, ITPR1-functional alterations by ATXs seem to have a pathogenic role, as they increase the apoptosis of Purkinje cells in animal models of ataxia [54]. This evidence supports the key role of calcium homeostasis regulation by ITPR1 in these neurological disorders even if the channel function is not directly altered.

2.2. *Huntington's Disease and Alzheimer's Disease*

To date, genetic mutations in the ITPR1 gene with a pathological relevance in human Huntington's Disease (HD) and Alzheimer's Disease (AD) have not been detected. However, both disorders are major examples of indirect involvement of ITPR1.

In HD, the causative mutation is the poliQ expansion of Huntingtin (Htt), although the cellular and molecular mechanisms of GABAergic neurons loss are not clearly understood [55]. Of note, the polyQ-Htt can bind ITPR1 with high affinity, sensitizing the receptor activity by IP3 [56,57]. Blocking the Htt–ITPR1 interaction in vivo was shown to regulate the abnormal calcium signaling in response to glutamate, protecting the neurons from death, and improving motor coordination [58], posing ITPR1 in a key position in HD pathophysiology and supporting the use of ITPR1-based therapies.

In AD, the pathogenic hypothesis of the beta-amyloid plaque has been extensively and historically investigated. However, in the last years, new and additional potential mechanisms have been suggested, including the dysregulation of calcium handling. In particular, ITPRs seem to have a key role in modulating calcium signals in AD [59]. Alterations in the ITPR function have been detected in cells derived from patients with AD already in 1994 [60,61]. Later, Ferreiro et al. demonstrated that antibody-aggregates are able to induce calcium release by ITPR in cortical neurons, leading to apoptosis, which was prevented by the ITPR inhibitor Xestopongin C [62].

2.3. Gillespie Syndrome

The Gillespie syndrome (GS) is a rare form of aniridia, cerebellar ataxia, and mental deficiency, described in 1965 by the American ophthalmologist Fredrick Gillespie [63]. Until 2016, its causative gene and mutations were unknown. Using a whole-exome sequencing approach, Gerber et al. identified several ITPR1 mutations in five GS-affected families [64]. In particular, the Authors detected truncating mutations in homozygous (Q1558*, R728*) or in composed heterozygous (G2102Valfs5/A2221Valfs23); the resultant truncated mutants were unable to generate a functional channel in a heterologous cell system. In the other two families, the Authors found one missense mutation (F2553L) and one deletion (K2563del) in the transmembrane domain. The latter, in addition to producing a dysfunctional channel, was able to exert a negative effect on the product derived from the wild type allele, with a dominant-negative action.

Later, next-generation sequencing approaches were used to study other GS families. The results evidenced novel missense mutations in the region of the calcium pore (N2543I), and in the regulatory domain (E2061G, E2061Q), further extending the ITPR1 mutations spectrum associated to GS [65,66].

2.4. Autism Spectrum Disorder

The Autism spectrum disorder (ASD) is a complex heterogeneous disorder with a poorly defined etiology and diagnosis criteria. Its high heritability, however, suggests a strong genetic component [67] and several genetic studies suggest that calcium homeostasis is a key determinant in its pathophysiology [68]. Recent studies demonstrate that IP_3-mediated calcium signals are significantly depressed in fibroblasts isolated from patients with ASD, identifying ITPR as a functional target in this disease [69]. These data are consistent with another study done in patients with autism in which a genetic variant of the oxytocin receptor (implicated in the etiology of ASD), causes a decline in the IP3/calcium signaling pathway in vitro [70].

2.5. Amyotrophic Lateral Sclerosis

Amyotrophic lateral sclerosis (ALS) is a condition characterized by a progressive degeneration of motor neurons in the brain and spinal cord. ITPR1 and ITPR2 are the main isoforms expressed in motor neurons [71]. ITPR2 mRNA levels are elevated in peripheral blood samples of patients with ALS [72] and studies done in human cells suggest that the pharmacological inhibition of ITPR1 is a potential strategy to prevent motor neuron deterioration in ALS [73].

3. ITPRs in Autoimmune Disorders

ITPRs are important for exocrine fluid secretion including saliva, pancreatic juice, and tear secretion [74]. Interestingly, anti-ITPR antibodies have been detected in sera from patients with Sjogren's syndrome (SS) [75], a chronic autoimmune disease involving lymphocytic infiltration and loss of secretory function in salivary and lacrimal glands [76]. A recent study demonstrates that the expression of ITPR2 and ITPR3 is significantly reduced in the salivary gland of SS patients, suggesting that deficits in ITPRs may underlie the secretory defect in SS [77].

Antibodies against ITPRs were also found in patients with rheumatoid arthritis and systemic lupus erythematosus, although the locations of the antigenic epitopes were different among the disease conditions [75].

4. ITPRs and Anhidrosis

Anhidrosis is the inability to sweat, which is responsible for heat tolerance; it is a rare disorder occurring even in the presence of morphologically normal eccrine glands, which are the main glands that respond to thermal stress with a high secretion rate. The whole-genome analysis of a family with anhidrosis and normal eccrine glands unveiled a novel missense mutation (G2498S) in ITPR type 2 [78]. This mutation occurs in the calcium pore-forming region. This association was corroborated by the observation of anhidrosis and hyperhidrosis in human pathologies linked to ITPR dysfunction; also, there was a marked reduction of sweat secretion in ITPR2$^{-/-}$ animals. Interestingly, ITPR2 inhibitors have the potential to reduce sweat production in hyperhidrosis, suggesting that ITPR2 is a potential pharmacological target in the treatment of sweat secretion conditions [78].

5. ITPRs and Cancer

Calcium has a key role in proliferation, differentiation, and migration; therefore, it is not surprising that ITPR, one of the main regulators of calcium handling, is involved in neoplastic transformation and progression [79]. Neck squamous cell carcinoma (HNSCC) was one of the first diseases connected to ITPR [80]; a whole-exome sequencing analysis of HNSCC patients revealed missense mutations affecting the ITPR3 gene, R64H, and R149L, both in the regulatory domain of the receptor [80]. Importantly, ITPR3 gene mutations were detectable only in metastatic or in recurrent tumors, but not in the respective primary tumors. This finding strongly suggests a role for ITPR3 in the metastatic process and malignant transformation, very significant if we take into account that the major problem related to HNSCC is given by recurrent metastases, which occur in more than half of the patients.

An increased expression of ITPR3 was detected in clear renal cell carcinoma compared to the unaffected part of the kidney [81]; ITPR3 silencing affected tumor growth, in vitro as well as in vivo, providing a direct proof of the involvement of this receptor in the carcinogenesis. An increased expression of ITPR3 has been also observed in cholangiocarcinoma [82] and in colorectal cancer [83]; in both cases the expression of ITPR3 correlated with the degree of neoplasia severity [82,83].

Alterations of ITPR1 and ITPR2 have been associated with the Sézary syndrome, a T-cell lymphoma with an aggressive clinical course. The analysis of gene mutations in 15 patients with the neoplastic syndrome unveiled somatic point mutations in ITPR1 including A95T in the regulatory domain and S2454F in the trans-membrane domain, and mutation in ITPR2, such as S2508L, in the trans-membrane domain [84]. These discoveries have important implications in considering ITPRs as new therapeutic targets in cancer.

6. Potential Role of ITPRs in Human Disease: Evidence from GWAS

While an evident role of ITPRs has been recognized for several human pathologies by identifying specific mutations, a potential role of this channel in other human conditions has been suggested by genome whole association studies (GWASs). Eleftherohorinou et al. have shown that a defective second messenger signaling could be involved in the predisposition to rheumatoid arthritis [85]. Specifically, alterations in ITPRs were proposed to be responsible for calcium signaling deregulations in this disease [85]. As revealed by another GWAS, the involvement of ITPR3 in the release of the macrophage migration inhibitory factor (MIF) confirmed the role of this receptor in rheumatoid arthritis [86]. In the same study, ITPR was also associated with type 1 diabetes mellitus [86], reflecting the similarity of genetic perturbations and the comparable immunological dysfunctions underlying these diseases, further corroborated by genetic analyses identifying ITPR3 as an independent risk locus in

Graves' disease [87] and allergic disorders including asthma, allergic rhinitis, atopic dermatitis [88,89], and airflow obstruction [90]. The involvement of ITPR3 in diabetes has been also confirmed by the significant recurrence of single nucleotides polymorphisms (SNPs) in the ITPR3 gene in diabetic American women [91], as well as in a Swedish nationwide study [92]. The latter study reported that a variation at rs2296336 (a SNP within ITPR3) might influence the risk of developing diabetes through an effect on alternative splicing. Moreover, rs3748079, a SNP located in the promoter region of ITPR3, has been associated with several autoimmune diseases including systemic lupus erythematosus, rheumatoid arthritis, and Graves' disease in a Japanese population [93], and the variant rs999943 of ITPR3 has been linked to obesity [94]. Equally important, ITPR1 has been associated in different GWASs with diabetic kidney disease [95] and obesity-related traits [96]. Of note, a recent GWAS in a Chinese population identified *ITPR2* as a susceptibility gene for the Kashin-Beck disease, a chronic osteochondropathy characterized by cartilage degeneration [97]; in this study, a significant association between the disease and nine SNPs of *ITPR2* was described. Interestingly, the regulatory role of ITPR2 in apoptosis is a possible contributor to the Kashin-Beck disease, since excessive chondrocyte apoptosis was found to be related to cartilage lesions in affected patients [98]. Moreover, a GWAS has revealed that the ITPR signaling pathway is genetically associated with epilepsy [99], and the anti-epileptic drug levetiracetum is known to act inhibiting the release of calcium by ITPRs, highlighting the relevance of enhanced ITPRs action in epilepsy [100].

Other association studies have underlined the role of ITPRs in the cardiovascular field. The association between gene expression and dilated cardiomyopathy (DCM) has been studied by assessing the presence of CpG sites in the proximity of gene-promoters, as an index of promoter methylation and consequent downregulation of transcription [101]; using this strategy, the CpG site "cg26395694" close to the ITPR1 locus (ENSG00000150995) has been shown to be significantly associated to DCM (*p*-value: 2.57E-02). More in general, ITPR3-mediated pathways have been also linked to ischemic heart disease [86] and coronary artery disease [102]. ITPR3 has been associated with the risk of developing coronary artery aneurism in Taiwanese children with Kawasaki disease [103], a multisystemic vasculitis that can result in coronary artery lesions and that had been linked to aberrant calcium signaling [104]. In a case-control study involving 93 Kawasaki disease patients and 680 healthy controls, the frequency of the rs2229634 T/T genotype was significantly higher in Kawasaki disease patients with coronary artery aneurism than in patients without coronary artery aneurism [103]. The key importance of ITPRs in cardiovascular medicine is confirmed by the crucial role of ITPRs in cardiogenesis [105–107]; ergo, it may be difficult to detect mutations causing severe heart defects by using genetic analyses of patient samples postnatally, especially if considering that ITPRs have been shown to be essential in very early embryogenesis and some mutations might cause lethality in utero [108,109].

An international GWAS identified ITPR1 between the novel loci associated with blood pressure in children and adolescents [110]. Finally, in the Hispanic population, ITPR1 was associated to the pathophysiology of childhood obesity [96], while ITPR3 was linked to body mass index variants conferring a high risk of extreme obesity [94].

The GWAS demonstrated an association of ITPR1–2 with different forms of cancer, especially breast cancer [111–113]. Other studies associated the expression level of ITPR3 with the aggressiveness of different types of tumors, including colorectal carcinoma, gastric cancers [114], and head and neck squamous cell carcinoma [80]. *ITPR3* variants were also found to be implied in cervical squamous cell carcinoma [115]. Interestingly, ITPR3 appears also to actively participate in cell death in several tissues and its increased activity was demonstrated to induce apoptosis in T lymphocytes [116,117]. These findings indicate that compounds aimed at controlling the ITPR activity may be useful as a therapeutic approach for modulating immune responses in cancer.

7. Conclusions

In this systematic review, we illustrated the association of ITPRs mutations with human disorders. The mutations of ITPRs reported in humans are summarized in Table 2 and represented in Figure 1. Throughout the analysis of current literature, the involvement of ITPRs in human disease appears to be under-investigated.

Table 2. Spectrum of IP3Rs mutations identified in humans.

Mutation	IP3R Isoform	Effect on Protein	Disease	Reference
5′ deletion	IP3R1	Downregulation	SCA15	[32]
1-48 exons deletion	IP3R1	Downregulation	SCA15-16	[33,34]
P1059L	IP3R1	Missense (ND)	SCA15	[35]
P1074L	IP3R1	Missense (ND)	SCA15	[35]
V494I	IP3R1	Missense (ND)	SCA15	[36]
V1553M	IP3R1	Missense (ND)	SCA29	[38]
N602D	IP3R1	Missense (ND)	SCA29	[38]
G2547A	IP3R1	Missense (ND)	SCA29	[39]
R269G	IP3R1	Missense (ND)	SCA29	[40]
K279E	IP3R1	Missense (ND)	SCA29	[40]
G2506R	IP3R1	Missense (ND)	SCA29	[40]
I2550T	IP3R1	Missense (ND)	SCA29	[40]
T1386M	IP3R1	Missense (ND)	SCA29	[40]
R36C	IP3R1	Gain-of-function Increase of IP3 binding affinity	SCA29	[41]
c.1207-2A-T	IP3R1	Splicing variant	SCA29	[42]
L1787P	IP3R1	Protein-instability*	Autosomal-recessive SCA	[43]
T267M	IP3R1	Missense (ND)	Sporadic infantile-onset-SCA	[44,45]
T594I	IP3R1	Missense (ND)	Sporadic infantile-onset-SCA	[44,45]
S277I	IP3R1	Missense (ND)	Sporadic infantile-onset-SCA	[44,45]
T267R	IP3R1	Missense (ND)	Sporadic infantile-onset-SCA	[44,45]
R269W	IP3R1	Missense (ND)	Congenital-ataxias	[46]
R241K	IP3R1	Missense (ND)	Congenital-ataxias	[46]
A280D	IP3R1	Missense (ND)	Congenital-ataxias	[46]
E512K	IP3R1	Missense (ND)	Congenital-ataxias	[46]
S1493D	IP3R1	Missense (ND)	Ataxic-cerebral-palsy	[47]
V2541A	IP3R1	Missense (ND)	Molecular-unassigned SCA	[48]
T2490M	IP3R1	Missense (ND)	Molecular-unassigned SCA	[48]
T2552P	IP3R1	Missense (ND)	Cerebellar-hypoplasia	[50]
I2550N	IP3R1	Missense (ND)	Cerebellar-hypoplasia	[51]
Q1558	IP3R1	Truncating-protein, no functional channel	Gillespie syndrome	[64]
R728	IP3R1	Truncating-protein, no functional channel	Gillespie syndrome	[64]
F2553L	IP3R1	Missense (ND)	Gillespie syndrome	[64]
K2563 deletion	IP3R1	Dysfunctional channel with dominant negative action	Gillespie syndrome	[64]
N2543I	IP3R1	Missense (ND)	Gillespie syndrome	[65]
E2061G	IP3R1	Missense (ND)	Gillespie syndrome	[66]
E2061Q	IP3R1	Missense (ND)	Gillespie syndrome	[66]
A95T	IP3R1	Missense (ND)	Sézary syndrome	[84]
S2454F	IP3R1	Missense (ND)	Sézary syndrome	[84]
S2508L	IP3R1	Missense (ND)	Sézary syndrome	[84]
G2498S	IP3R2	Missense: dysfunctional channel *	Anhidrosis	[78]
R64H	IP3R3	Missense (ND)	HNSCC	[80]
R149L	IP3R3	Missense (ND)	HNSCC	[80]

HNSCC: Head and neck squamous cell carcinoma; ND: Not determined; SCA: Spinocerebellar ataxia; * predicted effect on protein.

The currently known contribution of the receptor to the pathogenesis of human disease is only the top of the iceberg. The information about causative genetic alterations affecting ITPRs mainly come from the neurology-related fields, cancer fields, or rare disease field, where the genetic analysis is a more common approach included in diagnostic procedures. However, in several studies of large-scale genome analysis, ITPRs recurrently emerge as a susceptibility gene for several pathological conditions. This evidence confirms that only little is known about this channel, particularly in cardiac and vascular homeostasis or metabolism. The recent findings of the physical link between ER and mitochondria, mediated by a protein complex including ITPR, suggest a potential role of the receptor in the regulation of calcium-dependent mitochondrial metabolism [118–130]. The ability of ITPR to indirectly regulate mitochondrial energetic metabolism could have a significant impact on the health and homeostasis of the tissues strongly dependent on mitochondrial energetic production, such as cardiac and skeletal muscle. However, this aspect needs to be further explored.

The underestimated pathophysiological role of ITPR might also depend on the fact that the cellular context strongly affects the impact of ITPR alterations on calcium handling and the relative cell fate. A good example comes from a study in neuronal cells about the P1059L affecting the regulatory domain of ITPR1; this mutation increases the affinity of ITPR1 to IP3, altering the functional output of Purkinje cells, however, no differences were detected in calcium signaling between the wild type and the same mutant in B-cells [131]. The regulatory domain of ITPR is the target of several molecular partners whose expression and activity profile are different among the different cellular contexts. Therefore, the regulation around the P1059 residue of ITPR could be different—and/or of different impact—in Purkinje cells compared to other cells, such as B-cells. Nevertheless, the experiments performed in stable cell lines can alter the impact of ITPR alterations, as several adaptive pathways could affect the expression of ITPR regulatory proteins minimizing the effects of mutations. These observations encourage future studies on ITPR in the appropriate native cellular context, both in physiological and pathological conditions.

Author Contributions: Conceptualization, G.S.; data curation, M.B.M. and J.F.; writing—original draft preparation, J.G., A.L. and M.B.M.; writing—review and editing, J.F. and G.S. All authors have read and agreed to the published version of the manuscript.

References

1. Mikoshiba, K.; Changeux, J.P. Morphological and biochemical studies on isolated molecular and granular layers from bovine cerebellum. *Brain Res.* **1978**, *142*, 487–504. [CrossRef]
2. Mikoshiba, K.; Huchet, M.; Changeux, J.P. Biochemical and immunological studies on the P400 protein, a protein characteristic of the Purkinje cell from mouse and rat cerebellum. *Dev. Neurosci.* **1979**, *2*, 254–275. [CrossRef] [PubMed]
3. Crepel, F.; Dupont, J.L.; Gardette, R. Selective absence of calcium spikes in Purkinje cells of staggerer mutant mice in cerebellar slices maintained in vitro. *J. Physiol.* **1984**, *346*, 111–125. [CrossRef] [PubMed]
4. Maeda, N.; Niinobe, M.; Nakahira, K.; Mikoshiba, K. Purification and characterization of P400 protein, a glycoprotein characteristic of Purkinje cell, from mouse cerebellum. *J. Neurochem.* **1988**, *51*, 1724–1730. [CrossRef]
5. Furuichi, T.; Yoshikawa, S.; Miyawaki, A.; Wada, K.; Maeda, N.; Mikoshiba, K. Primary structure and functional expression of the inositol 1,4,5-trisphosphate-binding protein P400. *Nature* **1989**, *342*, 32–38. [CrossRef]
6. Furuichi, T.; Yoshikawa, S.; Mikoshiba, K. Nucleotide sequence of cDNA encoding P400 protein in the mouse cerebellum. *Nucleic Acids Res.* **1989**, *17*, 5385–5386. [CrossRef]
7. Iino, M. Biphasic Ca2+ dependence of inositol 1,4,5-trisphosphate-induced Ca release in smooth muscle cells of the guinea pig taenia caeci. *J. Gen. Physiol* **1990**, *95*, 1103–1122. [CrossRef]
8. Finch, E.A.; Turner, T.J.; Goldin, S.M. Calcium as a coagonist of inositol 1,4,5-trisphosphate-induced calcium release. *Science* **1991**, *252*, 443–446. [CrossRef]
9. Santulli, G.; Nakashima, R.; Yuan, Q.; Marks, A.R. Intracellular calcium release channels: An update. *J. Physiol.* **2017**, *595*, 3041–3051. [CrossRef]
10. Paknejad, N.; Hite, R.K. Structural basis for the regulation of inositol trisphosphate receptors by Ca(2+) and IP3. *Nat. Struct. Mol. Biol.* **2018**, *25*, 660–668. [CrossRef]
11. Belkacemi, A.; Hui, X.; Wardas, B.; Laschke, M.W.; Wissenbach, U.; Menger, M.D.; Lipp, P.; Beck, A.; Flockerzi, V. IP3 Receptor-Dependent Cytoplasmic Ca(2+) Signals Are Tightly Controlled by Cavbeta3. *Cell Rep.* **2018**, *22*, 1339–1349. [CrossRef] [PubMed]

12. Rong, Y.P.; Bultynck, G.; Aromolaran, A.S.; Zhong, F.; Parys, J.B.; De Smedt, H.; Mignery, G.A.; Roderick, HL.; Bootman, M.D.; Distelhorst, C.W. The BH4 domain of Bcl-2 inhibits ER calcium release and apoptosis by binding the regulatory and coupling domain of the IP3 receptor. *Proc. Natl. Acad. Sci. USA* **2009**, *106*, 14397–14402. [CrossRef] [PubMed]
13. Prole, D.L.; Taylor, C.W. Structure and Function of IP3 Receptors. *Cold Spring Harb Perspect Biol* **2019**, *11*. [CrossRef] [PubMed]
14. Lin, C.C.; Baek, K.; Lu, Z. Apo and InsP(3)-bound crystal structures of the ligand-binding domain of an InsP(3) receptor. *Nat. Struct Mol. Biol.* **2011**, *18*, 1172–1174. [CrossRef] [PubMed]
15. Seo, M.D.; Velamakanni, S.; Ishiyama, N.; Stathopulos, P.B.; Rossi, A.M.; Khan, S.A.; Dale, P.; Li, C.; Ames, J.B.; Ikura, M.; et al. Structural and functional conservation of key domains in InsP3 and ryanodine receptors. *Nature* **2012**, *483*, 108–112. [CrossRef]
16. Fan, G.; Baker, M.L.; Wang, Z.; Baker, M.R.; Sinyagovskiy, P.A.; Chiu, W.; Ludtke, S.J.; Serysheva, I.I. Gating machinery of InsP3R channels revealed by electron cryomicroscopy. *Nature* **2015**, *527*, 336–341. [CrossRef]
17. Chandran, A.; Chee, X.; Prole, D.L.; Rahman, T. Exploration of inositol 1,4,5-trisphosphate (IP3) regulated dynamics of N-terminal domain of IP3 receptor reveals early phase molecular events during receptor activation. *Sci. Rep.* **2019**, *9*, 2454. [CrossRef]
18. Hamada, K.; Miyatake, H.; Terauchi, A.; Mikoshiba, K. IP3-mediated gating mechanism of the IP3 receptor revealed by mutagenesis and X-ray crystallography. *Proc. Natl. Acad. Sci. USA* **2017**, *114*, 4661–4666. [CrossRef]
19. Lock, J.T.; Alzayady, K.J.; Yule, D.I.; Parker, I. All three IP3 receptor isoforms generate Ca(2+) puffs that display similar characteristics. *Sci. Signal.* **2018**, *11*, eaau0344. [CrossRef]
20. Thul, P.J.; Akesson, L.; Wiking, M.; Mahdessian, D.; Geladaki, A.; Ait Blal, H.; Alm, T.; Asplund, A.; Bjork, L.; Breckels, L.M.; et al. A subcellular map of the human proteome. *Science* **2017**, *356*, eaal3321. [CrossRef]
21. Chan, C.; Ooashi, N.; Akiyama, H.; Fukuda, T.; Inoue, M.; Matsu-Ura, T.; Shimogori, T.; Mikoshiba, K.; Kamiguchi, H. Inositol 1,4,5-Trisphosphate Receptor Type 3 Regulates Neuronal Growth Cone Sensitivity to Guidance Signals. *iScience* **2020**, *23*, 100963. [CrossRef] [PubMed]
22. Yuan, Q.; Yang, J.; Santulli, G.; Reiken, S.R.; Wronska, A.; Kim, M.M.; Osborne, B.W.; Lacampagne, A.; Yin, Y.; Marks, A.R. Maintenance of normal blood pressure is dependent on IP3R1-mediated regulation of eNOS. *Proc. Natl. Acad. Sci. USA* **2016**, *113*, 8532–8537. [CrossRef] [PubMed]
23. Perry, R.J.; Zhang, D.; Guerra, M.T.; Brill, A.L.; Goedeke, L.; Nasiri, A.R.; Rabin-Court, A.; Wang, Y.; Peng, L.; Dufour, S.; et al. Glucagon stimulates gluconeogenesis by INSP3R1-mediated hepatic lipolysis. *Nature* **2020**, *579*, 279–283. [CrossRef] [PubMed]
24. Santulli, G.; Xie, W.; Reiken, S.R.; Marks, A.R. Mitochondrial calcium overload is a key determinant in heart failure. *Proc. Natl. Acad. Sci. USA* **2015**, *112*, 11389–11394. [CrossRef]
25. Wang, Y.; Li, G.; Goode, J.; Paz, J.C.; Ouyang, K.; Screaton, R.; Fischer, W.H.; Chen, J.; Tabas, I.; Montminy, M. Inositol-1,4,5-trisphosphate receptor regulates hepatic gluconeogenesis in fasting and diabetes. *Nature* **2012**, *485*, 128–132. [CrossRef]
26. Kuchay, S.; Giorgi, C.; Simoneschi, D.; Pagan, J.; Missiroli, S.; Saraf, A.; Florens, L.; Washburn, M.P.; Collazo-Lorduy, A.; Castillo-Martin, M.; et al. PTEN counteracts FBXL2 to promote IP3R3- and Ca(2+)-mediated apoptosis limiting tumour growth. *Nature* **2017**, *546*, 554–558. [CrossRef]
27. Cheung, K.H.; Mei, L.; Mak, D.O.; Hayashi, I.; Iwatsubo, T.; Kang, D.E.; Foskett, J.K. Gain-of-function enhancement of IP3 receptor modal gating by familial Alzheimer's disease-linked presenilin mutants in human cells and mouse neurons. *Sci. Signal.* **2010**, *3*, ra22. [CrossRef]
28. Gambardella, J.; Trimarco, B.; Iaccarino, G.; Santulli, G. New Insights in Cardiac Calcium Handling and Excitation-Contraction Coupling. *Adv. Exp. Med. Biol* **2018**, *1067*, 373–385.
29. Huang, W.; Cane, M.C.; Mukherjee, R.; Szatmary, P.; Zhang, X.; Elliott, V.; Ouyang, Y.; Chvanov, M.; Latawiec, D.; Wen, L.; et al. Caffeine protects against experimental acute pancreatitis by inhibition of inositol 1,4,5-trisphosphate receptor-mediated Ca2+ release. *Gut* **2017**, *66*, 301–313. [CrossRef]
30. Maeda, N.; Niinobe, M.; Mikoshiba, K. A cerebellar Purkinje cell marker P400 protein is an inositol 1,4,5-trisphosphate (InsP3) receptor protein. Purification and characterization of InsP3 receptor complex. *EMBO J.* **1990**, *9*, 61–67. [CrossRef]

31. Hisatsune, C.; Mikoshiba, K. IP3 receptor mutations and brain diseases in human and rodents. *J. Neurochem.* **2017**, *141*, 790–807. [CrossRef] [PubMed]
32. van de Leemput, J.; Chandran, J.; Knight, M.A.; Holtzclaw, L.A.; Scholz, S.; Cookson, M.R.; Houlden, H.; Gwinn-Hardy, K.; Fung, H.C.; Lin, X.; et al. Deletion at ITPR1 underlies ataxia in mice and spinocerebellar ataxia 15 in humans. *PLoS Genet.* **2007**, *3*, e108. [CrossRef] [PubMed]
33. Marelli, C.; van de Leemput, J.; Johnson, J.O.; Tison, F.; Thauvin-Robinet, C.; Picard, F.; Tranchant, C.; Hernandez, D.G.; Huttin, B.; Boulliat, J.; et al. SCA15 due to large ITPR1 deletions in a cohort of 333 white families with dominant ataxia. *Arch. Neurol.* **2011**, *68*, 637–643. [CrossRef] [PubMed]
34. Novak, M.J.; Sweeney, M.G.; Li, A.; Treacy, C.; Chandrashekar, H.S.; Giunti, P.; Goold, R.G.; Davis, M.B.; Houlden, H.; Tabrizi, S.J. An ITPR1 gene deletion causes spinocerebellar ataxia 15/16: A genetic, clinical and radiological description. *Mov. Disord.* **2010**, *25*, 2176–2182. [CrossRef]
35. Hara, K.; Shiga, A.; Nozaki, H.; Mitsui, J.; Takahashi, Y.; Ishiguro, H.; Yomono, H.; Kurisaki, H.; Goto, J.; Ikeuchi, T.; et al. Total deletion and a missense mutation of ITPR1 in Japanese SCA15 families. *Neurology* **2008**, *71*, 547–551. [CrossRef]
36. Ganesamoorthy, D.; Bruno, D.L.; Schoumans, J.; Storey, E.; Delatycki, M.B.; Zhu, D.; Wei, M.K.; Nicholson, G.A.; McKinlay Gardner, R.J.; Slater, H.R. Development of a multiplex ligation-dependent probe amplification assay for diagnosis and estimation of the frequency of spinocerebellar ataxia type 15. *Clin. Chem.* **2009**, *55*, 1415–1418. [CrossRef]
37. Ando, H.; Hirose, M.; Mikoshiba, K. Aberrant IP3 receptor activities revealed by comprehensive analysis of pathological mutations causing spinocerebellar ataxia 29. *Proc. Natl. Acad. Sci. USA* **2018**, *115*, 12259–12264. [CrossRef]
38. Huang, L.; Chardon, J.W.; Carter, M.T.; Friend, K.L.; Dudding, T.E.; Schwartzentruber, J.; Zou, R.; Schofield, P.W.; Douglas, S.; Bulman, D.E.; et al. Missense mutations in ITPR1 cause autosomal dominant congenital nonprogressive spinocerebellar ataxia. *Orphanet. J. Rare Dis.* **2012**, *7*, 67. [CrossRef]
39. Gonzaga-Jauregui, C.; Harel, T.; Gambin, T.; Kousi, M.; Griffin, L.B.; Francescatto, L.; Ozes, B.; Karaca, E.; Jhangiani, S.N.; Bainbridge, M.N.; et al. Exome Sequence Analysis Suggests that Genetic Burden Contributes to Phenotypic Variability and Complex Neuropathy. *Cell Rep.* **2015**, *12*, 1169–1183. [CrossRef]
40. Zambonin, J.L.; Bellomo, A.; Ben-Pazi, H.; Everman, D.B.; Frazer, L.M.; Geraghty, M.T.; Harper, A.D.; Jones, J.R.; Kamien, B.; Kernohan, K.; et al. Spinocerebellar ataxia type 29 due to mutations in ITPR1: A case series and review of this emerging congenital ataxia. *Orphanet J. Rare. Dis.* **2017**, *12*, 121. [CrossRef]
41. Casey, J.P.; Hirouchi, T.; Hisatsune, C.; Lynch, B.; Murphy, R.; Dunne, A.M.; Miyamoto, A.; Ennis, S.; van der Spek, N.; O'Hici, B.; et al. A novel gain-of-function mutation in the ITPR1 suppressor domain causes spinocerebellar ataxia with altered Ca(2+) signal patterns. *J. Neurol.* **2017**, *264*, 1444–1453. [CrossRef] [PubMed]
42. Wang, L.; Hao, Y.; Yu, P.; Cao, Z.; Zhang, J.; Zhang, X.; Chen, Y.; Zhang, H.; Gu, W. Identification of a Splicing Mutation in ITPR1 via WES in a Chinese Early-Onset Spinocerebellar Ataxia Family. *Cerebellum* **2018**, *17*, 294–299. [CrossRef] [PubMed]
43. Klar, J.; Ali, Z.; Farooq, M.; Khan, K.; Wikstrom, J.; Iqbal, M.; Zulfiqar, S.; Faryal, S.; Baig, S.M.; Dahl, N. A missense variant in ITPR1 provides evidence for autosomal recessive SCA29 with asymptomatic cerebellar hypoplasia in carriers. *Eur J. Hum. Genet.* **2017**, *25*, 848–853. [CrossRef] [PubMed]
44. Sasaki, M.; Ohba, C.; Iai, M.; Hirabayashi, S.; Osaka, H.; Hiraide, T.; Saitsu, H.; Matsumoto, N. Sporadic infantile-onset spinocerebellar ataxia caused by missense mutations of the inositol 1,4,5-triphosphate receptor type 1 gene. *J. Neurol* **2015**, *262*, 1278–1284. [CrossRef]
45. Fogel, B.L.; Lee, H.; Deignan, J.L.; Strom, S.P.; Kantarci, S.; Wang, X.; Quintero-Rivera, F.; Vilain, E.; Grody, W.W.; Perlman, S.; et al. Exome sequencing in the clinical diagnosis of sporadic or familial cerebellar ataxia. *JAMA Neurol.* **2014**, *71*, 1237–1246. [CrossRef] [PubMed]
46. Barresi, S.; Niceta, M.; Alfieri, P.; Brankovic, V.; Piccini, G.; Bruselles, A.; Barone, M.R.; Cusmai, R.; Tartaglia, M.; Bertini, E.; et al. Mutations in the IRBIT domain of ITPR1 are a frequent cause of autosomal dominant nonprogressive congenital ataxia. *Clin. Genet.* **2017**, *91*, 86–91. [CrossRef]
47. Parolin Schnekenberg, R.; Perkins, E.M.; Miller, J.W.; Davies, W.I.; D'Adamo, M.C.; Pessia, M.; Fawcett, K.A.; Sims, D.; Gillard, E.; Hudspith, K.; et al. De novo point mutations in patients diagnosed with ataxic cerebral palsy. *Brain* **2015**, *138*, 1817–1832. [CrossRef]

48. Valencia, C.A.; Husami, A.; Holle, J.; Johnson, J.A.; Qian, Y.; Mathur, A.; Wei, C.; Indugula, S.R.; Zou, F.; Meng, H.; et al. Clinical Impact and Cost-Effectiveness of Whole Exome Sequencing as a Diagnostic Tool: A Pediatric Center's Experience. *Front. Pediatr.* **2015**, *3*, 67. [CrossRef]
49. Hsiao, C.T.; Liu, Y.T.; Liao, Y.C.; Hsu, T.Y.; Lee, Y.C.; Soong, B.W. Mutational analysis of ITPR1 in a Taiwanese cohort with cerebellar ataxias. *PLoS ONE* **2017**, *12*, e0187503. [CrossRef]
50. Hayashi, S.; Uehara, D.T.; Tanimoto, K.; Mizuno, S.; Chinen, Y.; Fukumura, S.; Takanashi, J.I.; Osaka, H.; Okamoto, N.; Inazawa, J. Comprehensive investigation of CASK mutations and other genetic etiologies in 41 patients with intellectual disability and microcephaly with pontine and cerebellar hypoplasia (MICPCH). *PLoS ONE* **2017**, *12*, e0181791. [CrossRef]
51. van Dijk, T.; Barth, P.; Reneman, L.; Appelhof, B.; Baas, F.; Poll-The, B.T. A de novo missense mutation in the inositol 1,4,5-triphosphate receptor type 1 gene causing severe pontine and cerebellar hypoplasia: Expanding the phenotype of ITPR1-related spinocerebellar ataxia's. *Am. J. Med. Genet. A* **2017**, *173*, 207–212. [CrossRef] [PubMed]
52. Chen, X.; Tang, T.S.; Tu, H.; Nelson, O.; Pook, M.; Hammer, R.; Nukina, N.; Bezprozvanny, I. Deranged calcium signaling and neurodegeneration in spinocerebellar ataxia type 3. *J. Neurosci.* **2008**, *28*, 12713–12724. [CrossRef] [PubMed]
53. Liu, J.; Tang, T.S.; Tu, H.; Nelson, O.; Herndon, E.; Huynh, D.P.; Pulst, S.M.; Bezprozvanny, I. Deranged calcium signaling and neurodegeneration in spinocerebellar ataxia type 2. *J. Neurosci.* **2009**, *29*, 9148–9162. [CrossRef] [PubMed]
54. Kasumu, A.W.; Hougaard, C.; Rode, F.; Jacobsen, T.A.; Sabatier, J.M.; Eriksen, B.L.; Strobaek, D.; Liang, X.; Egorova, P.; Vorontsova, D.; et al. Selective positive modulator of calcium-activated potassium channels exerts beneficial effects in a mouse model of spinocerebellar ataxia type 2. *Chem. Biol.* **2012**, *19*, 1340–1353. [CrossRef]
55. Vonsattel, J.P.; Myers, R.H.; Stevens, T.J.; Ferrante, R.J.; Bird, E.D.; Richardson, E.P. Jr. Neuropathological classification of Huntington's disease. *J. Neuropathol. Exp. Neurol.* **1985**, *44*, 559–577. [CrossRef]
56. Tang, T.S.; Tu, H.; Chan, E.Y.; Maximov, A.; Wang, Z.; Wellington, C.L.; Hayden, M.R.; Bezprozvanny, I. Huntingtin and huntingtin-associated protein 1 influence neuronal calcium signaling mediated by inositol-(1,4,5) triphosphate receptor type 1. *Neuron* **2003**, *39*, 227–239. [CrossRef]
57. Tang, T.S.; Tu, H.; Orban, P.C.; Chan, E.Y.; Hayden, M.R.; Bezprozvanny, I. HAP1 facilitates effects of mutant huntingtin on inositol 1,4,5-trisphosphate-induced Ca release in primary culture of striatal medium spiny neurons. *Eur. J. Neurosci.* **2004**, *20*, 1779–1787. [CrossRef]
58. Tang, T.S.; Guo, C.; Wang, H.; Chen, X.; Bezprozvanny, I. Neuroprotective effects of inositol 1,4,5-trisphosphate receptor C-terminal fragment in a Huntington's disease mouse model. *J. Neurosci.* **2009**, *29*, 1257–1266. [CrossRef]
59. Green, K.N.; Demuro, A.; Akbari, Y.; Hitt, B.D.; Smith, I.F.; Parker, I.; LaFerla, F.M. SERCA pump activity is physiologically regulated by presenilin and regulates amyloid beta production. *J. Cell Biol.* **2008**, *181*, 1107–1116. [CrossRef]
60. Ito, E.; Oka, K.; Etcheberrigaray, R.; Nelson, T.J.; McPhie, D.L.; Tofel-Grehl, B.; Gibson, G.E.; Alkon, D.L. Internal Ca2+ mobilization is altered in fibroblasts from patients with Alzheimer disease. *Proc. Natl. Acad. Sci. USA* **1994**, *91*, 534–538. [CrossRef]
61. Hirashima, N.; Etcheberrigaray, R.; Bergamaschi, S.; Racchi, M.; Battaini, F.; Binetti, G.; Govoni, S.; Alkon, D.L. Calcium responses in human fibroblasts: A diagnostic molecular profile for Alzheimer's disease. *Neurobiol. Aging* **1996**, *17*, 549–555. [CrossRef]
62. Ferreiro, E.; Oliveira, C.R.; Pereira, C. Involvement of endoplasmic reticulum Ca2+ release through ryanodine and inositol 1,4,5-triphosphate receptors in the neurotoxic effects induced by the amyloid-beta peptide. *J. Neurosci. Res.* **2004**, *76*, 872–880. [CrossRef] [PubMed]
63. Gillespie, F.D. Aniridia, Cerebellar Ataxia, and Oligophrenia in Siblings. *Arch. Ophthalmol.* **1965**, *73*, 338–341. [CrossRef] [PubMed]
64. Gerber, S.; Alzayady, K.J.; Burglen, L.; Bremond-Gignac, D.; Marchesin, V.; Roche, O.; Rio, M.; Funalot, B.; Calmon, R.; Durr, A.; et al. Recessive and Dominant De Novo ITPR1 Mutations Cause Gillespie Syndrome. *Am. J. Hum. Genet.* **2016**, *98*, 971–980. [CrossRef]

65. Dentici, M.L.; Barresi, S.; Nardella, M.; Bellacchio, E.; Alfieri, P.; Bruselles, A.; Pantaleoni, F.; Danieli, A.; Iarossi, G.; Cappa, M.; et al. Identification of novel and hotspot mutations in the channel domain of ITPR1 in two patients with Gillespie syndrome. *Gene* **2017**, *628*, 141–145. [CrossRef]
66. McEntagart, M.; Williamson, K.A.; Rainger, J.K.; Wheeler, A.; Seawright, A.; De Baere, E.; Verdin, H.; Bergendahl, L.T.; Quigley, A.; Rainger, J.; et al. A Restricted Repertoire of De Novo Mutations in ITPR1 Cause Gillespie Syndrome with Evidence for Dominant-Negative Effect. *Am. J. Hum. Genet.* **2016**, *98*, 981–992. [CrossRef]
67. Schmunk, G.; Gargus, J.J. Channelopathy pathogenesis in autism spectrum disorders. *Front. Genet.* **2013**, *4*, 222. [CrossRef]
68. Cross-Disorder Group of the Psychiatric Genomics, C. Identification of risk loci with shared effects on five major psychiatric disorders: A genome-wide analysis. *Lancet* **2013**, *381*, 1371–1379.
69. Schmunk, G.; Boubion, B.J.; Smith, I.F.; Parker, I.; Gargus, J.J. Shared functional defect in IP(3)R-mediated calcium signaling in diverse monogenic autism syndromes. *Transl. Psychiatry* **2015**, *5*, e643. [CrossRef]
70. Ma, W.J.; Hashii, M.; Munesue, T.; Hayashi, K.; Yagi, K.; Yamagishi, M.; Higashida, H.; Yokoyama, S. Non-synonymous single-nucleotide variations of the human oxytocin receptor gene and autism spectrum disorders: A case-control study in a Japanese population and functional analysis. *Mol. Autism* **2013**, *4*, 22. [CrossRef]
71. Van Den Bosch, L.; Verhoeven, K.; De Smedt, H.; Wuytack, F.; Missiaen, L.; Robberecht, W. Calcium handling proteins in isolated spinal motoneurons. *Life Sci.* **1999**, *65*, 1597–1606. [CrossRef]
72. van Es, M.A.; Van Vught, P.W.; Blauw, H.M.; Franke, L.; Saris, C.G.; Andersen, P.M.; Van Den Bosch, L.; de Jong, S.W.; van 't Slot, R.; Birve, A.; et al. ITPR2 as a susceptibility gene in sporadic amyotrophic lateral sclerosis: A genome-wide association study. *Lancet Neurol.* **2007**, *6*, 869–877. [CrossRef]
73. Kim, S.H.; Zhan, L.; Hanson, K.A.; Tibbetts, R.S. High-content RNAi screening identifies the Type 1 inositol triphosphate receptor as a modifier of TDP-43 localization and neurotoxicity. *Hum. Mol. Genet.* **2012**, *21*, 4845–4856. [CrossRef] [PubMed]
74. Futatsugi, A.; Nakamura, T.; Yamada, M.K.; Ebisui, E.; Nakamura, K.; Uchida, K.; Kitaguchi, T.; Takahashi-Iwanaga, H.; Noda, T.; Aruga, J.; et al. IP3 receptor types 2 and 3 mediate exocrine secretion underlying energy metabolism. *Science* **2005**, *309*, 2232–2234. [CrossRef]
75. Miyachi, K.; Iwai, M.; Asada, K.; Saito, I.; Hankins, R.; Mikoshiba, K. Inositol 1,4,5-trisphosphate receptors are autoantibody target antigens in patients with Sjogren's syndrome and other systemic rheumatic diseases. *Mod. Rheumatol.* **2007**, *17*, 137–143. [CrossRef]
76. Vivino, F.B. Sjogren's syndrome: Clinical aspects. *Clin. Immunol.* **2017**, *182*, 48–54. [CrossRef]
77. Teos, L.Y.; Zhang, Y.; Cotrim, A.P.; Swaim, W.; Won, J.H.; Ambrus, J.; Shen, L.; Bebris, L.; Grisius, M.; Jang, S.I.; et al. IP3R deficit underlies loss of salivary fluid secretion in Sjogren's Syndrome. *Sci. Rep.* **2015**, *5*, 13953. [CrossRef]
78. Klar, J.; Hisatsune, C.; Baig, S.M.; Tariq, M.; Johansson, A.C.; Rasool, M.; Malik, N.A.; Ameur, A.; Sugiura, K.; Feuk, L.; et al. Abolished InsP3R2 function inhibits sweat secretion in both humans and mice. *J. Clin. Invest.* **2014**, *124*, 4773–4780. [CrossRef]
79. Sneyers, F.; Rosa, N.; Bultynck, G. Type 3 IP3 receptors driving oncogenesis. *Cell Calcium* **2020**, *86*, 102141. [CrossRef]
80. Hedberg, M.L.; Goh, G.; Chiosea, S.I.; Bauman, J.E.; Freilino, M.L.; Zeng, Y.; Wang, L.; Diergaarde, B.B.; Gooding, W.E.; Lui, V.W.; et al. Genetic landscape of metastatic and recurrent head and neck squamous cell carcinoma. *J. Clin. Invest.* **2016**, *126*, 169–180. [CrossRef]
81. Rezuchova, I.; Hudecova, S.; Soltysova, A.; Matuskova, M.; Durinikova, E.; Chovancova, B.; Zuzcak, M.; Cihova, M.; Burikova, M.; Penesova, A.; et al. Type 3 inositol 1,4,5-trisphosphate receptor has antiapoptotic and proliferative role in cancer cells. *Cell Death Dis.* **2019**, *10*, 186. [CrossRef] [PubMed]
82. Ueasilamongkol, P.; Khamphaya, T.; Guerra, M.T.; Rodrigues, M.A.; Gomes, D.A.; Kong, Y.; Wei, W.; Jain, D.; Trampert, D.C.; Ananthanarayanan, M.; et al. Weerachayaphorn, J. Type 3 Inositol 1,4,5-Trisphosphate Receptor Is Increased and Enhances Malignant Properties in Cholangiocarcinoma. *Hepatology* **2020**, *71*, 583–599. [CrossRef] [PubMed]
83. Shibao, K.; Fiedler, M.J.; Nagata, J.; Minagawa, N.; Hirata, K.; Nakayama, Y.; Iwakiri, Y.; Nathanson, M.H.; Yamaguchi, K. The type III inositol 1,4,5-trisphosphate receptor is associated with aggressiveness of colorectal carcinoma. *Cell Calcium* **2010**, *48*, 315–323. [CrossRef] [PubMed]

84. Prasad, A.; Rabionet, R.; Espinet, B.; Zapata, L.; Puiggros, A.; Melero, C.; Puig, A.; Sarria-Trujillo, Y.; Ossowski, S.; Garcia-Muret, M.P.; et al. Identification of Gene Mutations and Fusion Genes in Patients with Sezary Syndrome. *J. Invest. Derm.* **2016**, *136*, 1490–1499. [CrossRef] [PubMed]
85. Eleftherohorinou, H.; Hoggart, C.J.; Wright, V.J.; Levin, M.; Coin, L.J. Pathway-driven gene stability selection of two rheumatoid arthritis GWAS identifies and validates new susceptibility genes in receptor mediated signalling pathways. *Hum. Mol. Genet.* **2011**, *20*, 3494–3506. [CrossRef] [PubMed]
86. Torkamani, A.; Topol, E.J.; Schork, N.J. Pathway analysis of seven common diseases assessed by genome-wide association. *Genomics* **2008**, *92*, 265–272. [CrossRef]
87. Nakabayashi, K.; Tajima, A.; Yamamoto, K.; Takahashi, A.; Hata, K.; Takashima, Y.; Koyanagi, M.; Nakaoka, H.; Akamizu, T.; Ishikawa, N.; et al. Identification of independent risk loci for Graves' disease within the MHC in the Japanese population. *J. Hum. Genet.* **2011**, *56*, 772–778. [CrossRef]
88. Ferreira, M.A.; Vonk, J.M.; Baurecht, H.; Marenholz, I.; Tian, C.; Hoffman, J.D.; Helmer, Q.; Tillander, A.; Ullemar, V.; van Dongen, J.; et al. Shared genetic origin of asthma, hay fever and eczema elucidates allergic disease biology. *Nat. Genet.* **2017**, *49*, 1752–1757. [CrossRef]
89. Kichaev, G.; Bhatia, G.; Loh, P.R.; Gazal, S.; Burch, K.; Freund, M.K.; Schoech, A.; Pasaniuc, B.; Price, A.L. Leveraging Polygenic Functional Enrichment to Improve GWAS Power. *Am. J. Hum. Genet.* **2019**, *104*, 65–75. [CrossRef]
90. Wilk, J.B.; Shrine, N.R.; Loehr, L.R.; Zhao, J.H.; Manichaikul, A.; Lopez, L.M.; Smith, A.V.; Heckbert, S.R.; Smolonska, J.; Tang, W.; et al. Genome-wide association studies identify CHRNA5/3 and HTR4 in the development of airflow obstruction. *Am. J. Respir. Crit. Care Med.* **2012**, *186*, 622–632. [CrossRef]
91. Reddy, M.V.; Wang, H.; Liu, S.; Bode, B.; Reed, J.C.; Steed, R.D.; Anderson, S.W.; Steed, L.; Hopkins, D.; She, J.X. Association between type 1 diabetes and GWAS SNPs in the southeast US Caucasian population. *Genes Immun.* **2011**, *12*, 208–212. [CrossRef] [PubMed]
92. Roach, J.C.; Deutsch, K.; Li, S.; Siegel, A.F.; Bekris, L.M.; Einhaus, D.C.; Sheridan, C.M.; Glusman, G.; Hood, L.; Lernmark, A.; et al. Swedish Childhood Diabetes Study, G.; Diabetes Incidence in Sweden Study, G. Genetic mapping at 3-kilobase resolution reveals inositol 1,4,5-triphosphate receptor 3 as a risk factor for type 1 diabetes in Sweden. *Am. J. Hum. Genet.* **2006**, *79*, 614–627. [CrossRef] [PubMed]
93. Oishi, T.; Iida, A.; Otsubo, S.; Kamatani, Y.; Usami, M.; Takei, T.; Uchida, K.; Tsuchiya, K.; Saito, S.; Ohnisi, Y.; et al. A functional SNP in the NKX2.5-binding site of ITPR3 promoter is associated with susceptibility to systemic lupus erythematosus in Japanese population. *J. Hum. Genet.* **2008**, *53*, 151–162. [CrossRef]
94. Cotsapas, C.; Speliotes, E.K.; Hatoum, I.J.; Greenawalt, D.M.; Dobrin, R.; Lum, P.Y.; Suver, C.; Chudin, E.; Kemp, D.; Reitman, M.; et al. Consortium, G. Common body mass index-associated variants confer risk of extreme obesity. *Hum. Mol. Genet.* **2009**, *18*, 3502–3507. [CrossRef] [PubMed]
95. Iyengar, S.K.; Sedor, J.R.; Freedman, B.I.; Kao, W.H.; Kretzler, M.; Keller, B.J.; Abboud, H.E.; Adler, S.G.; Best, L.G.; Bowden, D.W.; et al. Diabetes, Genome-Wide Association and Trans-ethnic Meta-Analysis for Advanced Diabetic Kidney Disease: Family Investigation of Nephropathy and Diabetes (FIND). *PLoS Genet.* **2015**, *11*, e1005352. [CrossRef] [PubMed]
96. Comuzzie, A.G.; Cole, S.A.; Laston, S.L.; Voruganti, V.S.; Haack, K.; Gibbs, R.A.; Butte, N.F. Novel genetic loci identified for the pathophysiology of childhood obesity in the Hispanic population. *PLoS ONE* **2012**, *7*, e51954. [CrossRef] [PubMed]
97. Zhang, F.; Wen, Y.; Guo, X.; Zhang, Y.; Wang, X.; Yang, T.; Shen, H.; Chen, X.; Tian, Q.; Deng, H.W. Genome-wide association study identifies ITPR2 as a susceptibility gene for Kashin-Beck disease in Han Chinese. *Arthritis Rheumatol.* **2015**, *67*, 176–181. [CrossRef]
98. Wang, S.J.; Guo, X.; Zuo, H.; Zhang, Y.G.; Xu, P.; Ping, Z.G.; Zhang, Z.; Geng, D. Chondrocyte apoptosis and expression of Bcl-2, Bax, Fas, and iNOS in articular cartilage in patients with Kashin-Beck disease. *J. Rheumatol.* **2006**, *33*, 615–619.
99. Mirza, N.; Appleton, R.; Burn, S.; Carr, D.; Crooks, D.; du Plessis, D.; Duncan, R.; Farah, J.O.; Josan, V.; Miyajima, F.; et al. Identifying the biological pathways underlying human focal epilepsy: From complexity to coherence to centrality. *Hum. Mol. Genet.* **2015**, *24*, 4306–4316. [CrossRef]
100. Nagarkatti, N.; Deshpande, L.S.; DeLorenzo, R.J. Levetiracetam inhibits both ryanodine and IP3 receptor activated calcium induced calcium release in hippocampal neurons in culture. *Neurosci. Lett.* **2008**, *436*, 289–293. [CrossRef]

101. Meder, B.; Haas, J.; Sedaghat-Hamedani, F.; Kayvanpour, E.; Frese, K.; Lai, A.; Nietsch, R.; Scheiner, C.; Mester, S.; Bordalo, D.M.; et al. Epigenome-Wide Association Study Identifies Cardiac Gene Patterning and a Novel Class of Biomarkers for Heart Failure. *Circulation* **2017**, *136*, 1528–1544. [CrossRef] [PubMed]
102. Consortium, C.A.D.; Deloukas, P.; Kanoni, S.; Willenborg, C.; Farrall, M.; Assimes, T.L.; Thompson, J.R.; Ingelsson, E.; Saleheen, D.; Erdmann, J.; et al. Large-scale association analysis identifies new risk loci for coronary artery disease. *Nat. Genet.* **2013**, *45*, 25–33.
103. Huang, Y.C.; Lin, Y.J.; Chang, J.S.; Chen, S.Y.; Wan, L.; Sheu, J.J.; Lai, C.H.; Lin, C.W.; Liu, S.P.; Chen, C.P.; et al. Single nucleotide polymorphism rs2229634 in the ITPR3 gene is associated with the risk of developing coronary artery aneurysm in children with Kawasaki disease. *Int J. Immunogenet.* **2010**, *37*, 439–443. [CrossRef] [PubMed]
104. Bijnens, J.; Missiaen, L.; Bultynck, G.; Parys, J.B. A critical appraisal of the role of intracellular Ca(2+)-signaling pathways in Kawasaki disease. *Cell Calcium* **2018**, *71*, 95–103. [CrossRef]
105. Nakazawa, M.; Uchida, K.; Aramaki, M.; Kodo, K.; Yamagishi, C.; Takahashi, T.; Mikoshiba, K.; Yamagishi, H. Inositol 1,4,5-trisphosphate receptors are essential for the development of the second heart field. *J. Mol. Cell Cardiol.* **2011**, *51*, 58–66. [CrossRef]
106. Uchida, K.; Aramaki, M.; Nakazawa, M.; Yamagishi, C.; Makino, S.; Fukuda, K.; Nakamura, T.; Takahashi, T.; Mikoshiba, K.; Yamagishi, H. Gene knock-outs of inositol 1,4,5-trisphosphate receptors types 1 and 2 result in perturbation of cardiogenesis. *PLoS ONE* **2010**, *5*, e12500. [CrossRef]
107. Uchida, K.; Nakazawa, M.; Yamagishi, C.; Mikoshiba, K.; Yamagishi, H. Type 1 and 3 inositol trisphosphate receptors are required for extra-embryonic vascular development. *Dev. Biol* **2016**, *418*, 89–97. [CrossRef]
108. Miyazaki, S.; Yuzaki, M.; Nakada, K.; Shirakawa, H.; Nakanishi, S.; Nakade, S.; Mikoshiba, K. Block of Ca2+ wave and Ca2+ oscillation by antibody to the inositol 1,4,5-trisphosphate receptor in fertilized hamster eggs. *Science* **1992**, *257*, 251–255. [CrossRef]
109. Saneyoshi, T.; Kume, S.; Amasaki, Y.; Mikoshiba, K. The Wnt/calcium pathway activates NF-AT and promotes ventral cell fate in Xenopus embryos. *Nature* **2002**, *417*, 295–299. [CrossRef]
110. Parmar, P.G.; Taal, H.R.; Timpson, N.J.; Thiering, E.; Lehtimaki, T.; Marinelli, M.; Lind, P.A.; Howe, L.D.; Verwoert, G.; Aalto, V.; et al. International Genome-Wide Association Study Consortium Identifies Novel Loci Associated With Blood Pressure in Children and Adolescents. *Circ. Cardiovasc. Genet.* **2016**, *9*, 266–278. [CrossRef]
111. Michailidou, K.; Beesley, J.; Lindstrom, S.; Canisius, S.; Dennis, J.; Lush, M.J.; Maranian, M.J.; Bolla, M.K.; Wang, Q.; Shah, M.; et al. Genome-wide association analysis of more than 120,000 individuals identifies 15 new susceptibility loci for breast cancer. *Nat. Genet.* **2015**, *47*, 373–380. [CrossRef] [PubMed]
112. Michailidou, K.; Lindstrom, S.; Dennis, J.; Beesley, J.; Hui, S.; Kar, S.; Lemacon, A.; Soucy, P.; Glubb, D.; Rostamianfar, A.; et al. Association analysis identifies 65 new breast cancer risk loci. *Nature* **2017**, *551*, 92–94. [CrossRef] [PubMed]
113. Lee, J.Y.; Kim, J.; Kim, S.W.; Park, S.K.; Ahn, S.H.; Lee, M.H.; Suh, Y.J.; Noh, D.Y.; Son, B.H.; Cho, Y.U.; et al. BRCA1/2-negative, high-risk breast cancers (BRCAX) for Asian women: Genetic susceptibility loci and their potential impacts. *Sci Rep.* **2018**, *8*, 15263. [CrossRef] [PubMed]
114. Sakakura, C.; Hagiwara, A.; Fukuda, K.; Shimomura, K.; Takagi, T.; Kin, S.; Nakase, Y.; Fujiyama, J.; Mikoshiba, K.; Okazaki, Y.; et al. Possible involvement of inositol 1,4,5-trisphosphate receptor type 3 (IP3R3) in the peritoneal dissemination of gastric cancers. *Anticancer Res.* **2003**, *23*, 3691–3697. [PubMed]
115. Yang, Y.C.; Chang, T.Y.; Chen, T.C.; Lin, W.S.; Chang, S.C.; Lee, Y.J. ITPR3 gene haplotype is associated with cervical squamous cell carcinoma risk in Taiwanese women. *Oncotarget* **2017**, *8*, 10085–10090. [CrossRef] [PubMed]
116. Blackshaw, S.; Sawa, A.; Sharp, A.H.; Ross, C.A.; Snyder, S.H.; Khan, A.A. Type 3 inositol 1,4,5-trisphosphate receptor modulates cell death. *FASEB J.* **2000**, *14*, 1375–1379.
117. Mendes, C.C.; Gomes, D.A.; Thompson, M.; Souto, N.C.; Goes, T.S.; Goes, A.M.; Rodrigues, M.A.; Gomez, M.V.; Nathanson, M.H.; Leite, M.F. The type III inositol 1,4,5-trisphosphate receptor preferentially transmits apoptotic Ca2+ signals into mitochondria. *J. Biol. Chem.* **2005**, *280*, 40892–40900. [CrossRef]
118. Bartok, A.; Weaver, D.; Golenar, T.; Nichtova, Z.; Katona, M.; Bansaghi, S.; Alzayady, K.J.; Thomas, V.K.; Ando, H.; Mikoshiba, K.; et al. IP3 receptor isoforms differently regulate ER-mitochondrial contacts and local calcium transfer. *Nat. Commun.* **2019**, *10*, 3726. [CrossRef]

119. Diaz-Vegas, A.R.; Cordova, A.; Valladares, D.; Llanos, P.; Hidalgo, C.; Gherardi, G.; De Stefani, D.; Mammucari, C.; Rizzuto, R.; Contreras-Ferrat, A.; et al. Mitochondrial Calcium Increase Induced by RyR1 and IP3R Channel Activation After Membrane Depolarization Regulates Skeletal Muscle Metabolism. *Front. Physiol.* **2018**, *9*, 791. [CrossRef]
120. Carreras-Sureda, A.; Jana, F.; Urra, H.; Durand, S.; Mortenson, D.E.; Sagredo, A.; Bustos, G.; Hazari, Y.; Ramos-Fernandez, E.; Sassano, M.L.; et al. Non-canonical function of IRE1alpha determines mitochondria-associated endoplasmic reticulum composition to control calcium transfer and bioenergetics. *Nature cell biology* **2019**, *21*, 755–767. [CrossRef]
121. Cardenas, C.; Muller, M.; McNeal, A.; Lovy, A.; Jana, F.; Bustos, G.; Urra, F.; Smith, N.; Molgo, J.; Diehl, J.A.; et al. Selective Vulnerability of Cancer Cells by Inhibition of Ca(2+) Transfer from Endoplasmic Reticulum to Mitochondria. *Cell Rep.* **2016**, *14*, 2313–2324. [CrossRef] [PubMed]
122. Arruda, A.P.; Pers, B.M.; Parlakgul, G.; Guney, E.; Inouye, K.; Hotamisligil, G.S. Chronic enrichment of hepatic endoplasmic reticulum-mitochondria contact leads to mitochondrial dysfunction in obesity. *Nat. Med.* **2014**, *20*, 1427–1435. [CrossRef] [PubMed]
123. Straub, S.V.; Giovannucci, D.R.; Yule, D.I. Calcium wave propagation in pancreatic acinar cells: Functional interaction of inositol 1,4,5-trisphosphate receptors, ryanodine receptors, and mitochondria. *J. Gen. Physiol.* **2000**, *116*, 547–560. [CrossRef] [PubMed]
124. Wiel, C.; Lallet-Daher, H.; Gitenay, D.; Gras, B.; Le Calve, B.; Augert, A.; Ferrand, M.; Prevarskaya, N.; Simonnet, H.; Vindrieux, D.; et al. Endoplasmic reticulum calcium release through ITPR2 channels leads to mitochondrial calcium accumulation and senescence. *Nat. Commun.* **2014**, *5*, 3792. [CrossRef]
125. Bononi, A.; Giorgi, C.; Patergnani, S.; Larson, D.; Verbruggen, K.; Tanji, M.; Pellegrini, L.; Signorato, V.; Olivetto, F.; Pastorino, S.; et al. BAP1 regulates IP3R3-mediated Ca(2+) flux to mitochondria suppressing cell transformation. *Nature* **2017**, *546*, 549–553. [CrossRef]
126. D'Eletto, M.; Rossin, F.; Occhigrossi, L.; Farrace, M.G.; Faccenda, D.; Desai, R.; Marchi, S.; Refolo, G.; Falasca, L.; Antonioli, M.; et al. Transglutaminase Type 2 Regulates ER-Mitochondria Contact Sites by Interacting with GRP75. *Cell Rep.* **2018**, *25*, 3573–3581. [CrossRef]
127. De Stefani, D.; Bononi, A.; Romagnoli, A.; Messina, A.; De Pinto, V.; Pinton, P.; Rizzuto, R. VDAC1 selectively transfers apoptotic Ca2+ signals to mitochondria. *Cell Death Differ.* **2012**, *19*, 267–273. [CrossRef]
128. Marchi, S.; Marinello, M.; Bononi, A.; Bonora, M.; Giorgi, C.; Rimessi, A.; Pinton, P. Selective modulation of subtype III IP(3)R by Akt regulates ER Ca(2)(+) release and apoptosis. *Cell Death Dis.* **2012**, *3*, e304. [CrossRef]
129. Suman, M.; Sharpe, J.A.; Bentham, R.B.; Kotiadis, V.N.; Menegollo, M.; Pignataro, V.; Molgo, J.; Muntoni, F.; Duchen, M.R.; Pegoraro, E.; et al. Inositol trisphosphate receptor-mediated Ca2+ signalling stimulates mitochondrial function and gene expression in core myopathy patients. *Hum. Mol. Genet.* **2018**, *27*, 2367–2382. [CrossRef]
130. Hohendanner, F.; Maxwell, J.T.; Blatter, L.A. Cytosolic and nuclear calcium signaling in atrial myocytes: IP3-mediated calcium release and the role of mitochondria. *Channels (Austin)* **2015**, *9*, 129–138. [CrossRef]
131. Yamazaki, H.; Nozaki, H.; Onodera, O.; Michikawa, T.; Nishizawa, M.; Mikoshiba, K. Functional characterization of the P1059L mutation in the inositol 1,4,5-trisphosphate receptor type 1 identified in a Japanese SCA15 family. *Biochem. Biophys. Res. Commun.* **2011**, *410*, 754–758. [CrossRef] [PubMed]

Permissions

All chapters in this book were first published by MDPI; hereby published with permission under the Creative Commons Attribution License or equivalent. Every chapter published in this book has been scrutinized by our experts. Their significance has been extensively debated. The topics covered herein carry significant findings which will fuel the growth of the discipline. They may even be implemented as practical applications or may be referred to as a beginning point for another development.

The contributors of this book come from diverse backgrounds, making this book a truly international effort. This book will bring forth new frontiers with its revolutionizing research information and detailed analysis of the nascent developments around the world.

We would like to thank all the contributing authors for lending their expertise to make the book truly unique. They have played a crucial role in the development of this book. Without their invaluable contributions this book wouldn't have been possible. They have made vital efforts to compile up to date information on the varied aspects of this subject to make this book a valuable addition to the collection of many professionals and students.

This book was conceptualized with the vision of imparting up-to-date information and advanced data in this field. To ensure the same, a matchless editorial board was set up. Every individual on the board went through rigorous rounds of assessment to prove their worth. After which they invested a large part of their time researching and compiling the most relevant data for our readers.

The editorial board has been involved in producing this book since its inception. They have spent rigorous hours researching and exploring the diverse topics which have resulted in the successful publishing of this book. They have passed on their knowledge of decades through this book. To expedite this challenging task, the publisher supported the team at every step. A small team of assistant editors was also appointed to further simplify the editing procedure and attain best results for the readers.

Apart from the editorial board, the designing team has also invested a significant amount of their time in understanding the subject and creating the most relevant covers. They scrutinized every image to scout for the most suitable representation of the subject and create an appropriate cover for the book.

The publishing team has been an ardent support to the editorial, designing and production team. Their endless efforts to recruit the best for this project, has resulted in the accomplishment of this book. They are a veteran in the field of academics and their pool of knowledge is as vast as their experience in printing. Their expertise and guidance has proved useful at every step. Their uncompromising quality standards have made this book an exceptional effort. Their encouragement from time to time has been an inspiration for everyone.

The publisher and the editorial board hope that this book will prove to be a valuable piece of knowledge for researchers, students, practitioners and scholars across the globe.

List of Contributors

Shi Hui Law, Vineet Kumar Mishra and Farzana Parveen
Department of Medical Laboratory Science and Biotechnology, College of Health Sciences, Kaohsiung Medical University, Kaohsiung 807378, Taiwan

Liang-Yin Ke
Department of Medical Laboratory Science and Biotechnology, College of Health Sciences, Kaohsiung Medical University, Kaohsiung 807378, Taiwan
Graduate Institute of Medicine, College of Medicine and Drug Development and Value Creation Research Center, Kaohsiung Medical University, Kaohsiung 807378, Taiwan
Center for Lipid Biosciences, Kaohsiung Medical University Hospital, Kaohsiung Medical University, Kaohsiung 807377, Taiwan

Hua-Chen Chan
Center for Lipid Biosciences, Kaohsiung Medical University Hospital, Kaohsiung Medical University, Kaohsiung 807377, Taiwan

Ye-Hsu Lu
Center for Lipid Biosciences, Kaohsiung Medical University Hospital, Kaohsiung Medical University, Kaohsiung 807377, Taiwan
Division of Cardiology, Department of International Medicine, Kaohsiung Medical University Hospital, Kaohsiung 807377, Taiwan

Chih-Sheng Chu
Center for Lipid Biosciences, Kaohsiung Medical University Hospital, Kaohsiung Medical University, Kaohsiung 807377, Taiwan
Division of Cardiology, Department of International Medicine, Kaohsiung Medical University Hospital, Kaohsiung 807377, Taiwan
Division of Cardiology, Department of Internal Medicine, Kaohsiung Municipal Ta-Tung Hospital, Kaohsiung 80145, Taiwan

Suho Jin and Seng Chan You
Department of Biomedical Informatics, Ajou University School of Medicine, Suwon 16499, Korea

Kristin Kostka and Christian Reich
Real World Solutions, IQVIA, Cambridge, MA 02139, USA

Jose D. Posada and Nigam H. Shah
Department of Medicine, School of Medicine, Stanford University, Stanford, CA 94305, USA

Yeesuk Kim
Department of Orthopaedic Surgery, College of Medicine, Hanyang University, Seoul 04763, Korea

Seung In Seo
Department of Internal Medicine, Kangdong Sacred Heart Hospital, Hallym University College of Medicine, Seoul 05355, Korea

Dong Yun Lee and Sang Joon Son
Department of Psychiatry, Ajou University School of Medicine, Suwon 16499, Korea

Sungwon Roh
Department of Psychiatry, College of Medicine, Hanyang University, Seoul 04763, Korea

Young-Hyo Lim
Division of Cardiology, Department of Internal Medicine, College of Medicine, Hanyang University, Seoul 04763, Korea

Sun Geu Chae
Department of Industrial Engineering, Hanyang University, Seoul 04763, Korea

UramJin
Department of Cardiology, Ajou University School of Medicine, Suwon 16499, Korea

Peter R. Rijnbeek
Department of Medical Informatics, Erasmus Medical Center, 3015 GD Rotterdam, The Netherlands

Rae Woong Park
Department of Biomedical Informatics, Ajou University School of Medicine, Suwon 16499, Korea
Department of Biomedical Sciences, Ajou University Graduate School of Medicine, Suwon 16499, Korea

Ahmed Ismaeel, Evlampia Papoutsi and Panagiotis Koutakis
Department of Nutrition, Food and Exercise Sciences, Florida State University, Tallahassee, FL 32306, USA

Marco E. Franco and Ramon Lavado
Department of Environmental Science, Baylor University, Waco, TX 76798, USA

George P. Casale, Matthew Fuglestad, Constance J. Mietus and Iraklis I. Pipinos
Department of Surgery, University of Nebraska at Medical Center, Omaha, NE 68198, USA

Gleb R. Haynatzki
Department of Biostatistics, University of Nebraska Medical Center, Omaha, NE 68198, USA

Robert S. Smith, William T. Bohannon and Ian Sawicki
Department of Surgery, Baylor Scott and White Hospital, Temple, TX 76508, USA

Giovanna Gallo and Andrea Berni
Department of Clinical and Molecular Medicine, School of Medicine and Psychology, Sapienza University of Rome, 00189 Rome, Italy

Massimo Volpe and Speranza Rubattu
Department of Clinical and Molecular Medicine, School of Medicine and Psychology, Sapienza University of Rome, 00189 Rome, Italy
IRCCS Neuromed, 86077 Pozzilli (Isernia), Italy

Maurizio Forte, Rosita Stanzione, Maria Cotugno, Franca Bianchi and Simona Marchitti
IRCCS Neuromed, 86077 Pozzilli (Isernia), Italy

Keiichi Odagiri, Akio Hakamata, Naoki Inui and Hiroshi Watanabe
Department of Clinical Pharmacology and Therapeutics, Hamamatsu University School of Medicine, 1-20-1 Handayama, Higashi-ku, Hamamatsu 431-3192, Japan

Naoki Katayama
Department of Clinical Pharmacology and Therapeutics, Hamamatsu University School of Medicine, 1-20-1 Handayama, Higashi-ku, Hamamatsu 431-3192, Japan
Department of Rehabilitation Medicine, Seirei Mikatahara General Hospital, 3453 Mikatahara-cho, Kita-ku, Hamamatsu 433-8558, Japan

Katsuya Yamauchi
Department of Rehabilitation Medicine, Hamamatsu University Hospital, 1-20-1 Handayama, Higashi-ku, Hamamatsu 431-3192, Japan

Aristides Tsatsakis
Center of Toxicology Science & Research, Medical School, University of Crete, 71003 Heraklion, Crete, Greece

Anca Oana Docea
Department of Toxicology, University of Medicine and Pharmacy of Craiova, 200349 Craiova, Romania

Daniela Calina and Laura-Maria Zamfira
Department of Clinical Pharmacy, University of Medicine and Pharmacy of Craiova, 200349 Craiova, Romania

Konstantinos Tsarouhas
Department of Cardiology, University Hospital of Larissa, 41221 Larissa, Greece

Radu Mitrut
Department of Pathology, University of Medicine and Pharmacy of Craiova, 200349 Craiova, Romania
Department of Cardiology, University and Emergency Hospital, 050098 Bucharest, Romania

Javad Sharifi-Rad
Zabol Medicinal Plants Research Center, Zabol University of Medical Sciences, Zabol 61615-585, Iran

Leda Kovatsi
Laboratory of Forensic Medicine and Toxicology, School of Medicine, Aristotle University of Thessaloniki, 54248 Thessaloniki, Greece

Vasileios Siokas and Efthimios Dardiotis
Department of Neurology, Stroke Unit, University of Thessaly, University Hospital of Larissa, 41221 Larissa, Greece

Nikolaos Drakoulis
Research Group of Clinical Pharmacology and Pharmacogenomics, Faculty of Pharmacy, School of Health Sciences, National and Kapodistrian University of Athens, 15771 Athens, Greece

George Lazopoulos
Department of Cardiothoracic Surgery, University General Hospital of Heraklion, University of Crete, Medical School, 71003 Heraklion, Crete, Greece

Christina Tsitsimpikou
Department of Hazardous Substances, Mixtures and Articles, General Chemical State Laboratory of Greece, 10431 Athens, Greece

Panayiotis Mitsias
Department of Neurology, School of Medicine, University of Crete, 71003 Heraklion, Greece
Comprehensive Stroke Center and Department of Neurology, Henry Ford Hospital, Detroit, MI 48202, USA

Monica Neagu
Department of Immunology, Victor Babes National Institute of Pathology, 050096 Bucharest, Romania
Department of Pathology, Colentina Clinical Hospital, 021183 Bucharest, Romania

Lisa-Marie Mauracher and Ingrid Pabinger
Clinical Division of Hematology and Hemostaseology, Department of Medicine I, Medical University of Vienna, 1090 Vienna, Austria

Nina Buchtele
Clinical Division of Hematology and Hemostaseology, Department of Medicine I, Medical University of Vienna, 1090 Vienna, Austria
Department of Clinical Pharmacology, Medical University of Vienna, 1090 Vienna, Austria

Christian Schorgenhofer and Bernd Jilma
Department of Clinical Pharmacology, Medical University of Vienna, 1090 Vienna, Austria

Christoph Weiser, Harald Herkner, Anne Merrelaar, Alexander O. Spiel and Michael Schwameis
Department of Emergency Medicine, Medical University of Vienna, 1090 Vienna, Austria

Lena Hell and Cihan Ay
Clinical Division of Hematology and Hemostaseology, Department of Medicine I, Medical University of Vienna, 1090 Vienna, Austria
I.M. Sechenov First Moscow State Medical University (Sechenov University), 119146 Moscow, Russia

Bettina Hieronimus and Kimber L. Stanhope
Department of Molecular Biosciences, School of Veterinary Medicine, University of California, Davis, CA 95616, USA

Steven C. Griffen and Lars Berglund
Department of Internal Medicine, School of Medicine, University of California, Davis, Sacramento, CA 95817, USA

Nancy L. Keim
United States Department of Agriculture, Western Human Nutrition Research Center, Davis, CA 95616, USA
Department of Nutrition, University of California, Davis, CA 95616, USA

Peter J. Havel
Department of Molecular Biosciences, School of Veterinary Medicine, University of California, Davis, CA 95616, USA
Department of Nutrition, University of California, Davis, CA 95616, USA

Andrew A. Bremer
Department of Pediatrics, School of Medicine, University of California, Davis, Sacramento, CA 95817, USA

Katsuyuki Nakajima
Department of Clinical Laboratory Medicine, Gunma University Graduate School of Medicine, Maebashi, Gunma 371-8510, Japan
Hidaka Hospital, Takasaki, Gunma 370-0001, Japan
General Internal Medicine, Kanazawa Medical University, Kanazawa 920-0265, Japan
Laboratory of Clinical Nutrition and Medicine, Kagawa Nutrition University, Tokyo 350-0288, Japan

Carmine Morisco
Dept. of Advanced Biomedical Science, Federico II University, 80131 Naples, Italy

Guido Iaccarino
Dept. of Advanced Biomedical Science, Federico II University, 80131 Naples, Italy
International Translational Research and Medical Education Consortium (ITME), 80131 Naples, Italy

Valeria Pascale, Rosa Finelli, Valeria Visco, Rocco Giannotti and Michele Ciccarelli
Dept. of Medicine, Surgery and Dentistry, University of Salerno, 8408 Baronissi, Italy

Angelo Massari and Enrico Coscioni
"San Giovanni di Dio e Ruggi d'Aragona" University Hospital, 84131 Salerno, Italy

Maddalena Illario
Health's Innovation, Campania Regional Government, 80132 Naples, Italy
Dept. of Public Health, Federico II University, 80131 Naples, Italy

Raluca M. Tat
Department of Anesthesia and Intensive Care I, "Iuliu Ha, tieganu" University of Medicine and Pharmacy, 400012 Cluj-Napoca, Romania

Adela Golea
Surgical Department of "Iuliu Ha, tieganu" University of Medicine and Pharmacy, 400012 Cluj-Napoca, Romania

Rodica Rahaian
Department of Immunology Laboratory, County Emergency Hospital, 400006 Cluj-Napoca, Romania

Stefan C. Vesa
Department of Pharmacology, Toxicology and Clinical Pharmacology, "Iuliu Ha, tieganu" University of Medicine and Pharmacy, 400012 Cluj-Napoca, Romania

Daniela Ionescu
Department of Anesthesia and Intensive Care I, "Iuliu Ha, tieganu" University of Medicine and Pharmacy, 400012 Cluj-Napoca, Romania
Outcome Research Consortium, Cleveland, OH 44195, USA

Agnieszka Maciejewska-Skrendo and Maciej Buryta
Department of Molecular Biology, Faculty of Physical Education, Gdansk University of Physical Education and Sport, 80-336 Gdansk, Poland

Wojciech Czarny and Pawel Król
Department of Anatomy and Anthropology, Faculty of Physical Education, University of Rzeszow, 35-310 Rzeszow, Poland

Michal Spieszny
Institute of Sports, Faculty of Physical Education, University of Physical Education and Sport, 31-571 Kraków, Poland

Petr Stastny and Miroslav Petr
Department of Sport Games, Faulty of Physical Education and Sport, Charles University, 162-52 Prague, Czech Republic

Krzysztof Safranow
Department of Biochemistry and Medical Chemistry, Pomeranian Medical University, 70-204 Szczecin, Poland

Marek Sawczuk
Unit of Physical Medicine, Faculty of Tourism and Recreation, Gdansk University of Physical Education and Sport, 80-336 Gdansk, Poland

Lukas Lanser, Gunter Weiss and Katharina Kurz
Department of Internal Medicine II, Medical University of Innsbruck, 6020 Innsbruck, Austria

Gerhard Polzl
Department of Internal Medicine III, Medical University of Innsbruck, 6020 Innsbruck, Austria

Dietmar Fuchs
Division of Biological Chemistry, Biocenter, Medical University of Innsbruck, 6020 Innsbruck, Austria

Maria-Angela Losi, Raffaele Izzo and Costantino Mancusi
Hypertension Research Center, University Federico II of Naples, I-80131 Naples, Italy
Department of Advanced Biomedical Sciences, University Federico II of Naples, I-80131 Naples, Italy

Wenyu Wang
College of Public Health, University of Oklahoma Health Sciences Center, Oklahoma City, OK 73104, USA

Giovanni de Simone
Hypertension Research Center, University Federico II of Naples, I-80131 Naples, Italy
Department of Advanced Biomedical Sciences, University Federico II of Naples, I-80131 Naples, Italy
Department of Medicine,Weill Cornell Medical College, New York, NY 10065, USA

Richard B. Devereux and Mary J. Roman
Department of Medicine, Weill Cornell Medical College, New York, NY 10065, USA

Elisa T. Lee
Center for American Indian Health Research, University of Oklahoma Health Sciences Center, Oklahoma City, OK 73126, USA

Barbara V. Howard
Medstar Health Research Institute, and Georgetown-Howard Universities Center for Translational Sciences, Washington, DC 20057, USA

John Ferrara
Department of Medicine, Einstein-Mount Sinai Diabetes Research Center (ES-DRC), Fleischer Institute for Diabetes and Metabolism, Albert Einstein College of Medicine, New York, NY 10461, USA

Jessica Gambardella
Department of Medicine, Einstein-Mount Sinai Diabetes Research Center (ES-DRC), Fleischer Institute for Diabetes and Metabolism, Albert Einstein College of Medicine, New York, NY 10461, USA
International Translational Research and Medical Education Consortium (ITME), 80100 Naples, Italy
Department of Advanced Biomedical Sciences, "Federico II" University, 80131 Naples, Italy

Angela Lombardi
Department of Medicine, Einstein-Mount Sinai Diabetes Research Center (ES-DRC), Fleischer Institute for Diabetes and Metabolism, Albert Einstein College of Medicine, New York, NY 10461, USA
Department of Microbiology and Immunology, Albert Einstein College of Medicine, New York, NY 10461, USA

Gaetano Santulli
Dept. of Medicine, Division of Cardiology, and Dept. of Molecular Pharmacology, Montefiore University Hospital, Fleischer Institute for Diabetes and Metabolism (FIDAM), Albert Einstein College of Medicine (AECOM), New York, NY 10461, USA
International Translational Research and Medical Education Consortium (ITME), 80100 Naples, Italy
Department of Advanced Biomedical Sciences, "Federico II" University, 80131 Naples, Italy
Department of Molecular Pharmacology, Wilf Family Cardiovascular Research Institute, Albert Einstein College of Medicine, New York, NY 10461, USA

Marco Bruno Morelli
Department of Medicine, Einstein-Mount Sinai Diabetes Research Center (ES-DRC), Fleischer Institute for Diabetes and Metabolism, Albert Einstein College of Medicine, New York, NY 10461, USA
Department of Molecular Pharmacology, Wilf Family Cardiovascular Research Institute, Albert Einstein College of Medicine, New York, NY 10461, USA

Index

Printed in the USA
CPSIA information can be obtained
at www.ICGtesting.com
JSHW051626061123
51533JS00005B/127

9 781639 277797